The Yeast Connection

A Medical Breakthrough

By William G. Crook, M.D.

Illustrated by Cynthia P. Crook

Vintage Books
A Division of Random House
New York

This book is dedicated with love to the most important person in my life—the one who, for over 40 years has patiently helped, supported and encouraged me—my wife, Betsy.

FIRST VINTAGE BOOKS EDITION,   October 1986

Published in the United States by Random House, Inc., New York, and simultaneously in Canada by Random House of Canada Limited, Toronto. Originally published by Professional Books, Jackson, Tennessee, in December 1983.

Library of Congress Cataloging-in-Publication Data

Crook, William G., (William Grant), 1917-
  The yeast connection.

  Reprint. Originally published: 2nd ed. Jackson,
Tenn.: Professional Books, © 1984.
  Includes bibliographies and index.
  1. Candidiasis—Complications and sequelae.
2. Candidiasis—Diet therapy.   3. Low-carbohydrate diet.
4. Allergy. I. Title. [DNLM: 1. Candidiasis—
complications—popular works.   2. Candidiasis—diet
therapy—popular works.   WC 470 C948y 1984]
RC123.C3C76   1986   616.9'69   86-40140
ISBN 0-394-74700-3 (pbk.)

Manufactured in the United States of America
40 39 38 37 36 35 34 33 32 31 30

What people are saying about *The Yeast Connection*:

"This new edition of *The Yeast Connection* represents a wonderful mix of scholarly dissertations from academic physicians and basic common sense clinical assessments from practicing doctors. All in all, it gives us simple solutions to complex questions."

> —Alan Scott Levin, M.D.
> Adjunct Associate Professor of
>   Immunology and Dermatology
> University of California, San Francisco
> School of Medicine

"The most fantastic medical book to hit the public in many a decade! It has . . . helped me get my patients well faster than any approach I've ever used."

> —Walter A. Ward, M.D.
> Past President, American Academy
>   of Otolaryngic Allergy
> Winston-Salem, North Carolina

"Beautifully written . . . a pleasure to read . . . instructive. Illustrations add enormously to the clarity and effectiveness of the text."

> —George E. Shambaugh, Jr., M.D.
> Professor Emeritus of
>   Otolaryngology
> Northwestern University

"It is time for all physicians and medical scientists to increase their understanding of the relationship between yeasts and human illness. . . . If one reviews the literature carefully, the supporting research is well documented."

> —James H. Brodsky, M.D.
> Instructor, Georgetown University
> School of Medicine

Acknowledgments

First, I thank C. Orian Truss, M.D. of Birmingham, Alabama. His brilliant pioneer observations on the *common yeast germ, Candida albicans,* alerted me to the possibility that candida could play an important role in causing health problems in many of my allergic patients . . . especially those with chemical sensitivity. I'm especially grateful to Dr. Truss for generously and patiently sharing his knowledge with me on countless occasions during the past seven years.

Special thanks are also due to Sidney M. Baker, M.D., Head of the Gesell Institute of Human Development, New Haven, Connecticut. During the past decade, Dr. Baker's observations and concepts have greatly influenced me and my work with my patients, including those with yeast-connected health problems.

I'm grateful to many other physicians who have shared their knowledge and experiences with me, including especially Doctors Robert Boxer, Cecil Bradley, Emanuel Cheraskin, Larry Dickey, John Gerrard, Hobart Feldman, Leo Galland, Zane Gard, Howard Hagglund, Harold Hedges, James Johnson, George Kroker, Alan Levin, Alan Lieberman, Richard Mabray, John Maclennan, Marshall Mandell, Joseph McGovern, Joseph Miller, Pamela Morford, David Morris, Lawrence Plumlee, James O'Shea, Robert Owen, Theron Randolph, Doris Rapp, William Rea, Phyllis Saifer, Douglas Sandberg, George Shambaugh, Don Sprague, Del Stigler, Robert Stroud, Morton Teich, Francis Waickman, Walter Ward, Edward Winger, Aubrey Worrell, Martin Zwerling, and the late Doctors Amos Christie, William Deamer and Frederic Speer.

I'm also grateful to Doctor Elmer Cranton and to Betty Flora. Each of these individuals carefully reviewed my entire manuscript and made constructive suggestions for improving it. Thanks are also due to other helpful consultants, including Doctor Dor Brown, Doctor John Curlin, and Pat Connolly.

Special appreciation is due Rebecca Davis who helped significantly with the diet sections of this book, and to Susan Karlgaard-Winfrey and Sally Karlgaard, R. N. who served as invaluable consultants, coordinators and collaborators in completing the book.

I also appreciate the charming and delightful art work of my daughter, Cynthia, whose pictures make "The Yeast Connection" easy to understand. Also to John Adams and the entire staff of ProtoType Graphics in Nashville for their skillful production services.

I'm grateful, also, to other members of my staff, Ditzi Brittain, Georgia Deaton, Brenda Harris, Brent Lay, Scott Marcon, Nancy Moss, Bettye Patterson, Charlotte Riggs, Nell Sellers, Therese Shelby, Denny Spencer, Alice Spragins, Maggie Spragins and Patrick Youngblood who have helped me in numerous ways in putting this book together.

Finally, I appreciate the suggestions of many candida "victims" who have taught me a lot about yeast-connected disease, including what helps them and what makes them worse. Included among these consultants are many of my own loyal patients as well as the patients of other physicians.

Foreword

It is time for all physicians and medical scientists to increase their understanding of the relationship between yeast and human illness. Many patients with yeast-related health disorders are being treated ineffectively just because their problem has gone unrecognized.

If one reviews the literature carefully, the supporting research is well documented. Antibiotics have been shown to inhibit both antibody synthesis and phagocytic activity, and thus may reduce the host resistance to invasion by *Candida albicans*.[1] Once established, candida components further depress immune function. Mannan, a carbohydrate component of candida, inhibits human lymphocyte proliferation.[2] Taking sera from women with recurrent vaginal candidiasis, Witkin and associates[3] were able to demonstrate a reduced or absent lymphocyte response to candida antigens. In another paper, Witkin thoroughly reviews the defective immune response in patients with recurrent candida infections.[4] The literature, therefore, clearly supports the theory that antibiotics can lead to candida overgrowth which suppresses immune function thereby predisposing one to recurrent infections.

There is much evidence to suggest that *C. albicans* is one of the most allergenic microbes.[5] Both immediate and delayed hypersensitivity reactions to candida are very common in the adult population. The relationship between yeast and urticaria has been established in a well-designed double blind trial.[6] The investigators estimate that in about 26% of patients with chronic urticaria, *C. albicans* sensitivity is an important factor. Significant clinical improvement was seen with anti-candida therapy and a low-yeast diet.

An increase in the population of *C. albicans* following antibiotic therapy or change in diet may also cause a chronic "irritable bowel" syndrome. This is ascribed to hypersensitivity to the organism or its metabolic products rather than actual infection.[5] *C. albicans* can cause allergic reactions in the large bowel and other mucous membranes.[7] The work of Holti[5] was so compelling that it was referenced in two of the most respected texts dealing with candida.[8,9]

The importance of the role of the intestinal tract in treating patients with recurrent vulvovaginal candidiasis has been nearly ignored. Vaginal candidiasis does not occur without the concomitant presence of *C. albicans* within the large bowel and a cure is unlikely as long as the vagina remains the only treatment target.[10]

Enteric candida undoubtedly play a greater role in human illness than has been previously suspected. A history of food and chemical intolerances is frequently seen in patients with a history of recurrent candida infections. There is increasing evidence that gut yeast may have a role in some cases of psoriasis.[11] Changes in mood and behavior related to yeast have been observed for over 30 years and are reviewed by Iwata.[12] Health professionals must take note of what is known about the yeast-human interaction. We must help our patients overcome this illness, which is probably, for most, iatrogenic in origin.

James H. Brodsky, M.D.
Chevy Chase, Maryland
Diplomate, American Board of Internal Medicine
Instructor, Georgetown University School of Medicine
American College of Physicians
American Society of Internal Medicine

References

1. Selig MS: Mechanisms by which antibiotics increase the incidence and severity of candidiasis and alter the immunological defenses. Bacteriol Rev, 30:442-459, 1966.
2. Nelson RD, Herron MJ, McCormack RJ, et al: Two mechanisms of inhibition of human lymphocyte proliferation by soluble yeast mannan polysaccharide. Infect Immun, 43:1041-1046, 1984
3. Witkin SS, Yu IR, Ledger WJ: Inhibition of Candida albicans-induced lymphocyte proliferation by lymphocytes and sera from women with recurrent vaginitis. Am J Obstet Gynecol, 147:809-811, 1983.
4. Witkin SS: Defective immune responses in patients with recurrent candidiasis. Infections in Medicine, pp. 129-132, May/June 1985.
5. Holti G: Candida allergy. *Symposium on Candida Infections*, pp. 73-81, 1966.

6. James J and Warrin RP: An assessment of the role of Candida albicans and food yeasts in chronic urticaria. Br J Derm, 84:227-237, 1971.
7. Alexander JG: Allergy in the gastrointestinal tract. Lancet, 2:1264, 1975.
8. Odds FC: *Candida and Candidosis*. Baltimore, University Park Press, 1979, p. 140.
9. Rippon JW: *Medical Mycology*. Second edition. Philadelphia, WB Saunders Co, 1982, p. 499.
10. Miles MR, Olsen L, Rogers A: Recurrent vaginal candidiasis; importance of an intestinal reservoir. JAMA, 238:1836-1837, 1977.
11. Rosenberg EW, Belew PW, Skinner RB, Crutcher N: Response to: Crohn's disease and psoriasis. New Eng J Med, 308:101, 1983.
12. Iwata K: A review of the literature on drunken symptoms due to yeasts in the gastrointestinal tract, in Iwata K (ed): *Yeasts and Yeast-Like Microorganisms in Medical Science*. Tokyo, University of Tokyo Press, 1976, pp. 260-268.

Preface
to the Third Edition

I finished medical school in 1942 and returned to my home town to practice in 1949. Beginning in 1955, I learned from the late Frederic Speer, M.D. and the late Albert Rowe, Sr., M.D. that many tired, irritable children and adults with multiple complaints would improve when they stopped eating common foods, including milk, corn, wheat, egg and chocolate.

Soon afterward, pioneer allergist Theron Randolph, M.D. taught me that many people with allergies and other chronic health problems suffered from the "chemical susceptibility" problem. And I learned that exposure to tobacco smoke, perfumes, colognes and petrochemicals would cause troublesome (and at times disabling) symptoms in such patients.

Through the decade of the '60s and '70s, my interest grew in chronic illness caused by adverse reactions to foods and chemicals. So did my interest in nutrition, including vitamin and mineral deficiencies, and the adverse effects of sugar.

In the fall of 1979, I learned from C. Orian Truss, M.D. of the relationship of *Candida albicans*, a common yeast, to many chronic illnesses. Then, following the recommendations of Dr. Truss, I began treating some of my difficult patients with a special diet and the safe, antifungal medication, *nystatin*. Nearly all were adults with complex health problems, including headache, fatigue, depression, irritability, digestive disorders, respiratory disorders, joint pains, skin rashes, menstrual disorders, loss of sex interest, recurrent bladder and vaginal infections and sensitivity to chemical odors and additives. Almost without exception, they improved. And some improved dramatically.

Since that time, I've become increasingly interested in *Candida albicans* and its relationship to human illness. And using a candida-control treatment program, I've been able to help hundreds of my adult patients with chronic health problems. Many of these patients felt "sick all over" and had struggled for years to overcome their health disorders.

Moreover, during the past several years, a number of my pediatric patients with chronic health problems, including hyperactive behavior, autism and recurrent ear disorders, have been helped by a similar program.

Yet, I've continued to be interested in factors other than yeasts which play a role in causing health problems in my patients. These include adverse reactions to specific foods, inhalants and chemicals, nutritional deficiencies and psychological factors.

But my recognition of "the yeast connection" has changed my life and my practice and has enabled me to help many, many patients conquer previously disabling illness.

This revised and expanded third edition contains many of the materials found in the previous editions. However, as I've learned new things, I've made appropriate changes and additions. These include: changes in the questions and answers section; deletion of some of the material relating to formaldehyde and mold control in your home; *complete revision of my dietary recommendations in Section B.*

You'll find my new recommendations and instructions a lot easier to follow. Moreover, since many people with candida-related health disorders are not allergic to yeasts, I suggest that you challenge with yeast (7-10 days after you begin your diet) to find out if yeast-containing foods bother you.

I added a brief, but important new chapter (38) entitled, "What You Should Do If You Aren't Improving."

I also made many changes in Section E. For example, in Chapter 34, I revised and updated my list of sources of information. Then I completely rewrote Chapter 35 ("What You Can Do If Your Physician Is Unaware of The Yeast Connection"). Included in this chapter is a new list of support groups, along with more specific suggestions to help you if you experience trouble in locating a physician.

Chapter 36 has been expanded to provide a more comprehensive report of the 1983 Birmingham Conference and to include, also, a report of many of the presentations at the 1985 San Francisco Conference. Appropriate additions and deletions have also been made in Chapter 37, "Potpourri."

I then added many pages of new information entitled, "THE YEAST CONNECTION UPDATE."

Included in this section is a discussion of the research studies of C. Orian Truss, M.D. which may explain how candida can make you sick. Also included is information about the recent scientific studies of Steven S. Witkin, Ph.D. (Cornell University Medical College) which describe "defects in cellular immunity" in patients who've received broad-spectrum antibiotics. Witkin also noted that many patients with yeast-related immunological problems "exhibited . . . . endocrine dysfunctions."

I discuss further the candida immunoglobulin studies which may help physicians determine more accurately the role of *Candida albicans* in making their patients sick. Included, also, are materials about other laboratory studies which may help identify viral infections and hormonal dysfunction in individuals who feel "sick all over" and who have failed to find help.

If your health problems are yeast connected, you'll usually develop nutritional deficiencies. Such deficiencies may be generalized and appear to especially involve the essential fatty acids, vitamins, magnesium and other minerals. To provide you with more information about nutrition, I interviewed Leo Galland, M.D. of New York City and included his comments, along with an extensive discussion of the essential fatty acids based on the clinical and laboratory studies of Dr. Galland and Dr. Sidney M. Baker.

Everyone today is worried about AIDS. And AIDS victims nearly always develop candidiasis because their immune systems have been weakened. To provide you with more information about AIDS and the yeast connection, I interviewed immunologist Alan Levin, M.D. of San Francisco and incorporated his comments.

Recently I've received many favorable reports about a nonprescription medication (caprylic acid). It is available in a number of different products, including Capricin®, Caprystatin®, Candistat-300®, Caprylate Plus® and Kaprycidin-A®. I briefly discuss these products and include information I've obtained from physicians who are using them.

I included my response to the skeptics who feel that the yeast/human illness hypothesis is "speculative" and "unproven." I then added more material on both old and new subjects that will interest you. These include especially PMS, sexual dysfunction, suicidal depression, mitral valve prolapse, silver/mercury dental fillings and the fascinating story of "the tomato effect."

Finally, I included material which will tell you about the International Health Foundation which has been established with a number of goals including helping people with chronic health disorders, especially those related to *Candida albicans*.

This book is designed to make "The Yeast Connection" easily understood by individuals with chronic health problems. It is also directed toward physicians and other professionals who are interested or involved in treating patients with these disorders.

I hope it will interest the public, including leaders in the field of business, labor, government and the media because I sincerely feel that recognition and appropriate management of yeast-connected illness can play a major role in what I recently referred to as "The Coming Revolution in Medicine."

This revolution can also save patients, the government, business and industry (including the health insurance industry) billions of dollars.

A Special Message For The Physician

I hope *The Yeast Connection* will interest you—even though you may feel that the candida-human illness hypothesis is "speculative" and "unproven". You may also feel that double blind (and other scientific) studies to document this hypothesis should be carried out and reviewed by competent institutional review boards.

I can understand such feelings. During the 40 years since I finished medical school, I've seen many therapies which were thought to be "the real thing" turn out to be inappropriate, worthless—or even dangerous.

For example, in the '40s and '50s, radiation therapy was used for many conditions including "enlarged thymus", facial acne, hypertrophic adenoid tissue, and fungal scalp infections. Yet, physicians subsequently learned that such therapy was inappropriate. Morever, they also discovered that head and neck radiation in children sometimes led to the development of malignant thyroid disease.

During the '50s, (along with most of my pediatric peers), I prescribed tetracycline for countless young children with respiratory infections. Then a decade later, I found that many of my tetracycline-treated youngsters' permanent teeth had become yellow and gray.

On the other hand, I've been fascinated by the story of James

Lind who, in the 1740s, prevented scurvy in English sailors by giving them limes. Yet, not until 1929 (when Nobel prize winner Albert Szent-Györgi isolated vitamin C) did we know why limes were effective.

I was similarly fascinated by the story of Ignace Semmelweiss, the young Viennese doctor who, in 1845, discovered a simple cure for dreaded "child-bed fever": handwashing before carrying out pelvic examinations of women in labor. Yet, because Semmelweiss' superiors objected to his "unscientific anecdotal observations", he was fired. Moreover, his hypothesis was rejected by the medical establishment for over twenty-five years.

In my opinion, the role of *Candida albicans* in making millions of people develop health problems resembles, in many ways, the observations of Lind and Semmelweiss. The hypothesis was proposed by C. Orian Truss, M.D. of Birmingham, Alabama and based on his clinical (anecdotal) observations. Moreover, Truss devised a simple treatment program which helped his patients before he understood the scientific mechanisms involved.

Although many questions remain unanswered, new clinical and laboratory studies are now explaining how and why candida causes symptoms in remote parts of the body. I hope you'll look at the observations of Iwata, Truss, Rosenberg, Witkin, Baker and Galland (Chapters 31, 36, 38, and 40 and 43 of the Update), and the unpublished candida immunoglobulin studies now being carried out by several other investigators. (Chapters 37 and 40 of the Update).

I am aware that THE YEAST CONNECTION has been "picked up" by many chronically ill people whose health problems may be related to other—or even more—significant causes. Moreover, as Ray C. Wunderlich, M.D. of St. Petersburg, Florida pointed out recently,

> "Desirable at all times, is a balanced approach that holds a healthy respect of *Candida albicans*—. At the same time, one does not wish to overlook the many other health departures that invite the candida syndrome. Those who suspect that they have symptoms—due to candida overgrowth, must not plunge headlong into a quest for a "magic bullet". Best and most long lasting health will be fostered by careful inquiry into yeast, but also, into psychological, nutritional, allergic, degenerative and toxic factors."

I agree.

Are Your Health Problems Yeast Connected?

	YES	NO
1. Have you taken repeated "rounds" of antibiotic drugs?	☐	☐
2. Have you been troubled by premenstrual tension, abdominal pain, menstrual problems, vaginitis, prostatitis, or loss of sexual interest?	☐	☐
3. Does exposure to tobacco, perfume and other chemical odors provoke moderate to severe symptoms?	☐	☐
4. Do you crave sugar, breads or alcoholic beverages?	☐	☐
5. Are you bothered by recurrent digestive symptoms?	☐	☐
6. Are you bothered by fatigue, depression, poor memory, or "nerves"?	☐	☐
7. Are you bothered by hives, psoriasis, or other chronic skin rashes?	☐	☐
8. Have you ever taken birth control pills?	☐	☐
9. Are you bothered by headaches, muscle and joint pains or incoordination?	☐	☐
10. Do you feel bad all over, yet the cause hasn't been found?	☐	☐

If you have 3 or 4 "yes" answers, yeasts *possibly* play a role in causing your symptoms.
If you have 5 or 6 "yes" answers, yeasts *probably* play a role in causing your symptoms.
If you have 7 or more "yes" answers, your symptoms are *almost certainly* yeast-connected.

Copyright ©1983, William G. Crook, M.D.

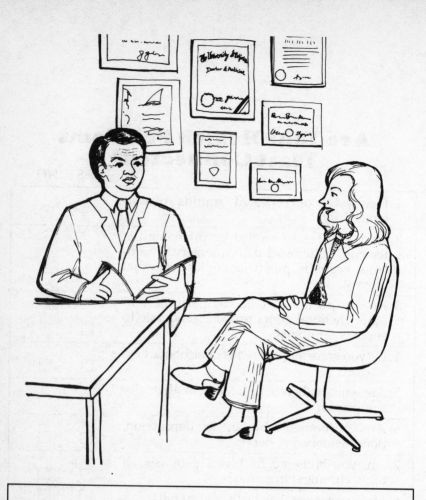

Before assuming your symptoms are caused or triggered by the common yeast germ, *Candida albicans*, go to your physician for a careful history and physical examination and appropriate laboratory studies or tests. An examination is important because many other disorders can cause similar symptoms.

However, if a careful check-up doesn't reveal the cause for your symptoms, and your medical history (as described in this book) is "typical," it's possible or even probable that your health problems are yeast connected.

What This Book Is All About

If you (or your child) are bothered by . . .

- Extreme fatigue or lethargy (the feeling of being drained)
- Depression
- Inability to concentrate
- Headaches
- Skin problems (such as hives, athlete's foot, fungous infection of the nails, jock itch, psoriasis or other chronic skin rashes)
- Gastrointestinal symptoms (especially constipation, abdominal pain, diarrhea, gas or bloating)
- Symptoms involving your reproductive organs
- Muscular and nervous system symptoms (including aching or swelling in your muscles and joints, numbness, burning or tingling, muscle weakness or paralysis)
- Respiratory symptoms
- Hyperactivity and recurrent ear problems . . .

go to your doctor for a careful checkup, including a history and physical examination, complete blood count, urinalysis, and tuberculin test. Depending on the nature and duration of your complaints and the findings on your initial examination, your physician may feel that other tests and studies are necessary.

However, if you've already been examined, tested and studied by your physician (. . . or by many physicians . . .) and the cause of your symptoms hasn't been identified, *reading this book could change your life*. Here's why: It's possible . . . or even probable . . . that toxins from the common yeast, *Candida albicans*, could be playing an important role in making you sick.

Yeast-connected health problems occur in people of all ages and both sexes. However, women are more apt to be affected. Yeasts are especially apt to play a role in causing your health problems if you:

1. Feel bad "all over," yet the cause can't be identified and treatment of many kinds hasn't helped.
2. Have taken prolonged courses of broad-spectrum antibiotic drugs, including the tetracyclines (Sumycin®, Panmycin®, Vibramycin®, Minocin®, etc.), ampicillin, amoxicillin, the cephalosporins (Keflex®, Ceclor®, etc.), and sulfonamide drugs, including Septra® and Bactrim®.
3. Have consumed diets containing a lot of yeast and sugar.
4. Crave sweets, breads or alcoholic beverages.
5. Notice that sweets make your symptoms worse or give you a "pick-up," followed by a "let-down."
6. Have symptoms of hypoglycemia.
7. Have taken birth control pills, prednisone, Decadron® or other corticosteroid drugs.
8. Have had multiple pregnancies.
9. Have been troubled by recurrent problems related to your reproductive organs, including abdominal pain, vaginal infection or discomfort, premenstrual tension, menstrual irregularities, prostatitis or impotence.
10. Are bothered by persistent or recurrent symptoms involving your digestive and nervous systems.
11. Have been bothered by persistent or recurrent athlete's foot, fungous infection of the nails or "jock itch."
12. Feel bad on damp days or in moldy places.
13. Are made ill when exposed to perfumes, tobacco smoke and other chemicals.

This book is written for patients, professionals, para-professionals, and the public. **Section A** explains why yeast-connected illness develops and how it can be suspected and identified. This section also deals with treatment, and a question and answer format discusses the use of diet and antifungal medication.

Diet plays a major role in the successful management of yeast-connected illness. **Section B** includes a discussion of the foods you should and should not eat. Illustrations and menus make the dietary instructions easier to follow.

Section C emphasizes that "unwellness" or ill health is rarely (if ever) due only to yeasts (or to any other single cause). Instead, illness develops because of a web of interacting causes. Accordingly, individuals with yeast-connected illness (and the professionals and para-professionals who work with them) must pay attention to the many other factors which determine whether a person is sick or well. Simple illustrations are again used to clarify concepts and instructions.

Section D discusses the many manifestations of yeast-connected illness. Featured in this section is an extensive discussion of yeast-connected illness in women, men, young children and teenagers. Also featured is a discussion of the relationship of yeasts to a number of supposedly incurable diseases, including multiple sclerosis and psoriasis.

In **Section E** you'll find suggestions that may help you overcome your yeast-connected health problems. Many items listed are "routine" instructions and their listing in this section serves as a reminder or check list. Others are based on suggestions I've obtained from many sources, including my patients and other professionals.

Section F is new information entitled, "The Yeast Connection Update."

The Yeast Connection . . . A Vicious Cycle

Antibiotics, especially broad spectrum antibiotics, kill "friendly germs" while they're killing enemies. And when friendly germs are knocked out, yeasts (*Candida albicans*) multiply.

Birth control pills, cortisone and other drugs stimulate yeast growth. So do diets rich in sugar.

Toxins from large numbers of yeasts weaken your immune system. Your immune system is also affected adversely by nutritional deficiencies and sugar consumption, and by exposure to environmental molds and chemicals (such as formaldehyde, petrochemicals, perfume and tobacco),

When your immune system is compromised, you're apt to develop respiratory, digestive and other symptoms and "feel bad all over." And you may develop adverse reactions to additional foods, inhalants and chemicals. As a part of these reactions, mucous membranes swell and you develop infections that a strong immune system would ordinarily conquer.

THE YEAST CONNECTION . . . A VICIOUS CYCLE

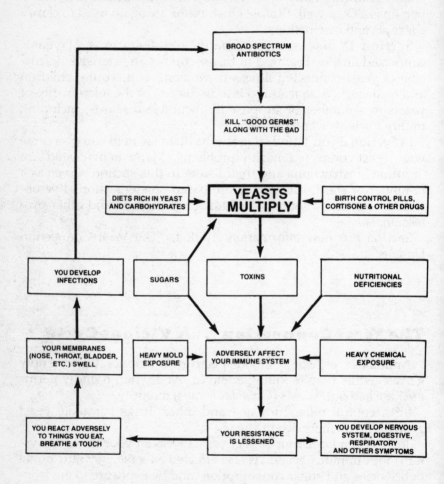

Table Of Contents

SECTION A:
How You Suspect, Identify and Treat Yeast-Connected Illness

SECTION B:
To Control Candida, You Must Change Your Diet

SECTION C:
Keeping Candida Under Control
Requires More Than Medication and a Special Diet

SECTION D:
Manifestations of Yeast-Connected Illness

SECTION E:
Other Helpful Information

SECTION F:
The Yeast Connection Update

"Sit down before a fact, as a little child, be prepared to give up every preconceived notion, follow humbly wherever and to whatever abyss nature leads or you shall learn nothing."

Thomas Huxley

"It is very unscientific not to have an open mind."

E. William Rosenberg, M.D.

Section
A

How you suspect, identify and treat yeast-connected illness.

What are yeasts?

Yeasts are single cell fungi which belong to the vegetable kingdom. And like their "cousins" the molds, they live all around you. And one family of yeasts, "Candida albicans", normally lives in your body and more especially in your intestines and other parts of your digestive tract.

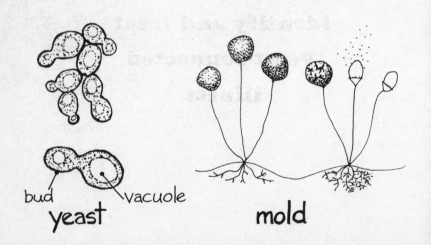

bud   vacuole
yeast   mold

What Are Yeasts?

In his book, *Medical Mycology,*[2] John Willard Rippon, Ph.D. said in effect:

> "Yeasts (including *Candida albicans*) are mild mannered creatures incapable of producing infection in the normal healthy individual. They only cause trouble in the person with weakened defenses.
> . . . "The severity of the disease will depend on how weak a person's resistance is, rather than on any disease-producing properties exhibited by the fungus . . . . Because of its rapid ability to make itself at home on mucous membranes (the medical term is "colonize") and take advantage of many types of host alterations, the clinical manifestations of candida infection are exceedingly variable . . . . *Candida albicans accounts for the vast majority of diseases caused by the yeast."*

In his continuing discussion, Dr. Rippon tells about the different types and classifications of the various yeasts, including common brewer's and baker's yeasts, as well as the yeasts found in beer, ale and wine. Still other yeasts are lactose fermenters and are associated with the preparation of fermented milk beverages.

Hippocrates described one type of yeast infection, *thrush*, in debilitated patients and the presence of this clinical condition has been recognized for centuries. Galen described it as a common occurence in children, particularly sickly children. Textbooks of pediatrics in the 1700s also described thrush and in the 1800s it was first noted to be acquired through passage of the baby through the mother's womb.

A confusing number of different names have been applied to this same yeast organism we know as *Candida albicans*. These have included '*Oidium albicans*', '*Saccaromyces albicans*' and '*Monilia albicans*'. Apparently different observers in different countries developed their own pet names.

According to Rippon, vaginal yeast infection (candidiasis) was first described by Wilkinson in 1849. Systemic disease caused by candida was described in a debilitated patient in 1861 and on a number of occasions thereafter during the 19th century.

Candida infections of the nails were first described in 1904, skin disease in 1907, and candida cystitis in 1910. Chronic mucocutaneous disease was probably first described in 1909. By the early 1940s, it thus became evident that candidiasis was the most variable of the fungous infections. Statistically it was a common infecting agent of the skin, mucosa and vagina; yet it was rarely found to cause serious systemic disease.

In his continuing discussion, Rippon commented,

> "A revival of interest in systemic candidiasis took place after 1940. The occurrence of candidiasis as a sequel to the use of antibacterial antibiotics, particularly broad spectrum antibiotics, evoked a great surge of research . . . Presently, candida is recognized as one of the most frequently encountered fungal opportunists and is now regarded as the commonest cause of serious fungal disease."

Another recent informative book, *Candida and Candidosis*,[3] by British microbiologist F.C. Odds, comprehensively covers *Candida albicans* and other candida species. According to Dr. Odds, 200 to 300 scientific articles on candida appear annually and his book lists 2,265 references. Serious students of yeast-connected illness will find this book to be a treasure house of information.

Yet, in spite of these thousands of scientific articles on *Candida albicans*, until the first paper by C. Orian Truss, M.D.[†], there were only occasional references in the medical literature[††] suggesting that usually harmless yeast organisms could be related to so many different medical disorders.

[†] Presented at the Eighth Annual Scientific Symposium of the Academy of Orthomolecular Psychiatry held in Toronto, April 30–May 1, 1977, and published in the *Journal of Orthomolecular Psychiatry*, 7:17–37, 1978 (Publications office: 2231 Broad Street, Saskatchewan, Canada). Two subsequent papers in the same journal extended and clarified Truss' brilliant pioneer observations and concepts. All three of these papers are reprinted in the book, THE MISSING DIAGNOSIS, published by Truss in January, 1983. (Information about ordering this book can be obtained by writing to: THE MISSING DIAGNOSIS, P.O. Box 26508, Birmingham, Alabama 35226.)

[††] In November, 1983, Drs. Lawrence Dickey and Francis Waickman pointed out that Alfred V. Zamm, M.D. of Kingston, New York, had published original observations on the role of *Candida albicans* in chronic urticaria and other allergies and diseases of obscure cause. Dr. Zamm's recommended program of management included a yeast free diet and a therapeutic trial of nystatin. His observations were presented in part at the annual meeting of the Society for Clinical Ecology in Chicago December 12, 1970, and were subsequently published in a series of articles in CUTIS (January and February, 1972 and May, 1973) and in the book CLINICAL ECOLOGY (see Reading List—Chapter 47).

A Typical Patient, Janet, Tells Her Story

During the past 7 years, I've seen hundreds of patients (especially young women) with yeast-connected health problems. Here's a typical story as recorded by 33-year-old Janet:†

"I'm ready to find out if it's 'all in my head' and my symptoms are due to 'just getting older' or whether there's something that's really making me feel sick.

"All my childhood, I suffered with stomach problems which were usually blamed on 'nerves.' But when my children developed allergies, I began to suspect that allergies were part of my trouble, too.

"After my first child was born (1976), I was troubled by painful aches in my fingers and knees for 2 or 3 months. When my mother suggested I quit dipping the baby's diapers and quit using Clorox® , the aches went away.

"About a year later, I developed a strange swelling in my ankles and feet which caused enough pain to prevent walking. I couldn't even get my shoes on. So I went to an orthopedic surgeon (my dad, a physician, was out of the country). Although he found no reason for the swelling, he did give me medicine. Gradually the swelling subsided.

"I began having headaches, dizziness, nausea, sore throat and earaches in the fall of 1980. My doctor put me on several antihistamines and intermittent antibiotics. But because I hate to depend on medicine, in the fall of 1981, I decided to eliminate coffee, tea, milk, orange juice, colas and chocolate because of food-induced reactions I'd seen in my children.

"Food elimination helped to some degree, but during the winter and spring I was troubled by persistent night cough and a tickle in my throat. I took another round of antibiotics which helped temporarily, but then my symptoms returned.

"Last summer, after a short exposure to paint, I felt sick with generalized aching, symptoms of a cold and hurting in my chest. From time to

†This patient was reported in my recent article in the *Journal of the Tennessee State Medical Association.*[1]

time, I would develop what seemed like the flu but it would only last one day. As I tried to figure it out, I remembered that I had used Clorox® and Comet® .

"On the last two occasions when I've had my teeth filled, the reaction I experienced scared me and my dentist, too. Injections of Lidocaine® to deaden my gum made me tingle and feel light-headed, confused and fatigued. Codeine also caused adverse effects.

"This spring, I've developed bladder problems; two infections and frequent urination. I've also been unable to empty my bladder without hard pushing. These symptoms took me to a urologist who diagnosed it as 'a small urethra and spasm'. He dilated me and gave me medicine. Incidentally, frequent urination had been a part of my life, but not the pressure. (I have even wet the bed since I've been married.)

"I also am bothered by nervousness, fatigue, puffiness of my fingers, bloating, excessive weight gain and breast soreness during the week before my period."

When I first saw Janet on July 10, 1982, she looked tired, and dark circles under her eyes accentuated the appearance of fatigue. Her nasal membranes appeared swollen and lavender in color, and a transverse crease extended across her nose. A review of her diet showed that while she ate some "good foods," she "loved sweets," including sugar-sweetened cereals, ice cream, Mountain Dew® and Oreo® cookies.

A further review of Janet's history revealed that she had taken antibiotics on five occasions during the last year. Moreover, she had been treated for vaginal yeast infection on four occasions in less than 12 months. Other symptoms included swelling, weight gain, breast soreness, loss of sexual feeling and increased fatigue during the week before the beginning of her menstrual period.

Because of Janet's respiratory symptoms, I carried out limited allergy testing to the common inhalants. Much to my surprise, there were no significant reactions. So because her history strongly suggested yeast-related illness, I prescribed nystatin, 1-million units (¼ teaspoon of powder) four times a day, and a yeast-free, low-carbohydrate diet. Two weeks after beginning treatment, Janet reported:

"I'm much better. My ears are better, my night cough and bladder symptoms are gone. My energy level has improved significantly and I no longer feel bloated."

Nystatin and dietary treatment were continued, and a yeast-free vitamin/mineral preparation was added along with supplemental essential fatty acids, calcium lactate and magnesium oxide.

In the ensuing months, Janet steadily improved. However, she would notice a flareup of her symptoms whenever she ate foods containing sugar or yeast, or when she was exposed to chemicals. She also found that a dose of ½ teaspoon of nystatin, 4 times a day, was needed for maximal symptom relief; when she cut the dose in half, her generalized aching returned.

At a follow-up visit on March 8, 1983, eight months after starting on her treatment program, Janet reported:

> "I've had an excellent winter. I'm symptom-free and well, except when I cheat on my diet."

Janet moved to an adjoining state in 1985 and I haven't seen her as a patient since that time. However, in June, 1986, during a phone visit, she commented,

> "I've felt almost completely well a good part of the time. My serious problems of four years ago are, happily, a thing of the past. Yet, I've found I must watch my diet and cannot consume junk foods. Also, if I eat bread, my ring finger turns black. One thing I feel has helped me during the past year is moving away from a farm community and the many agricultural chemicals which were spread around.
>
> "I've experimented with my nystatin and gradually cut my dose down. Yet, I still require one tablet a day. If I don't take it, I can tell the difference . . . my fatigue symptoms return."

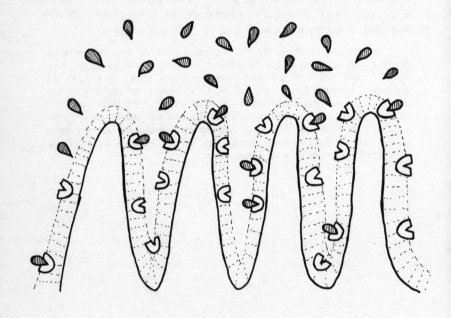

♥ Attacker

♡ Defender

♥ Immune Complex

⬚ Intestinal Membrane

Yeast Germs Naturally Live In Your Body

3

About Your Immune System And How Yeasts Make You Sick

How A Strong Immune System Protects You

Your immune system includes *antibodies* and many different kinds of *white blood cells*. These defenders might be compared to your Army, Navy, Marines, Air Force, police and secret service. Using many marvelous methods, they first recognize your enemies. Then they neutralize, conquer or eliminate them.

Fortifications or mechanical barriers (including your skin and mucous membranes) help keep invaders out. Your mucous membranes ("MM's") line the interior cavities and passageways of your body. Just below their surfaces are mucus-secreting glands which work like plastic "squeeze bottles." These glands help protect your delicate membranes by coating them with mucus. And when bacteria, viruses, chemicals or other substances try to invade or penetrate, the mucus provides a mechanical barrier.

Your MM's are also coated or "painted" with many different *antibodies*, including "secretory IgA" (a special type of gamma globulin or *immunoglobulin* . . . one of your immune system's important soldiers). When your lining membranes become inflamed, other *immunoglobulins*, including IgG, are found in the secretions.

The surface area of your intestinal membrane is as large as a tennis court. But rather than being flat, it looks like the coast of Norway. When yeasts, toxins or other enemies (*antigens*) try to break through your MM's, your defenders (*antibodies*) combine with them. The resulting antigen/antibody complexes on the surface of your MM's are known as *immune complexes*.

9

Yeast Germs Normally Live In Your Body

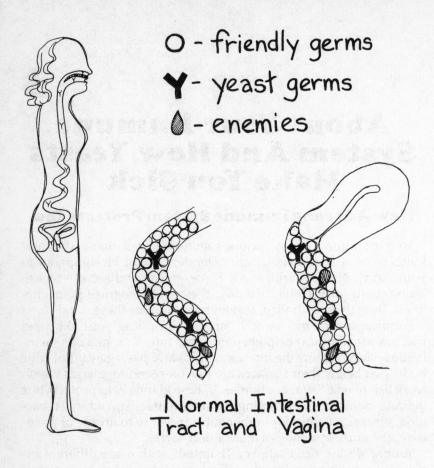

O – friendly germs

Y – yeast germs

◊ – enemies

Normal Intestinal
Tract and Vagina

A few families of yeast germs normally live on your mucuous membranes, along with billions of friendly germs. (Yeasts especially feel at home in the warm, dark recesses of your digestive tract and your vagina.) Unfriendly bacteria, viruses, allergens and other enemies also find their way into these and other membrane-lined passageways and cavities, including your respiratory tract. But when your immune system is strong, they aren't able to get through into your deeper tissues or blood stream and make you sick.

When Yeasts Multiply
They Weaken Your Immune System

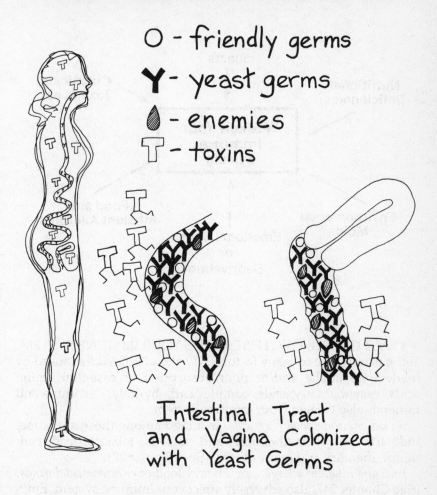

O - friendly germs

Y - yeast germs

🌢 - enemies

T - toxins

Intestinal Tract
and Vagina Colonized
with Yeast Germs

When you take antibiotics, especially if you take them repeatedly, many of the friendly germs in your body (especially those in your digestive tract) are "wiped out." Since yeasts aren't harmed by these antibiotics, they spread out and raise large families (the medical term is "colonization").

When yeasts multiply, they put out toxins which circulate through your body, weaken your defenders and make you sick.

11

Yeasts Are Only One Of The Factors Which Weaken Your Immune System

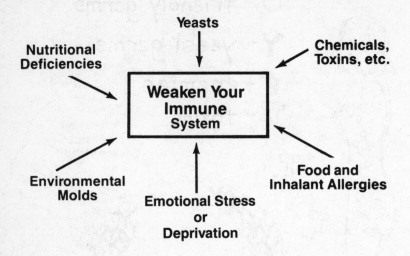

YEAST OVERGROWTH WEAKENS YOUR IMMUNE SYSTEM. Yet, it is only one of many factors. *Nutritional deficiencies* caused by inadequate intake and/or poor absorption of essential amino acids, essential fatty acids, complex carbohydrates, vitamins and minerals also weaken your immune system.

So do *environmental chemicals.* Included among these are home, industrial and farm chemicals and poisons, tobacco, lead, cadmium, mercury and many others. (See Chapter 22).

Food and inhalant allergies, or a heavy load of *environmental molds,* (See Chapter 24), also adversely affect your immune system. Emotional stress or deprivation may also weaken your immune system[†].

---

†Such a relationship has been described by Ronald J. Glasser and Norman Cousins (see Chapter 24), and in the recent book, PSYCHONEUROIMMUNOLOGY, edited by Robert Ader with a foreword by Robert Good (Academic Press, 1981).

When Your Immune System Is Weak, You Develop Health Problems

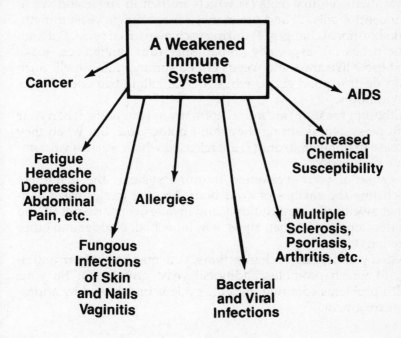

A Weakened Immune System

Cancer

AIDS

Fatigue
Headache
Depression
Abdominal
Pain, etc.

Allergies

Increased
Chemical
Susceptibility

Multiple
Sclerosis,
Psoriasis,
Arthritis, etc.

Fungous
Infections
of Skin
and Nails
Vaginitis

Bacterial
and Viral
Infections

When your immune system is weak, you're apt to complain of fatigue, headache and depression, and develop yeast or fungous infections of your skin, nails or vagina. You're also apt to develop allergies and become more susceptible to infections.

You may be troubled by multiple sclerosis, psoriasis or other serious disorders and show an increased susceptibility to chemicals.

When a person's immune system isn't functioning properly, other even more serious disorders may develop, including cancer[†] and the acquired immune deficiency syndrome . . . "AIDS".[†]

[†]Could either of these disorders be yeast-connected? I do not know. Yet it is logical to assume that they could be because they occur in persons with weakened immune systems. For a further discussion of the relationship of *Candida albicans* to AIDS, see Chapter 41, Update.

Many Different Things Encourage Yeast Growth.

Twentieth century diets (1) which are rich in sugar and yeast, birth control pills (2) and pregnancy (3) encourage yeast growth. So do hormonal changes (4) during each menstrual cycle. But antibiotic drugs (5), especially "broad spectrum" antibiotics, make yeast grow like grass and weeds after a summer rainy spell. Such drugs destroy good germs while they're killing bad ones. Yeasts then multiply.

Although yeasts (6) are found normally in your body, when your immune system is strong they don't bother you. But when they increase in number, toxins (7) are released which weaken your immune system (8).

Because of your weakened immune system, the defenders which line the cavities of your body become ineffective. Membranes swell and germs multiply and invade deeper tissues (9). So you develop nose, throat, sinus, ear, bronchial, bladder and other infections (10).

When you develop such infections, you may be given an antibiotic (5) which promotes additional yeast growth (6). So your health problems continue until the cycle is interrupted by appropriate treatment.

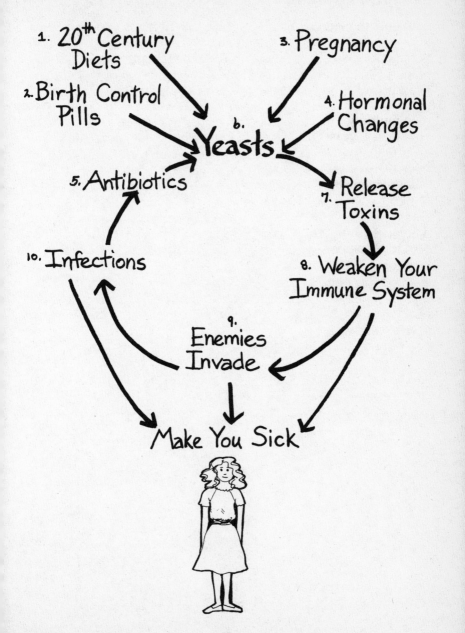

1. 20th Century Diets

2. Birth Control Pills

3. Pregnancy

4. Hormonal Changes

5. Antibiotics

6. Yeasts

7. Release Toxins

8. Weaken Your Immune System

9. Enemies Invade

10. Infections

Make You Sick

4

You Can Suspect That Candida Plays A Role In Making You Sick If . . .

you've taken antibiotics for acne

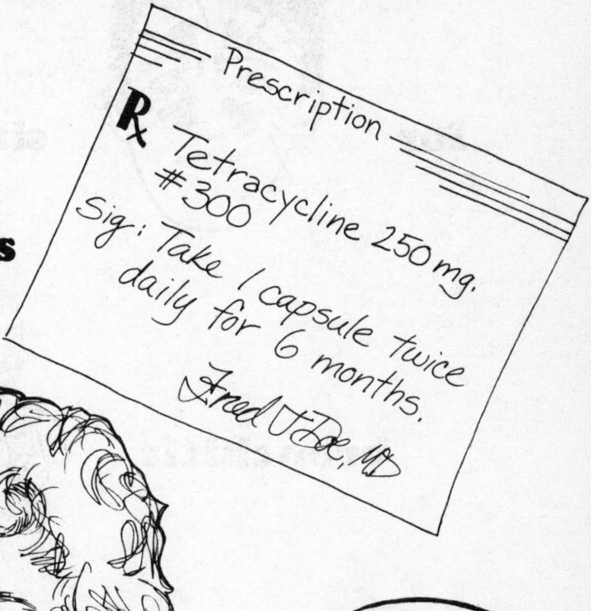

Prescription

℞ Tetracycline 250 mg.
#300

Sig: Take 1 capsule twice daily for 6 months.

Fred U Doe, MD

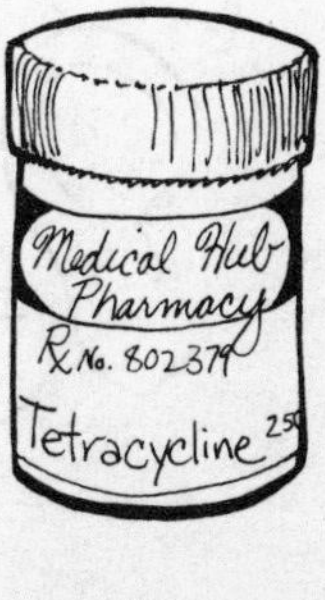

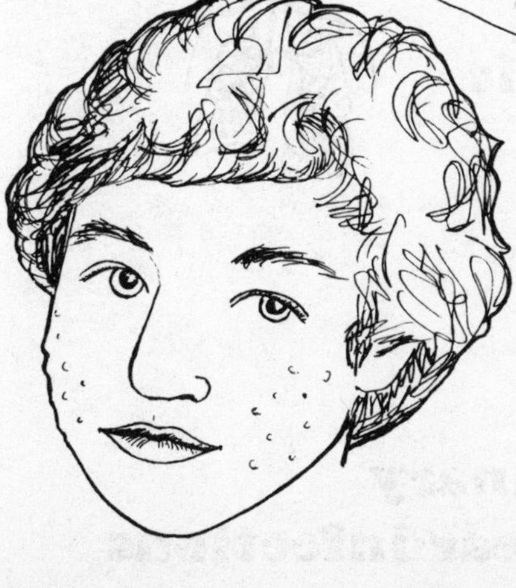

Medical Hub Pharmacy
Rx No. 802379
Tetracycline 250

or prolonged or repeated courses of antibiotics

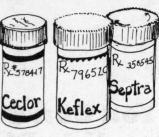

for 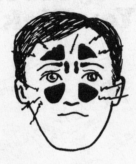 **sinusitis**

bronchitis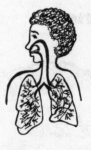

 **urinary or ear infections**

you've taken birth control pills[†]

or have been pregnant[†]

---

†Birth control pills and pregnancy stimulate growth of the yeast germ.

you've taken cortisone, prednisone or other corticosteroids

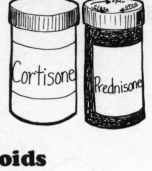

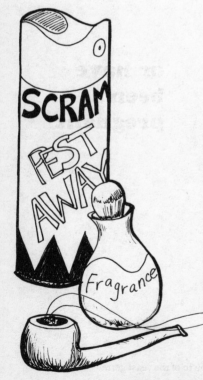

or your symptoms are aggravated by tobacco smoke, perfumes, diesel fumes and other chemical odors

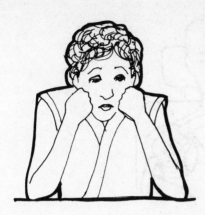

you feel tired, lethargic, drained or depressed

you're bothered by all sorts of other nervous system symptoms, including poor memory, feelings of unreality, irritability, headache or inability to concentrate

When **is** my next appointment ???

or . . .

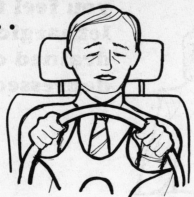

inappropriate drowsiness

numbness, tingling and muscle weakness

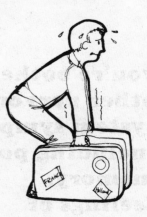

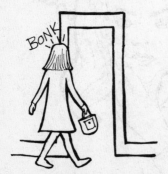

incoordination

you've been troubled by recurrent vaginal yeast infections or other disorders involving the sex organs or urinary system

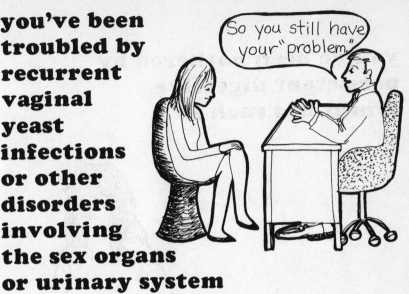

So you still have your "problem."

or athlete's foot, jock itch and other fungous infections of the skin

you've been bothered by
persistent digestive
symptoms such as

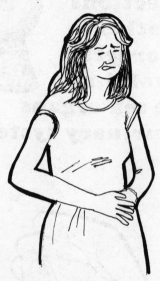

heartburn,
indigestion,
bloating,
abdominal pain,
gas,
constipation,
diarrhea,

you're bothered by other
troublesome symptoms such as
pain or swelling
of your joints,
nasal congestion,
recurrent sore
throats, cough,

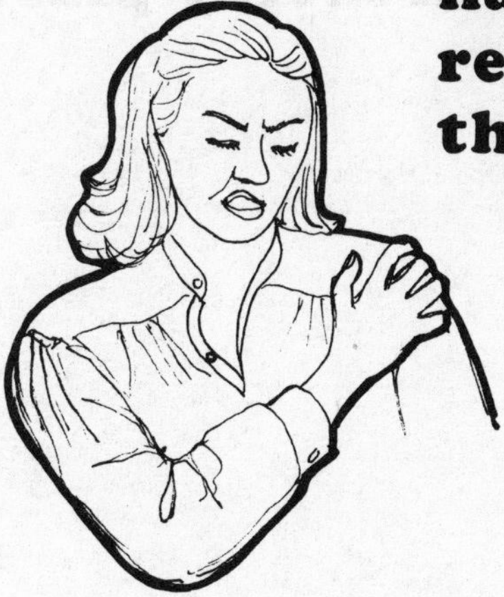

pain or tightness
in your chest,
spots in front
of your eyes,
or blurred
vision, fluid
in your ears
or just
feeling "lousy"

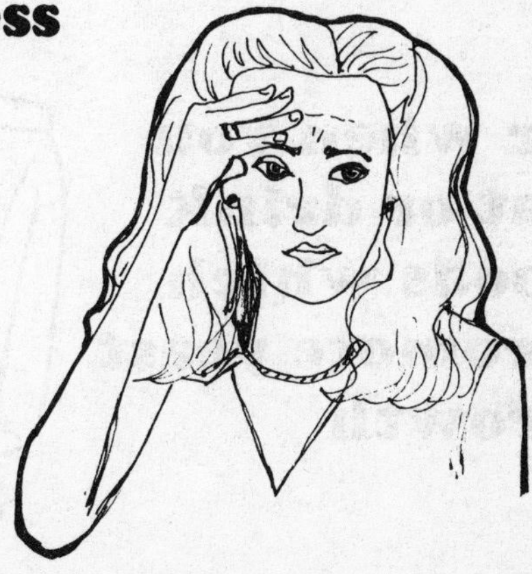

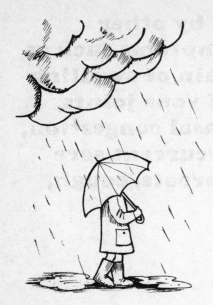

your symptoms flare up on damp days or in moldy places

or when you eat or drink foods which promote yeast growth

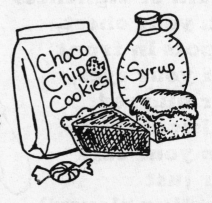

5

Identifying The Candida Problem

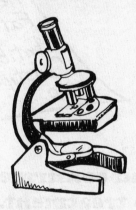

**Do tests help?
No . . .
or not much.†**

**Here's why: Candida germs
live in every person's body . . .
especially on the mucous
membranes. Accordingly
vaginal and other smears
and cultures for Candida don't
help.**

---

† New laboratory tests are now available which help confirm the diagnosis of an immune system disorder related to *Candida albicans*. (See Chapter 40, Update).

Therefore the diagnosis is suspected from your history

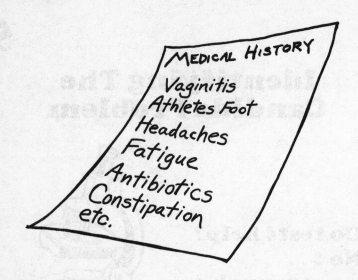

MEDICAL HISTORY

Vaginitis
Athletes Foot
Headaches
Fatigue
Antibiotics
Constipation
etc.

and confirmed by your response to treatment.

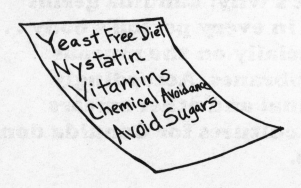

Yeast Free Diet
Nystatin
Vitamins
Chemical Avoidance
Avoid Sugars

6

Candida Questionnaire And Score Sheet

This questionnaire is designed for adults and the scoring system isn't appropriate for children. It lists factors in your medical history which promote the growth of *Candida albicans* (Section A), and symptoms commonly found in individuals with yeast-connected illness (Section B and C).

For each "Yes" answer in Section A, circle the Point Score in that section. Total your score and record it in the box at the end of the section. Then move on to Sections B and C and score as directed.

Filling out and scoring this questionnaire should help you and your physician evaluate the possible role of candida in contributing to your health problems. Yet it will not provide an automatic "Yes" or "No" answer.

SECTION A: HISTORY

1. Have you taken tetracyclines (Sumycin® , Panmycin® , Vibramycin® , Minocin® , etc.) or other antibiotics for acne for 1 month (or longer)?	35
2. Have you, at any time in your life, taken other "broad spectrum" antibiotics† for respiratory, urinary or other infections (for 2 months or longer, or in shorter courses 4 or more times in a 1-year period?)	35
3. Have you taken a broad spectrum antibiotic drug†— even a single course?	6
4. Have you, at any time in your life, been bothered by persistent prostatitis, vaginitis or other problems affecting your reproductive organs?	25
5. Have you been pregnant . . .	
2 or more times?	5
1 time?	3
6. Have you taken birth control pills . . .	
For more than 2 years?	15
For 6 months to 2 years?	8
7. Have you taken prednisone, Decadron® or other cortisone-type drugs . . .	
For more than 2 weeks	15
For 2 weeks or less?	6
8. Does exposure to perfumes, insecticides, fabric shop odors and other chemicals provoke . . .	
Moderate to severe symptoms?	20
Mild symptoms?	5
9. Are your symptoms worse on damp, muggy days or in moldy places?	20
10. Have you had athlete's foot, ring worm, "jock itch" or other chronic fungous infections of the skin or nails? Have such infections been . . .	
Severe or persistent?	20
Mild to moderate?	10
11. Do you crave sugar?	10

---

†Including Keflex,® ampicillin, amoxicillin, Ceclor,® Bactrim® and Septra®. Such antibiotics kill off "good germs" while they're killing off those which cause infection.

12. Do you crave breads?	10
13. Do you crave alcoholic beverages?	10
14. Does tobacco smoke *really* bother you?	10
Total Score, Section A........................	_____

SECTION B: MAJOR SYMPTOMS

For each of your symptoms, enter the appropriate figure in the Point Score column:

If a symptom is *occasional or mild* ....score 3 points
If a symptom is *frequent and/or moderately severe* ....score 6 points
If a symptom is *severe and/or disabling* ....score 9 points
Add total score and record it in the box at the end of this section.

	Point Score
1. Fatigue or lethargy	
2. Feeling of being "drained"	
3. Depression	
4. Poor memory	
5. Feeling "spacy" or "unreal"	
6. Inability to make decisions	
7. Numbness, burning or tingling	
8. Headache	
9. Muscle aches	
10. Muscle weakness or paralysis	
11. Pain and/or swelling in joints	
12. Abdominal pain	
13. Constipation and/or diarrhea	
14. Bloating, belching or intestinal gas	
15. Troublesome vaginal burning, itching or discharge	
16. Prostatitis	
17. Impotence	
18. Loss of sexual desire or feeling	
19. Endometriosis or infertility	

20. Cramps and/or other menstrual irregularities	
21. Premenstrual tension	
22. Attacks of anxiety or crying	
23. Cold hands or feet and/or chilliness	
24. Shaking or irritable when hungry	

Total Score, Section B . . . . ._____

SECTION C: OTHER SYMPTOMS†

For each of your symptoms, enter the appropriate figure in the Point Score column:

If a symptom is *occasional or mild* . . . . .score 1 point
If a symptom is *frequent and/or moderately severe* . . . .score 2 points
If a symptom is *severe and/or disabling* . . . . .score 3 points
Add total score and record it in the box at the end of this section.

Point Score

1. Drowsiness	
2. Irritability or jitteriness	
3. Incoordination	
4. Inability to concentrate	
5. Frequent mood swings	
6. Insomnia	
7. Dizziness/loss of balance	
8. Pressure above ears . . . feeling of head swelling	
9. Tendency to bruise easily	
10. Chronic rashes or itching	
11. Numbness, tingling	
12. Indigestion or heartburn	
13. Food sensitivity or intolerance	
14. Mucus in stools	
15. Rectal itching	

---

†While the symptoms in this section commonly occur in people with yeast-connected illness they are also found in other individuals.

16. Dry mouth or throat
17. Rash or blisters in mouth
18. Bad breath
19. Foot, hair or body odor not relieved by washing
20. Nasal congestion or post nasal drip
21. Nasal itching
22. Sore throat
23. Laryngitis, loss of voice
24. Cough or recurrent bronchitis
25. Pain or tightness in chest
26. Wheezing or shortness of breath
27. Urinary frequency or urgency
28. Burning on urination
29. Spots in front of eyes or erratic vision
30. Burning or tearing of eyes
31. Recurrent infections or fluid in ears
32. Ear pain or deafness

Total Score, Section C . . . . ._____

Total Score, Section A . . . . ._____

Total Score, Section B . . . . ._____

GRAND TOTAL SCORE . . . . ._____

The Grand Total Score will help you and your physician decide if your health problems are yeast-connected. Scores in women will run higher as 7 items in the questionnaire apply exclusively to women, while only 2 apply exclusively to men.

Yeast-connected health problems are almost certainly present in women with scores *over 180,* and in men with scores *over 140.*

Yeast-connected health problems are probably present in women with scores *over 120,* and in men with scores *over 90.*

Yeast-connected health problems are possibly present in women with scores *over 60,* and in men with scores *over 40.*

With scores of less than 60 in women and 40 in men, yeasts are less apt to cause health problems.

7

Treating Your Candida Problem

If I have a Candida problem how do I get rid of it?

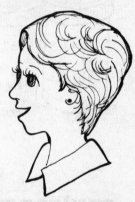

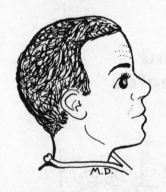

you avoid foods which promote yeast growth

and you take medication which helps rid your body of yeast germs

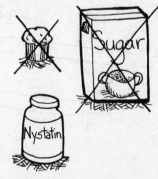

**you also need
to avoid birth
control pills,
antibiotics**

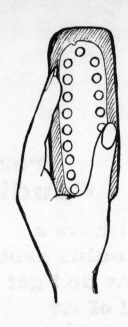

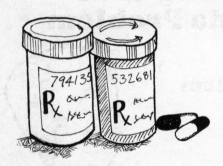

**and
environmental molds**

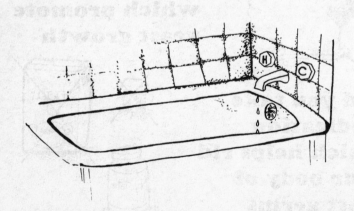

**you also need
to take other
steps to improve
your health**

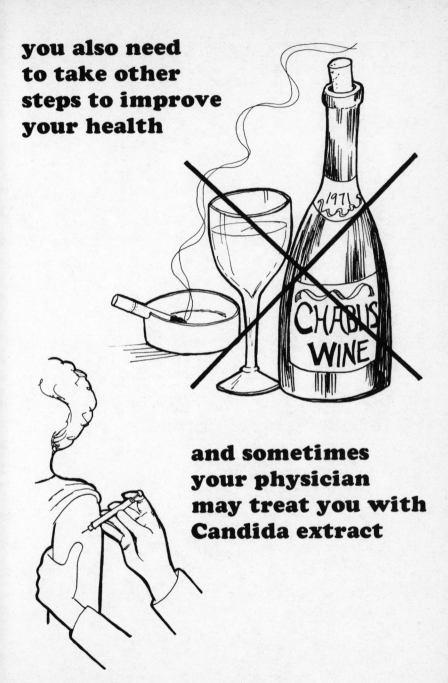

**and sometimes
your physician
may treat you with
Candida extract**

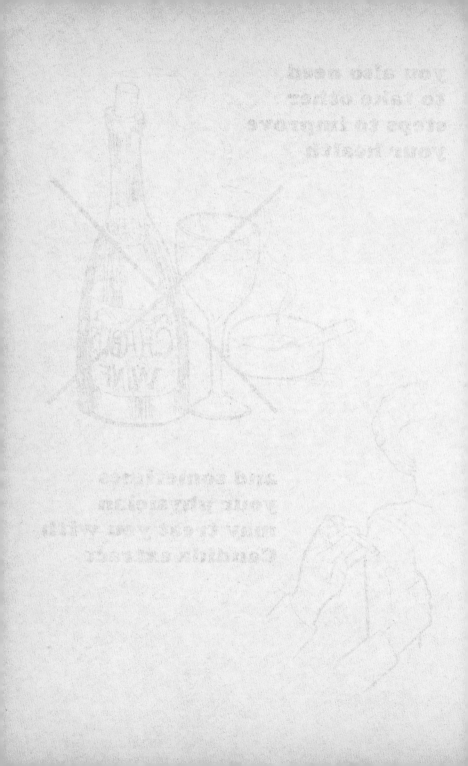

8

Overcoming Yeast-Connected Illness... Questions And Answers

(Q) Tell me more about "The Yeast Connection." And how can you tell if yeasts play a significant role in causing my health problems?

(A) If you're tired and feel bad all over, especially if your fatigue isn't relieved by a night's rest . . .

(Q) That's me. I feel "drained" . . . no matter how much rest I get.

(A) And if you're bothered by all sorts of other peculiar nervous system symptoms . . .

(Q) Like feeling spaced out, jittery and nervous . . . and forgetful? Sometimes I go to the pantry or refrigerator to get something and when I get there I've forgotten what I was looking for . . .

(A) Those are typical symptoms. Here are other symptoms that suggest candida: Problems with digestion, including diarrhea, bloating, gas and constipation.

(Q) Constipation!! I was *never* constipated until the last couple of years. But now, even though I eat tons of prunes and bran, I stay constipated. And gas . . . that's become really embarrassing. What other symptoms? . . .

(A) Those involving your reproductive organs, including severe menstrual cramps, menstrual irregularities and premenstrual tension.

(Q) You mean it could have something to do with my being hard to get along with and feeling like a stuffed sausage the week before my period starts? My husband can't stand me and I can't stand myself.

(A) Yes. And some of my candida patients tell me they gain 3 or 4 pounds during the week before their period and lose it after their period starts.

(Q) Does candida bother only women? I'm wondering if my husband has this problem. He's tired, grumpy and irritable, and is forever treating his jock itch and athlete's foot with powder. He's also visited a urologist because of prostate trouble.

(A) Sound like he may have the problem too. Recent research by a number of professionals, including Patricia Lucas, Ph.D.[4] suggests that candida *is* a low grade infection which can be transmitted by close association. Moreover, your husband's symptoms certainly suggest that he could have the problem, too. (See Chapters 34 and 42 of the Update)

(Q) OK . . ., you suspect the candida problem from my history. How do you go about making a positive diagnosis . . . do tests help?

(A) No . . . or not much. Here's why: Candida germs are present in everyone's body . . . yours included. They live on your mucous membranes, in your digestive tract[†] and in your vagina, even if you aren't troubled by digestive symptoms or vaginitis. Accordingly, smears and cultures which show candida don't help.

(Q) If tests don't help, what do you do? How can you make a positive diagnosis of a candida problem? Or how can you rule it out?

(A) If a careful history, physical examination and appropriate diagnostic tests and studies rule out other causes for your symptoms, I prescribe an anticandida treatment program and note your response. I call this a "therapeutic trial."

---

†Research studies to determine the level of candida in the stool are now being carried out in several medical centers. Perhaps objective laboratory data which will help in the diagnosis of the patient with candida-related illness may be available in the near future.

(Q) "Therapeutic trial?" . . . Tell me more about it . . . What does it consist of?

(A) It's a treatment program designed to *discourage* the growth of candida in your body, especially in your digestive tract and in your vagina. The program consists of two main parts . . . a special diet† and nystatin or other antifungal medication. Let's talk about your diet first. You'll be able to eat plenty of good foods while avoiding foods of low nutritional quality. *Before starting your diet, read your instructions carefully. Get the cooperation of other family members, prepare your menus, go shopping. Then begin.*

(Q) What foods can I eat?

(A) During the early weeks of your diet, feature vegetables . . . . especially asparagus, broccoli, cabbage, cucumbers, peppers, greens of all kinds, lettuce, okra, beans and squash (see Chapter 11). Also, eat some good protein foods, including fish (especially salmon and mackerel) and other seafood, chicken, lean beef and eggs. You should also consume some unrefined vegetable oils, including linseed, safflower, soy, walnut and corn. Also, small amounts of butter. You can eat some . . . but not too large a quantity . . . of the high carbohydrate vegetables and the grains.

(Q) What foods should I avoid?

(A) Candies, cakes, ice cream, soft drinks and sugar-containing foods of all sorts. Also honey, maple syrup and carob.

(Q) No way! I'm a sugar addict. I can't live without sweets.

(A) I'm not surprised. Sugar craving occurs commonly in people with the candida problem. So what you're saying makes me suspect candida even more.

(Q) How about fructose, and honey, and corn syrup? Are they as bad as ordinary table sugar?

(A) Yes. Just as bad, and they encourage the growth of yeasts . . . like rain makes grass, weeds and mushrooms grow.

(Q) What foods besides sweets should I avoid?

(A) Foods that contain yeast . . . especially raised breads, moldy cheeses, vinegar and other condiments, mushrooms, yeast-containing vitamins and alcoholic beverages (see Chapter 11). Although yeasty foods don't encourage candida growth, people with candida-related disorders are often allergic to all food and beverage yeasts, whether "live" or "dead" (cooked).

(Q) How will I know if I'm allergic to yeasty foods?

(A) If you're feeling better after following your diet for 7 to 10 days, eat some pure baker's yeast or brewer's yeast and see what happens. If you show no reaction, eat a yeasty food for three successive days. If there's still no reaction, you can consume yeast-containing foods in limited quantities. However, I suggest that you rotate them.

(Q) How about nuts, seeds and sprouts? Are they OK to eat on the diet?

(A) Such food substances are loaded with important essential nutrients, including minerals, vitamins, protein and essential fatty acids (see also Chapter 17). I recommend them. Yet, sprouts, seeds and nuts . . . . especially peanuts[†] . . . . usually contain molds. So they could disagree with you . . . . especially if you find you're allergic to the yeast-containing foods.

(Q) What can I drink?

(A) Water.

(Q) Water . . . you mean the stuff that comes out of the tap and nothing else?

(A) Yes . . . I mean water . . . during the first week or two. And since the water you drink is often loaded with chemicals, I recommend filtered water or bottled spring water. Then if you find you aren't allergic to yeasts in your diet, you can add teas, especially herb teas, on a rotated basis.

(Q) How about coffee and diet drinks?

(A) If you aren't allergic to yeasts, a cup or two of coffee a day is probably OK . . . but don't use sugar or the "whitener" in it. And the packets of artifical sweeteners also contain dextrose

---

[†]Most peanuts and peanut products are contaminated with the mold, *Aspergillus flavus*.

or corn sugar. So avoid them. Instead, you can use small amounts of liquid saccharin (Sweeta® or Fasweet®).

About the diet drinks. Sugar-free drinks don't promote the growth of candida. And an occasional one is probably OK. But they're loaded with phosphates, coloring, flavorings, and additives that could disagree with you. I don't recommend them.

(Q) What other foods must I avoid?

(A) Most boxed, canned, processed and packaged foods. Here's why: Such foods usually contain hidden ingredients, including sugar, dextrose, corn syrup and/or yeast. They also often contain hydrogenated or partially hydrogenated vegetable oils . . . a type of fat which may aggravate your health problems (see also Chapter 17).

(Q) Anything else?

(A) Yes. During the first three weeks avoid fruits completely. Although fruits contain complex carbohydrates, they're quickly converted into sugar and may encourage the growth of candida. After three weeks, if you're improving, try a fruit and see if you tolerate it without developing symptoms, but don't go overboard.

(Q) Let's talk about other carbohydrates. I see that I must avoid sugar completely and for the first three weeks I should also avoid fruits. But I'm wondering if I'll need to limit the good complex carbohydrates, including those in potatoes, yams, beans, corn, whole wheat, brown rice and oats.

(A) That's a hard question to answer. And you'll run into different opinions . . . even from the experts. Here are my suggestions: During the first few weeks of your diet, fill up on the low-carbohydrate vegetables (see list in Chapter 11). Include some, but not too large a helping of the high carbohydrate vegetables and grains (see list in Chapter 11). However, it's important for you to rotate them.

(Q) Rotate them? . . . Please explain.

(A) Food allergies and intolerances occur commonly in people with candida-related health problems. And if you eat a food every day you increase your chances of developing an allergy to that food. So eat potatoes on Monday, yams on Tuesday, lima beans on Wednesday and corn on Thursday. Then on Friday, you can eat potatoes again, and so on.

As you improve, you can try eating larger portions of potatoes, yams, corn, whole wheat, brown rice and other complex carbohydrates on a rotated basis. Remember, such foods contain many essential nutrients.

(Q) We've talked about my husband. Now I'd like to talk about my children. My 6-year-old son is hyperactive and keeps a cold. He has been given numerous rounds of antibiotics. And my year-old baby is experiencing many health problems. One cold after another, five ear infections, and a month ago tubes were put in his ears. His nose stays congested and he's irritable and restless. Do you think the anticandida program will help them?

(A) Yes. Although I've treated more adults than children with candida-related illness during the past year, I've found that candida plays an important role in causing health problems in many of my pediatric patients. (See Chapter 29).

Naturally, before putting your children on an anticandida treatment program, I need to examine them and carefully review their histories, because factors other than candida can play a role in causing the health problems you describe. For example, inhalant allergies, hidden food allergies and nutritional deficiencies may contribute to health disorders in children of all ages.

(Q) Suppose they were put on the anticandida program. What sort of diet restrictions would you recommend?

(A) I restrict sugar and other refined carbohydrates in all of my pediatric patients, even those in whom I don't suspect candida. My own observations,[5A,B,C] as well as those of Cheraskin,[6] Prinz[7] and others[8A,B,C] make me feel that sugar may bother both children and adults. Such individuals tend to develop emotional and behavior problems and suffer from recurrent respiratory infections. So keep your children off sugar and corn syrup, maple syrup and honey. *Do not limit their good complex carbohydrates*.

Offer them a variety of nutritious foods, including meats, eggs, vegetables, whole grains, nuts, seeds, fresh fruits and some dairy products, if they aren't allergic to milk. In infants still taking a formula, I prescribe a special soy formula which contains no corn syrup or other refined carbohydrates. And I use cereal grains, fruits and vegetables to supply the child's carbohydrate needs.

(Q) Would my children need to avoid yeast-containing foods?

(A) Possibly. You can find out by completely avoiding such foods for 7 to 10 days and then challenging and noting symptoms.

(Q) How about fruit juices?

(A) Fruit juices are loaded with yeasts. In addition, they're quickly converted into sugar. So offer your child water or vegetable juices and avoid fruit juices during the first 7-10 days of the diet; then use them sparingly . . . whole fruit is better.

(Q) OK. Back to my own situation. Other than following the diet, what else should I do?

(A) You'll need a medication which helps eradicate or control the yeast organisms in your digestive tract. Nystatin is the medication I usually prescribe for my patients with yeast-connected health problems.

(Q) What kind of medicine is nystatin?

(A) Nystatin is an antifungal drug which kills yeasts and yeast-like fungi. Yet it doesn't affect bacteria and other germs. (See, also, the story of nystatin, Chapter 43, Update).

(Q) What form does nystatin come in? Is it available on prescription?

(A) Nystatin is available on prescription in 500,000 unit oral tablets. These tablets are marketed by Lederle under the brand name, Nilstat® , and by Squibb under the brand name, Mycostatin® . Nystatin is also available in liquid oral suspensions, vaginal tablets and suppositories,† and topical

---

†Women with yeast-connected health problems should take appropriate steps to control candida in the vagina—*even if they are NOT bothered by vaginal symptoms.* Effective preparations include Mycelex G® , Monistat-7® and Gyne-Lotrimin® creams and suppositories. Yogurt douches are also effective as are intravaginal preparations of nystatin. (See also Chapter 34).

powders. Generic preparations of nystatin are also available.

Still another form, chemically-pure nystatin powder, is manufactured by The American Cyanamid Company, Lederle division. Pharmacists, hospitals, clinics and physicians can obtain information about nystatin powder by calling 1-800-LEDERLE (see Chapter 43).

(Q) What form of nystatin do you recommend?

(A) Although nystatin tablets are convenient and easy to obtain on prescription, I usually recommend the powder. Here's why:

1. Yeasts live in your digestive tract, from your mouth to your rectum. Accordingly, the powder helps you get rid of yeast in your upper digestive tract, as well as in your intestines.

2. The powder contains no food coloring, chemicals, dye or other similar ingredients which may cause reactions in chemically-sensitive patients.

3. The powder is more economical.

(Q) Do precautions need to be taken in storing the powder?

(A) Yes. The powder should be refrigerated. In talking to a representative from the manufacturer, she commented, "We ship the powder through ordinary channels and it does not lose significant potency in several days without refrigeration. However, potency is more apt to be retained when the powder is refrigerated."

(Q) How should I take the powder?

(A) Here's a method used by many physicians: Add the prescribed dose to 3 ounces of water. Take a large mouthful and swish it around before swallowing. Then drink the rest of the dose.

Here's another way I like better. Dump the nystatin powder on your tongue and let it gradually dissolve in your mouth. I prefer this method and feel it is more effective. I realize the powder has a bitter taste, but not as bitter as many other medicines. Moreover, the taste soon goes away.

Some of my patients say, "At work or especially when I'm travelling, I find it inconvenient or impossible to take nystatin powder during the day. So I like the tablets during the day and the powder for my morning and evening doses."

Recently, I've advised all my patients to use the nystatin powder for 2 of their 4 doses, and the capsules (or tablets) for the other doses. Here's why: The antifungal action of the powder in the mouth, esophagus and stomach is important. Yet, since studies show that candida growth is heavier in the lower bowels, the nystatin in capsules (or tablets) should reach this part of the digestive tract in higher concentration than the powder.

(Q) Are dye-free tablets or capsules of nystatin available that I could use in place of the powder for my daytime dose of nystatin?

(A) Although dye-free tablets aren't manufactured by the large pharmaceutical firms, some pharmacists prepare and dispense nystatin powder in dye-free capsules.

(Q) If nystatin helps me, how long will I need to take it?

(A) This will depend on your response. You'll need to take it for many, many months . . . or until you're well. And some of my patients have required nystatin for a year or longer. Try to be patient.

(Q) Does nystatin often cause adverse reactions . . . or side effects?

(A) Nystatin is an unusually safe medicine . . . as safe or safer than most drugs physicians prescribe for their patients. According to the *Physician's Desk Reference*[9] (which gives information on over 2500 prescription drugs), "Nystatin is virtually non-toxic and non-sensitizing and is well tolerated by all age groups, even on prolonged administration."

Here's a major reason for the safety of nystatin . . . *very little is absorbed from the intestinal tract*. Accordingly, it helps the person with yeast-related health problems by killing candida in the digestive tract.

Nevertheless, it disagrees with some patients and may cause digestive symptoms or skin rashes. In addition, some individuals develop other symptoms, including headache, fatigue and flu-like symptoms, especially during the first few days of treatment. Fortunately, these symptoms usually subside within several days, even though the medication is continued.

(Q) What causes these symptoms? Do they develop because of an allergy to the nystatin?

(A) Although scientists haven't yet determined the mechanism of these reactions, many experts believe they occur when your body absorbs large quantities of killed yeast germs. Somewhat similar reactions to the killing off of other harmful micro-organisms were first described almost 100 years ago and are sometimes referred to as "Herxheimer" reactions.

A physician consultant who has suffered from candida-related illness commented, "As long as nystatin causes symptoms, it's probably killing candida. And in my experience, most patients who develop such symptoms can take nystatin at a reduced dose, if symptoms are intolerable. Then, as they improve, they can usually take larger doses."

(Q) Could reactions to nystatin make it necessary for me to stop the drug or change the dose?

(A) Yes, but before I give up on nystatin, I instruct my patients to experiment with the dose, as the proper dose of nystatin must be determined by trial and error. Moreover, the correct dose varies from patient to patient.

Most of my patients improve when they take 500,000 to 1,000,000 units (1 or 2 tablets or 1/8 to 1/4 teaspoon of the powder) of nystatin four times a day. However, some patients require 4 to 8 tablets or 1/2 to 1 teaspoon of the powder four times a day. And a rare patient requires an even larger dose. By contrast, an occasional patient does well on a dose of 1/16 teaspoonful (or less) given 4 times a day.

Now, I'd like to repeat and clarify my comments about reactions.

Many of my patients show a temporary worsening of symptoms after starting to take nystatin.

Such symptoms aren't normally caused by an allergic reaction to the nystatin. Instead, they indicate that the nystatin is killing the candida and the patient may need either a bigger dose or a smaller dose.

Symptoms of too big a dose include flushing, fever and flu-like symptoms. By contrast, fatigue, headache, depression and digestive upsets are common underdose symptoms that will often improve on a bigger dose. Either type of reaction usually subsides in 4 to 7 days, even though the medication is continued.

An occasional patient has developed headaches, depression, fatigue, muscle aching, vomiting, diarrhea or skin rashes. Usually, these symptoms occur during the first week of treatment.

However, such reactions may rarely occur in patients who have been taking nystatin for several months without previous adverse effects.

When nystatin reactions persist, I usually discontinue it for 3 weeks. During this period, I prescribe a strict diet and products containing acidophilus and other friendly bacteria. Some of my patients have also found that eating garlic or taking odorless aged garlic extract (Kyolic) is effective in controlling candida.

In many patients I recommend other nonprescription anti-yeast products including caprylic acid (See Chapter 43 update) and citrus seed extract. Then depending on the patient's response, I may again try nystatin.

In other patients, especially those with severe problems, I now prescribe Diflucan (fluconazole).

(Q) Diflucan?

(A) Yes . . . Diflucan . . . a drug which was used extensively in Europe in the 1980's without significant unfavorable side effects.

Diflucan was first licensed by the Federal Drug Administration (FDA) in the spring of 1990 for use in the United States. However, the initial recommendations by the manufacturer (Pfizer-Roerig) focused mainly on using Diflucan in treating patients with severe depression of the immune system, including those with AIDS and cancer.

During the past several years, word of the effectiveness of Diflucan in treating patients with Chronic Fatigue Syndrome and related disorders spread to many physicians.

And in November 1993, William C. Steere, Jr., CEO of Pfizer, said that in early August Pfizer received an "approval" letter from the FDA for the use of Diflucan in the treatment of vaginal candidiasis.

"In U.S. clinical trials, which included more than 800 women with vaginal candidiasis, a single 150 mg. oral Diflucan tablet proved to be well tolerated and as effective as seven days of intravaginal therapy.

"In the 57 countries where Diflucan is already available for vaginal candidiasis, more than 9 million women have received single dose treatment."

(Q) What kind of medicine is Diflucan? How does it differ from nystatin?

(A) Like nystatin, Diflucan is an antifungal drug which kills yeast and yeast-like fungi. Like nystatin, it doesen't affect bacteria or other germs.

(Q) Would I need a prescription? What form does Diflucan come in?

(A) Yes. You'd need a prescription from a licensed M.D. or D.O. Diflucan is available in 50, 100 and 200 mg. tablets.

(Q) What is the usual dose? How long would I need to take it?

(A) The dose and duration of therapy depends on the severity of your health problems. Patients with mild problems may respond to 100 mgs. a day for a week, then one tablet every two to seven days.

Individuals with more severe problems may require 200 to 400 to 600 mgs. daily for a month—or many months. When improvement occurs, medication can be taken less frequently or discontinued.

(Q) Please tell me more about possible side effects.

(A) In responding I'd like to cite the experiences of Sidney M. Baker, M.D., a Connecticut physician who commented recently: "I started using Diflucan before it was on the market in the U.S. and I have now prescribed it for over 1000 patients. *I have not seen a single significant toxic effect—even in children.* I've seen only a handful of gastrointestinal disturbances . . . some of them persisting for a while after the patient stops the medication. I've also seen a few people who claim they were getting dizzy and lightheaded and had to stop."

"But this is only a handful and it's amazing considering that one is bound to see a certain amount of "die-off" with any antifungal drug.

"When I first started using Diflucan I did so cautiously and used 50 mgs. once a day. Now I give patients 200 mgs. a day for a month. If this program doesn't provide them with significant help, a yeast problem isn't apt to be their main difficulty."

(Q) Have other physicians seen similar favorable results?

(A) Yes. Here are other reports I've received. Charles S. Resseger, D.O., an Ohio physician commented: "I've now treated over 1000 people with Diflucan ranging up to 600 mgs. a day for up to 18 months. *I've never yet seen any adverse reaction other than an occasional mild one after four months of therapy.* (emphasis added) Usually patients who experience adverse reactions are taking more than 100 mgs. a day.

Phillip K. Nelson, M.D., a Florida gynecologist commented: "I've had the opportunity of working with patients with CFIDS (Chronic Fatigue-Immune Deficiency Syndrome) over the past two years and seeing their response to both diet and antifungals has been impressive.

"That is not to say that all CFIDS patients will benefit from this approach but certainly many do and with this illness we accept improvement from many sources.

"Many people have trouble sticking to the diet completely, but even avoidance of simple sugars has been a great help. I've been using Diflucan more than nystatin. I found that an initial dose of 200 mgs. followed by 100 mgs. weekly for several months has apparently succeeded in clearing the gut of candida when combined with carbohydrate restriction.

"This same regimen has helped many of my patients who have recurrent candida vaginitis. I think most experts agree that vaginal candidiasis has a bowel reservoir."

(Q) Are there still other prescription antiyeast medications?

(A) Yes. Ketoconazole. This drug was licensed by the Federal

Drug Administration (FDA) in 1981 and is marketed in this country by the Janssen Company under the name Nizoral.

Nizoral is a potent valuable drug and like nystatin is absorbed from the intestinal tract and transported by the circulation to various parts of the body.

(Q) What is the usual dose? How does Nizoral compare with Diflucan? Are there side effects?

(A) The usual dose: One 200 mg. tablet, once or twice daily. Because Nizoral can adversely affect the liver in a rare patient, the manufacturers state, "It is important to carry out liver function tests before treatment and at periodic intervals during treatment (monthly or more frequently), particularly in patients who will be on prolonged therapy who have a history of liver disease."

Nizoral may also transiently inhibit testosterone production in men and adrenal cortisol production in people of both sexes.

(Q) Since Nizoral causes these side effects, is it worth the risk?

(A) In some patients the answer would be "yes." These would include people with obvious yeast related health problems who did not respond to Diflucan or nystatin. And some physicians, including Allan Levin of California prefer Nizoral to other antiyeast medications. Also Nizoral is less expensive.

(Q) Are there still other prescription antiyeast medications?

(A) Yes, Sporanox (itraconazole). After extensive research trials in the U.S. and other countries this drug which might be called a "cousin" of Diflucan and Nizoral was released for use in the U.S. by the Janssen Company early in 1993.

(Q) What is the dose?

(A) The usual dose: Two 100 mg. capsules once or twice daily with meals.

(Q) What are the indications for Sporanox?

(A) Generally similar to those for Diflucan. According to a January 1993 report in Antimicrobial Agents in Chemotherapy,

Sporanox is safe and effective in treating women with acute candida vaginitis.
One third of the patients who received a 3-day course of treatment reported mild side effects, including nausea and headache.
However, none of these reactions were severe enough to require that the therapy be discontinued.

(Q) Does Sporanox possess other advantages?

(A) Possibly. According to studies published by Janssen, this medication would appear to be especially useful in treating fungus infection of the nails.

(Q) What else will I need to do to overcome my yeast problem?

(A) Molds and yeasts are kin to each other. So you should lessen your exposure to molds in any and every way you can, both at home and in your work place.
Here's why: Molds you breathe can trigger your symptoms.

(Q) What can I do to avoid molds and get rid of them?

(A) Learn as much as you can about where molds are found and take steps to avoid them. Common sources of airborne molds include bathrooms, damp basements, carpeting, poorly ventilated closets, old upholstered furniture, humidifiers, decaying leaves, stored fruits and vegetables, old wallpaper and home air ducts. (See Chapter 9 for a discussion of environmental molds.)

(Q) Could a candida (yeast) vaccine help me?

(A) Possibly. In some of my patients, the yeast vaccine has worked like a miracle in relieving symptoms. Apparently, it helps by stimulating the immune system. (For a further discussion on the use of candida extracts or vaccines in diagnosis and treatment, see Chapter 34 and 40.)

(Q) What else do I need to do?

(A) Many things. Here's why: When you're sick or don't feel well, your health problems are nearly always due to a variety of causes rather than a single one. And although taking anticandida medication and avoiding sugar and yeast-containing foods will help you regain your health, you'll also need to pay attention to many other factors. (A more complete discussion of some of the causes of illness can be found in Section C.)

You are what you eat. And you need to eat a variety of wholesome foods, including proteins, complex carbohydrates and essential fats and oils. I also prescribe nutritional supplements, including vitamins and minerals.

You must also avoid poisons and pollutants, including those which contaminate the air, soil and water; and you must limit your intake of nutritionally poor foods, including sugar, white flour and hardened vegetable oil.

If you're allergic to foods and inhalants you must receive appropriate treatment for those sensitivities. You also need a favorable environment, including fresh air, sunlight, pure water and the loving support of those around you.

A few final words: Although your health disorder is yeast connected, we're treating your immune system and not just *Candida albicans.* So be patient. Your problems didn't develop overnight and they won't go away in a few days, or a few weeks or months. Yet, if you're like most of my patients, be of good cheer! *You will get well.*

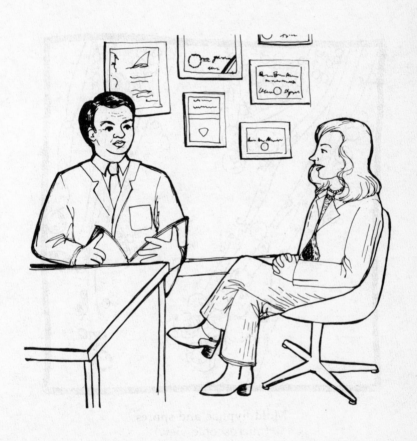

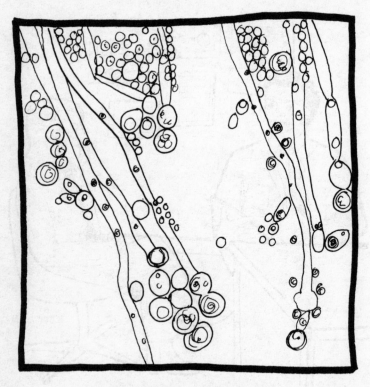

Mold hyphae and spores
(microscopic view)

9

More About Yeasts, Molds And Other Fungi

If candida plays a role in making you sick, eating or breathing other yeasts and molds will aggravate your symptoms. So you should learn about yeasts and molds and take steps to avoid them.

Yeasts and molds are members of the vegetable kingdom. Generally speaking, yeasts are oval or elliptical single-celled organisms. By contrast, molds form colonies and each cell grows long, intertwining, hair-like branches called "hyphae."

However, identifying a particular yeast or mold isn't easy. Here's why: Sometimes these little plants can change from a mold to a yeast, and back again.

Yeasts and molds live all around us. They commonly grow on fruits and vegetables, especially dried fruits and grapes. They're also found in the soil, air and water. Some outdoor molds die when snow covers the ground. Yet, even in the wintertime, mold spores live in the soil.

Mold spores float in the air like pollen. So you can breathe them and they may be deposited in your lungs, as well as in your nose and throat.

Some molds are found on decomposing plants, leather, cloth, rubber, wood and paper products. Others grow outdoors on vegetation.

Conditions that promote mold growth can be summarized in two words: *Dampness* and *darkness*. Accordingly, if you want to control molds around you, change the conditions that favor their growth. Sometimes you can accomplish this by using a dehumidifier, especially in damp basements or closets. You can also destroy molds by applying a boric solution. A low-wattage bulb burning in a closet will lessen the mold population. And an electric heat lamp designed to dry out dark closets is available from Damp Chaser Electronics, Inc., Hendersonville, NC 28739.

If you're sensitive to molds, get rid of the mold catchers in your home. And there are many of these, including old books, upholstered furniture and flower pots. Washing, airing and sunning will help retard mold growth on your bed clothing, pillows, mattress pads and rugs.

Besides candida and air-borne molds, other yeasts and fungi are found in foods you eat every day. Among the more obvious of these foods are mushrooms, aged cheeses and alcoholic beverages. Yeasts are also found in fermented beverages and in baked goods that rise. They also grow quickly in fruit juices and foods that ferment easily.

Yeast growth in your body is also encouraged or stimulated by medications of various types, including especially antibiotics, birth control pills and the corticosteroid group of drugs.

Sources Of Mold In Homes

Damp basements—especially those with dirt floors—encourage mold growth. (Moisture tends to evaporate from the floor; this draws additional soil water into the house by capillary action.)

Bathrooms provide a comfortable home for molds. They love every nook and cranny. They'll grow in your bathtub drain and on wash cloths, damp towels, crevices or cracks in the wall covering.

Closets, drawers or hampers often promote mold growth, especially when you load them up with clothing you've worn that hasn't been laundered. (Perspiration encourages mold growth as do shoes saturated with perspiration.)

Mattresses and other bedding sometimes become mold infested. Mold growth can be lessened by washing the mattress pads frequently.

Carpets of all kinds encourage mold growth, especially shag carpets. You can lessen mold exposure by using throw rugs. (Wash them often!)

Old upholstered furniture, bedding, pillows, rags, sleeping bags or other items, particularly those made from natural fibers.

Old newspapers, books or magazines.

Flower pots and dried or decaying plant materials.

Houses, especially those in shaded areas or near rivers or streams, tend to collect mold. Shrubs or vines planted close to your house retain moisture and tend to encourage mold growth.

Humidifiers, especially vaporizers, encourage mold growth.

Kitchens that are inadequately ventilated. The area between the kitchen sink and the wall, around the bottom of the cold water pipe, wood chopping boards marred from use and rotting fruits and vegetables are all locations molds favor. Other sites include the rubber gasket that seals the refrigerator door and the surplus water tray located in the bottom of self-defrosting refrigerators.

Decaying leaves, compost, lawn clippings or hay. Raking or mowing the grass launches millions of mold spores and fragments into the air.

Some wallpapers contain chemical mold-retardants. However, these chemicals may "outgas" and cause symptoms in some chemically sensitive individuals.

Fruits or vegetables stored in a basement or cellar. Potatoes, carrots and other root vegetables begin to mold soon after they're taken from the ground.

Controlling Yeasts And Molds

Avoid molds at home and at work

One of my patients with severe health problems related to candida was improving on a treatment program which included nystatin and a low-carbohydrate, yeast-free diet. At one of her recheck visits, she came in with this story:

> "I know I felt worse in damp weather or when I went to my moldy basement. I also noted that if I worked in the kitchen for more than a few minutes, I would develop a headache and feel 'spaced out' and depressed. So with my husband's help, I did some detective work. We found heavy mold growth under the sink. My husband cleaned it out and now the kitchen doesn't bother me."

Another patient, a physician, suffered from severe, incapacitating depression. Many mornings he found it impossible to get out of bed or to carry out any useful work. Although he realized that going to the basement or other moldy places aggravated his symptoms, he had not associated his severe symptoms with molds in his home.

Then he was hospitalized because of a bleeding ulcer. Even though he was seriously ill and four pints of blood were necessary for therapy, he was amazed to find that while in the hospital his fatigue and depression vanished. He commented,

> "I felt better than I had felt since I played football in college . . . lots of energy, no depression, and I was able to think clearly."

Following recovery, he returned to his home and, within 2 to 3 days, his symptoms of fatigue and depression returned. When he stayed out of his home for 3 days on a trip, his symptoms disappeared.

On testing with candida extract, his symptoms of depression and mental dullness were provoked by the initial test dose and blocked or neutralized when he was given a different dose.

One of my patients was interviewed recently by Mary Reed, Features Editor of *The Jackson Sun*. In a special article on yeast-connected health problems, published on May 26, 1983, Mary wrote:

> "Marilyn Smith's problems started about 15 years ago when she started taking birth control pills, but they really got bad after her third child was born four years ago. The problem progressed over the years until Marilyn thought she was having a nervous breakdown.
>
> "Besides having joint swelling and other arthritic symptoms, Mrs. Smith would become emotional, get migraine headaches, get dizzy and faint. Her colon and stomach would hurt so much she could hardly walk.
>
> "Marilyn commented, 'I've cried for days and days at a time. My family thought I was losing my mind. It's just horrid.'
>
> "Today, she knows her allergies to yeast and some other foods were the cause of her problems. If she eats white potatoes, she'll get a headache almost immediately. Like other patients, *even smelling yeast or mold brings on symptoms*. Recently, she walked into a school cafeteria where yeast cinnamon rolls were baking and she just started crying.
>
> "Now that she avoids yeast-containing foods, processed sugar and places like bakeries and greenhouses (which have a lot of mold in the air), Marilyn's life has changed. 'When I found out I wasn't crazy, it was so wonderful'."

Three of my patients work at the local office of the Social Security Administration and are bothered by many candida-related symptoms. Recently, one of them commented,

"The office I work in makes me sick. It's full of mold. The roof leaked last year and the whole building is damp. We've even found mold on records in the filing cabinet. I feel much better on weekends when I'm at home. Then when I go back to the office my symptoms return."

Two of my patients who work in a restaurant featuring pizza noted their symptoms gradually became worse while working there. On weekends off or vacation, symptoms would improve.

If your home or work place is loaded with molds, your yeast-connected health problems may bother you until you take measures to lessen your exposure to molds. And you may even need to change jobs or find another place to live.

Avoid antibiotics

If you develop a bacterial pneumonia, meningitis or a severe kidney infection, you'll need to be treated with an antibiotic drug to help your body combat the invading bacteria. But if you do not have such a disorder (even if you run a fever), you may not need such medication. If you're bothered by yeast-related illness, take antibiotics only when absolutely necessary, since antibiotics promote the growth of the yeast germ in your body.

Some 80 to 90 percent of respiratory infections are caused by viruses and such illnesses aren't helped by antibiotics. So if you come down with a fever, cough or cold, don't pressure your physician to give you an antibiotic unless he finds it essential.

When antibiotics are necessary, I usually prescribe penicillin or erythromycin rather then Keflex®, Ceclor®, ampicillin, amoxicillin, Septra®, Bactrim®, or other "broad-spectrum" antibiotics. Here's why: penicillin and erythromycin attack mainly the "strep" and pneumonia germs found in the nose, throat and lungs. (However, they, too, may activate either vaginal or digestive tract yeast.) By contrast, the broad-spectrum drugs kill these same organisms and also destroy many normal bacteria. And when such bacteria are wiped out, yeasts are apt to take their place.

I also usually prescribe nystatin along with the antibiotic. Nystatin is, of course, indicated in patients with immune system problems related to candida. *However, even in patients in whom such a relationship is uncertain, especially children with recurrent ear and/or urinary tract infections,* I prescribe nystatin along with the antibiotic. And I discontinue the antibiotic drug as soon as is feasible, depending on the type and duration of the infection.

How about patients who develop infections of the kidney or bladder which require that an antibiotic drug be used in treatment? In discussing such drugs, several urologists have commented, "Most urinary tract infections will respond to the nitrofurantoin drugs, Furadantin® and Macrodantin®. These drugs do not promote the growth of yeast germs." (For a more detailed discussion of these drugs, see Chapter 29.)

I feel that antibiotics are often used when they aren't needed in the treatment of women with urinary tract symptoms. Because such individuals complain of painful and frequent urination, both the physician and the patient assumes the symptoms are caused by cystitis . . . a bacterial infection.

In patients of this type, the symptoms may be due to the generalized candida infection in the vulvovaginal area, giving rise to urethritis. And the use of antibiotic drugs in this condition serves only to aggravate further the yeast infection that is the actual cause of the discomfort.

I've also seen a number of patients with severe yeast-related illness who give a history of taking daily doses of sulfonamide or other antibacterial drugs for months or years to prevent recurrent urinary tract (or ear) infections. Although such drugs may suppress the germs which cause these infections, they also encourage the growth of candida. And the resulting health problems are often worse than those the antibacterial drugs were used to prevent. (See also, Chapter 29)

I also take a dim view of the long-term use of tetracyclines for acne because I've seen so many patients with severe yeast-connected illness who gave a history of such a treatment program.

Avoid "the pill"

Hormone pills containing both estrogens and progesterone have been widely used during the past two decades for contraception. They are also used commonly in treating women with menstrual cramps and a variety of menstrual irregularities. *Avoidance of the birth control pill is mandatory if chronic candidiasis is to be successfully controlled.*

The progesterone component of these pills causes changes in the vaginal mucous membrane which makes it easier for ever-present yeasts to multiply and cause not only vaginitis, but associated systemic symptoms, including irritability, fatigue and depression. Other mechanisms may also be involved in producing these symptoms, including changes in hormonal function.

Pure estrogen pills which are frequently prescribed for women during and after menopause do not encourage the growth of yeasts.

Treat your home with formaldehyde vapors?

One of my patients (I'll call her Susan) commented,

> "I'm sensitive to all sorts of chemicals. Yet, mold exposure causes severe symptoms, including depression and fatigue. My house is killing me and I can't afford to move. What can I do?"

Getting rid of molds isn't easy. Yet, there are steps which may help. One of these is the use of formaldehyde, a substance which causes both toxic and allergic reactions in many people, including individuals with yeast-connected illness.

In his book, *Dr. Mandell's 5-Day Allergy Relief System*,[10] (in a section entitled, "Steps To Take If Mold Is A Problem," pages 232-234), Dr. Mandell described a method of using formaldehyde. Using this method was "highly successful" in getting rid of molds; the beneficial effects lasted for approximately two months.

Because Susan was troubled both by severe chemical sensitivity and mold sensitivity, I was really on the fence. And it was hard for me to tell her what to do. So in concluding my discussion with her, I made these comments and suggestions:

1. Move out of your moldy house if you can. Even though you feel you can't afford to move, it's something you should consider.

2. Get mold cultures and colony counts on different rooms in your home (you can obtain information about such studies from Mould Service, c/o Sherry A. Rogers, M.D., 2800 West Genesee Street, Syracuse, NY 13219, and from Hollister-Stier Laboratories, P.O. Box 19957, Atlanta, GA 30325).

3. If the mold counts in your house are high, spend a night or two away from your home in a room which is less apt to be contaminated with molds or chemicals, and see if you can notice a difference.

4. Purchase and use one or more dehumidifiers in your home, especially in the rooms that seem to be loaded with mold.
5. Allergy testing, followed by treatment with mold extracts may help lessen your sensitivity.
6. Get a knowledgeable carpenter or building contractor to take a look at your home and see if he can recommend structural changes which can prevent moisture and prohibit or significantly reduce mold growth.
7. If nothing else works, you may want to consider treating your home with formaldehyde. However, because chemical fumes bother you, I can't recommend such a program with enthusiasm. Yet, if you can't move and can leave home for a few days while someone else does the work, you may want to consider it.

Section B

To control Candida, you must change your diet.

A Special Note on Candida Control Diets

As you read my comments on pages 67–77, you'll see that my diet recommendations change significantly after the early hardback editions of this book were published (1983–1985). You'll also learn that the observations of other physicians who treat patients with candida-related disorders vary.

This expanded, updated third paperback edition of *The Yeast Connection* was first published in October 1986. In my diet recommendations I continued to emphasize the importance of avoiding poor quality foods—especially those containing sugar, corn syrup and hydrogenated or partially hydrogenated fats.

During 1987 and 1988, I learned that food allergies were present, (almost without exception) in every person with a candida-related health problem. And to provide you with better information in this printing of the book, I again revised and updated my diet recommendations on pages 77–80.

You can obtain even more information in *The Yeast Connection Cookbook—A Guide to Good Nutrition and Better Health*. Features of this 384-page book include:

1. Over 225 kitchen and family tested recipes.
2. Diets which contain more complex carbohydrates.
3. A discussion of food allergies and how to manage them.
4. Information about food contaminants and how to find safe foods.

This new book was designed to be a "companion" to *The Yeast Connection*.

10

Introduction

To obtain adequate nutrition, you need proteins, fats (oils) and carbohydrates. According to the Food and Nutrition Board of the National Academy of Sciences, at least 50 to 100 grams (200 to 400 calories) of digestible carbohydrates per day are desirable to offset undesirable metabolic responses. Although this board made no distinction between *refined* and *unrefined* carbohydrates, a number of research studies, including those by Cheraskin and Ringsdorf,[11] show that unrefined carbohydrates (vegetables, fruits and whole grains) promote health. By contrast, their studies indicate that refined carbohydrates (cane, beet and corn sugars and syrups, and white flour) promote disease, including dental caries, high blood pressure, emotional disorders and susceptibility to infection.

I met Cheraskin over 10 years ago at a medical meeting in Miami and became one of his fans. I began following the Cheraskin-Ringsdorf recommendations in prescribing diets for my patients. And I urged them to eat more vegetables, fruits and whole grains along with a variety of other wholesome foods, including nuts and seeds, some dairy products, eggs and meats, especially chicken and fish.

About the same time, I began to notice that *children who consumed diets loaded with sugar and corn syrup became irritable, nervous and hyperactive.* And when these foods were removed from their diets, their symptoms would improve. Also, many of my adult patients would comment,

> "When I cut down on my sweets and other junk food, I feel better . . .
> less nervousness, irritability and fatigue."

At the same meeting where I met Cheraskin, I had dinner with the late Nathan Pritikin, the Californian who reported that diets containing 80% complex carbohydrates (400 or more grams of complex carbohydrate per day) would help people with all sorts of health disorders. Included among these were high blood pressure, hardening of the arteries and adult onset diabetes.

A couple of years later, Pritikin asked me to serve as a member of the Advisory Board of the Pritikin Research Foundation. I visited the Pritikin center in California twice and was impressed with the "fantastic" results obtained by many people I met who had followed the Pritikin program.

Soon thereafter, my good friend, Jacksonian H. A. ("Rich") Richardson who had suffered from the severe and persistent chest pain called "angina", learned of the Pritikin program. One of his sons commented,

> "Dad had to take nitroglycerin every day. His pain bothered him even at rest and during the night. He had to sit up in bed. He couldn't sleep."

Complete heart studies, including catheterization at the Ochsner Clinic in New Orleans, showed complete blockage of one of Rich's major arteries and 60 to 90 percent blockage of the others. Open heart surgery was initially recommended (in 1975). Yet the severity of Rich's heart disease was such that he was subsequently told,

> "You'd be a poor operative risk."

So Rich kept taking his nitroglycerin and his pain continued. About a year later, Rich and his wife, Rosemary, read a report in an Atlanta paper about the Pritikin program. They went to California, spent a month eating the high carbohydrate diet and started walking. Today, 11 years later, 73-year-old Rich walks three to six miles a day and works almost 12 hours a day, six days a week, running a highly successful business. He takes no medicine and experiences no pain unless he walks too fast up a hill. One of his sons commented,

> "Every person who works for dad has to push to keep up with him!"

Soon afterward, an across-the-street neighbor, Turner Bridges (then age 69), was told by his physician,

> "You have diabetes. And your cholesterol is too high . . . over 250."

On a modified Pritikin diet, Turner's diabetes has vanished and his cholesterol has fallen to 165. Turner travels, plays golf regularly (no golf cart) and enjoys better health than many men half his age.

For over 10 years, I've admired Roger Williams, Ph.D. of the University of Texas in Austin, Ross Hume Hall, Ph.D. of McMasters University in Hamilton, Ontario, and author Beatrice Trum Hunter of Hillsboro, New Hampshire. These professionals have stressed the importance of nutritious, wholesome, truly natural foods, including vegetables, fruits and whole grains. And I've read their books from cover to cover several times.

Each of these professionals say in effect,

> "Avoid fabricated and processed foods of all sorts, especially those containing sugar, processed fat, food coloring and other additives."

Moreover, I've been impressed by the growing interest of both professionals and non-professionals in diets containing less meat, eggs and fat-laden dairy products, and featuring more vegetables, fruits and grains. For example, Jane Brody, award-winning science writer and personal health columnist of *The New York Times*, and author of *Jane Brody's Nutrition Book*[12], commented,

> "Even if you have no interest in vegetarianism, *there's no reason why you should have animal protein at every meal or even every day.*"

Then, in January, 1986, I saw an interview with an executive of the American Cancer Society on one of the evening news shows. And he said, in effect,

> "If you want to decrease your chances of developing cancer, you'll have to change your diet. Eat, especially, more cabbage, broccoli, brussel sprouts, cauliflower and other vegetables and cut down on your high fat meats."

In March, 1986, I received a brochure from Scott M. Grundy, M.D., Ph.D., Professor of Internal Medicine and Biochemistry, University of Texas Health Science Center, Dallas, TX 75235. This brochure provided information about a new Center for Human Nutrition which was established at the University of Texas Health Science Center in Dallas in 1981. The Center's program will study especially the role of nutrition in the prevention of disease and in optimising mental and physical health in people of all ages and both sexes including expectant mothers, children and older people.

So during the first half of the '80s, the nutritional recommendations of Roger Williams, Pritikin and some of the other pioneers I cited had come into the mainstream.

Moreover, in my own practice, I had, for a long time, been pleased and often astounded over the favorable reports I received from my own patients and their families who had changed their diets. A typical example: Angela M. commented,

> "Tommy's behavior has improved tremendously since we 'cleaned up his diet.' What's more, my husband and I feel a lot better . . . less fatigue and irritability, fewer headaches and muscle aches. The whole family is doing better."

So in discussing diets with my candida patients during the years 1979 through 1983, I said:

> "Avoid all sugars, corn syrup, maple syrup, honey and refined carbohydrates, including white flour and white rice. Also avoid junk foods and all yeast-containing foods and beverages. Feature the good carbohydrates, including vegetables of all kinds, whole grains (from your health food store) and fruits. You can also eat seafood, lean meats and some butter and eggs."

Carrying out these dietary instructions enabled most of my patients to improve. Yet, some would report a flare-up in symptoms after eating a banana or other fruits, and several of my patients reported,

> "When I eat too many carbohydrates, even the 'good ones', my symptoms flare."

One patient, Lynn, who suffered with severe fatigue, bloating, abdominal stress and other candida-connected health problems, had this to say,

> "If I eat fruits or grains, I develop immediate symptoms."

Here's still more: In March 1983, I met Betty Flora who commented,

> "Stopping all gluten-containing foods (wheat, rye, barley and oats) and all fruits was an important factor in helping me conquer my yeast-connected health problems."

Moreover, other physicians who were treating patients with yeast-connected health disorders commented,

> "Avoiding sugar and other refined carbohydrates is absolutely essential, if a person with a candida problem is to improve. In addition, some patients must temporarily restrict all carbohydrates, including the good ones. . . . at least, until they improve."

Accordingly, in the first edition of THE YEAST CONNECTION,

I included two diets. . . . the Candida Control Diet and the Low-Carbohydrate Diet. The Candida Control Diet eliminated sugars, syrups, yeast-containing foods and beverages, and junk foods, and allowed all vegetables, fruits and grains.

The Low-Carbohydrate Diet also recommended avoiding sugars, syrups and yeast-containing foods and beverages. In addition, it limited the intake of all carbohydrates, including potatoes, sweet potatoes, wheat, corn (and other grains) and fruits.

Not long after the first edition of THE YEAST CONNECTION came out in December, 1983, I ran into my long-time friend, Pat Connolly, Curator of the Price-Pottenger Foundation, who said in effect, "Your book is wonderful! And your daughter's illustrations are lovely. BUT, we wish you hadn't included all those fruits in the diets you recommend. In our experience, the carbohydrates found in fruits and milk promote yeast growth. That's why we feel they must be avoided during the early weeks of the diet, until the patient improves."

Then, in early 1984, I received a letter from John A. Henderson, M.D. of San Diego who commented,

> "In this office we restrict milk because of the lactose content as well as the presence of molds. *Candida albicans* may not be able to ferment lactose but in individuals who break the lactose down into glucose and fructose, yeasts thrive on both of these sugars. There are approximately 12 grams of lactose in every eight ounces of milk and I hardly see the rationale for permitting candida patients to use milk in their diets."

To get more information about milk, fruits and other carbohydrates in contributing to candida growth, on several occasions during the winter of 1983-1984 I interviewed John W. Rippon, Ph.D. of the University of Chicago and an authority on yeasts and molds. Here's an edited transcript of our conversations:

Crook: John, I need your help. I'd especially like to ask you about carbohydrates in the diet. . . . what foods are OK for the person with a candida problem and which foods should be avoided?

Rippon: Yeasts thrive on the simple carbohydrates. These include cane sugar, beet sugar, honey, corn syrup, maple syrup and molasses. *In addition, eating fruits promotes yeast growth*. Here's why: Fruits are loaded with fructose; in spite of their fiber content, fruits are readily converted to fructose and other simple sugars in the intestinal tract, thereby encouraging the growth of *Candida albicans*.

Crook: How about the grains and the potatoes and the other high carbohydrate vegetables? Do they promote yeast growth?

Rippon: No. And I base this opinion on what I know about the nutrition of the yeast organism. (Incidentally, this is well summarized in the book by Frank C. Odds,[†] a British mycologist.) The whole grains are difficult to digest, and whole wheat, brown rice and other whole grains are digested only slowly. Accordingly, they don't seem to be broken down to the point where yeasts can easily ferment them.

There really isn't any experimental evidence I could find on the subject except that grains, by themselves, aren't utilizable by yeasts. This is why, in making beer, you have to predigest the wheat, rice or other grain product using malt which has an enzyme, diastase, in it. So it would seem to me that whole grains would be against the metabolism of yeasts in contrast to the fruits.

Crook: How about peas, beans and other legumes?

Rippon: They don't contain a large percentage of utilizable carbohydrate, so shouldn't cause trouble. To repeat, it's the short chain, utilizable carbohydrates such as those found in sugar, honey, corn syrup, maple syrup and fruits which cause the trouble.

When you eat fruits, you produce carbon dioxide. We've had patients who so overindulged in fruits and got so gassy that they had to come into the hospital. Gas produced by beans is a different sort of gas. It is methane produced by bacteria rather than carbon dioxide which comes from yeasts.

White flour products which are easier to break down than whole wheat products may be more conducive to yeast growth than whole grain products.

Crook: How about mushrooms, brewer's yeast, moldy cheese and other yeast-containing products which often cause trouble? Do they do this by encouraging the growth of candida?

Rippon: No. Eating yeast or mold-containing foods doesn't promote the growth and multiplication of candida. So reactions to yeast-containing foods or beverages must be caused by an allergy to yeast products.

Crook: How about milk?

---

†Dr. Odds is the author of the comprehensive book, CANDIDA AND CANDIDOSIS, Baltimore, University Park Press, 1979.

Rippon: Milk does contain significant amounts of the simple carbohydrate, lactose, and intestinal bacteria and enzymes from the pancreas break the lactose down and, in so doing, provide simple sugars for the candida to thrive on. So until your patients with candidiasis improve, I feel it's best for them to avoid milk. Yet, some patients may tolerate sugar-free, fruit-free yogurt preparations.

Because of these important changes in dietary recommendations (plus other new developments), I began revising THE YEAST CONNECTION within a few weeks after the first edition came off the press. And in mid-summer, 1984, an expanded second edition was published which included the changes I've just discussed.

Yet, during the next two years, answering the question, "What diets should I follow to conquer my yeast-related health problems," continued to challenge me. And to obtain more information, I listened to my patients (and the hundreds of people who wrote to me). In addition, I "picked the brains" of my knowledgeable and experienced colleagues. The question of yeast-containing foods seemed especially to bother a lot of people. For example, Mary M. commented:

> "Dr. Crook, your book has helped me a lot and I follow most of your recommendations. But I find that avoiding all those foods you say I need to avoid . . . especially those that may contain some yeasts and molds . . . is almost impossible.
>
> "I know that when I cheat and eat sweets I feel terrible . . . tired, irritable and spaced out. But I've found I can eat left-overs, nuts, mushrooms, breads, cheeses and other yeast-containing foods without developing symptoms."

In addition, a number of my friends in the health food industry were concerned by what they felt was a blanket indictment of yeasts, and Bob M. commented:

> "Yeast is a nutritious substance. It contains a lot of essential nutrients. It also gives bread its good taste. It helps our bodies assimilate zinc and other minerals in the wheat. *Does everyone with a candida problem really need to avoid all yeast-containing foods?*"

To learn more about yeasts and molds in the diet, in the spring and summer of 1985, I again interviewed John Rippon, Ph.D. (See also Chapter 44, Update.) Here's an edited abstract of our conversation:

Crook: John, I'd again like to pick your brain. I'm especially interested in what you think about the consumption of yeasty foods by the person with a candida-related health problem.

Rippon: There are countless families of yeasts. All too frequently, both physicians and the public are using the general term "yeast" to include everything.

What I'm referring to is simply this: when you say a person has a "yeast problem," you tend to infer that all yeasts are bad. So some yeasts that may be harmless are made guilty by inference, and that isn't necessarily true.

Crook: Might you compare this situation to the person who is "pollen sensitive," and although inhaling grass pollen causes sneezing and nasal congestion, tree pollen causes no symptoms?

Rippon: That's right, that's exactly right, that's a very good analogy.

Crook: And if a person is sensitive to a grain such as corn, he may not be sensitive to barley or rice?

Rippon: Exactly. *Even though your patient has symptoms caused by* Candida albicans, *this does not necessarily mean he will have problems with other kinds of yeasts.*

Crook: In the patient with chronic candidiasis, is it reasonable during the first week of a treatment program to avoid food yeasts in case the person is allergic to yeast?

Rippon: Yes. I think this is a reasonable approach. Then when the patient challenges with yeast, he can see if he develops symptoms. And if he doesn't react to yeast challenges, he won't need to avoid the yeast-containing foods. This will make the diet easier for him to follow.

Crook: I'm delighted to get this information from you. And let me repeat it to make sure I understand: *Eating a yeast-containing food doesn't make candida organisms multiply. So when my patients develop symptoms, they do so because they're allergic to yeast products.*

Rippon: Exactly.

While we're talking about yeasts, I'd like to point out that the yeast cell, as you know, is composed of cytoplasm and cell walls. Moreover, some people may be allergic to the cell wall and show no reactions whatsoever to the cytoplasm. Incidentally, the cell wall is usually the most reactive part of the yeast organism.

Crook: How about the difference between live yeasts and dead yeasts? And are the yeasts in beer and wine live yeasts?

Rippon: Well, they were live, but after treatment and filtering you do not have live yeasts. Moreover, beer and wine yeasts contain essentially no cell wall, and so they may not cause problems.

To continue a little bit in response to your questions. In yeast breads, you have the whole yeast inside the bread, which contains both the cytoplasm and the cell wall. And your whole yeast organism is inside the bread. When the yeast is baked, you change many of the characteristics. As a result, a person may react differently between the heated and processed yeast found in bread and yeast which hasn't been similarly treated.

Crook: I'd like to learn a little more about the different families and catagories of yeasts.

Rippon: There are hundreds of them. Of course, the one we deal with most in foods and beverages are the *servicia* or *saccharomyces*, which are found in beer, wine and breads, as well as in brewer's yeast and baker's yeast. They are all the same.

Crook: And whether a yeast is "dead or alive" depends on whether food has been cooked?

Rippon: That's right. And as we discussed before, in the beer and wine you have yeast protein, but you won't have yeast cell wall. And in breads you have both the protein and the cell wall, but the cell wall yeast may be altered by the baking process. So there are all sorts of possibilities and ramifications.

Crook: How about other species of candida, more especially *Candida utilis*?

Rippon: It is a member of the candida family, but it's found in the soil and it isn't found in people. And it is only very distantly related to *Candida albicans* and shouldn't be in the same category. So a person could be sensitive to *Candida albicans* and not sensitive to *Candida utilis*.

A second question that concerned me related to nuts and seeds . . . also sprouts. And because these foods are apt to contain mold, a few of my colleagues felt they should be avoided.

Yet, if a person isn't allergic to yeasts and molds, I recommend them. And even if you react to the yeast challenge, I still recommend that you try nuts and see if they agree . . . especially freshly-shelled nuts. However, if yeasts and/or molds bother you, avoid peanuts[†] and pistachios as they're usually loaded with molds.

Moreover, I've been impressed by the comments of the late Henry Schroeder, M.D. of Dartmouth College, a recognized authority on trace minerals, who commented:

> "Nuts . . . contain adequate or surplus amounts of all the trace elements; coming from seeds; they contain the elements needed for the growth of the seed until the plant forms roots . . . *The essential trace elements are much more important than the vitamins. They cannot be synthesized, as can the vitamins . . . Without them, life would cease to exist."* (Schroeder, H.: *The Poisons Around Us*, Bloomington, Indiana University Press, 1974, pp. 118-119. Published in *Prevention*, July, 1975.)

Still another question which has concerned me relates to the carbohydrate content of the diet. As I've already pointed out, I had, for many years, been a "high carbohydrate" person and I never liked restricting the good carbohydrates. Moreover, low-carbohydrate diets were hard for people to follow. In addition, such diets caused a number of people to develop problems, including excessive weight loss.

Here, again, to obtain further information, in the spring of 1986 I consulted a number of my colleagues. Here are their comments:

Sidney Baker, M.D.: "I do not encourage my patients to restrict any complex carbohydrates. However, some of my patients have found, on their own, they must limit some of these carbohydrates."

Morton Teich, M.D.: "We avoid all sugars. In addition, we recommend that, during the initial phase of the diet, total carbohydrates be restricted to some degree. However, we allow fruits and grains at all times."

Don Mannerberg, M.D.: "I have my patients avoid sugars, but I do not restrict the complex carbohydrates."

Leo Galland, M.D.: "I ask all my patients to avoid sugar. However, I do not restrict the complex carbohydrates in most patients. An occasional patient seems to do better when the carbohydrate content is temporarily kept in the neighborhood of 60 grams a day. As the patient improves, it is increased."

Nick Nonas, M.D.: "We generally tend to prescribe a low-carbohydrate diet, but we don't eliminate fruits completely."

[†]I'm especially concerned about peanut products which often are contaminated with aflatoxin-producing *aspergillus flavus*.

Pam Morford, M.D.: "We initially prescribe low-carbohydrate diets (60 to 80 grams) in many of our patients. If a patient improves, they usually find they can increase their carbohydrate intake."

Phyllis Saifer, M.D.: "We've had problems with a low-carbohydrate diet and we feel such a diet should not be continued for long periods of time. In regard to yeast-containing foods, if a person is allergic to yeast we avoid them. If not, they can tolerate them on a rotated basis."

Ken Gerdes, M.D.: "We feel a low-carbohydrate diet (about 60-80 grams) is important during the first week of treatment. Then, as a patient improves, the complex carbohydrate content can be increased on a trial and error basis. However, some people seem to require a low-carbohydrate diet for longer periods of time, if they are to do well. We try to add grains like buckwheat to increase the fiber in the diet."

John Rippon, Ph.D.: "I do not feel that vegetables or grains should be restricted. They provide fiber and other important nutrients. In addition, a person's diet affects the bacterial flora, and the carbohydrates feed the lactobacilli and keep the candida in check. I strongly disagree with diets (in treating patients with yeast-related illness) which sharply limit the intake of all carbohydrates. My own feeling is that we should de-emphasize the intake of proteins and fats and emphasize the intake of carbohydrates."

Food allergies in the person with a yeast-connected health problem.

Candida related health problems and food allergies go "hand-in-hand." In a questionnaire and telephone survey of 25 knowledgeable and experienced physicians, each respondent said, "All of my patients with candida-related health problems are troubled by food sensitivities."

Why do individuals with CRC develop food hypersensitivities? Here's a probable explanation. Research studies by W. Allen Walker, Professor of Pediatrics, Harvard Medical School, show that the lining of the intestinal tract (the mucosal barrier) can be adversely affected through many different mechanisms.

Walker does not mention the possible role of candida in causing food allergies. Yet, the observations of both practicing physicians and researchers suggests that candida overgrowth in the gut may harm the mucosal barrier. This may lead to the absorption of incompletely digested food molecules which may then cause food allergies.

The most frequent food offenders in my patients—and in the experience of other physicians—are yeast, wheat, milk, corn, eggs and legumes. However, *any food may cause an adverse reaction.* Such reactions are divided into two general types:

A. Obvious food allergies with prompt reactions.

B. Hidden food allergies with delayed or masked reactions.

Obvious food allergies are usually caused by uncommonly eaten foods, including shrimp, cashew nuts, strawberries and lobster. However, they also can be caused by eggs, peanuts, and other commonly eaten foods.

Hidden food allergies are usually caused by foods you eat every day—especially milk, corn, wheat, sugar, yeast and citrus. (For a further discussion of food allergies, see pages 121–124 of this book and *The Yeast Connection Cookbook* pages 84–104.)

How do you know if you're sensitive to a food? With an obvious allergy, identifying the offender presents no problem. By contrast, detecting a hidden food allergy requires organization and planning before you get started. Here's what you do:

1. Avoid a food or foods you suspect completely for five to seven days. Keep a diet diary for three days before you omit the suspected food or foods. Continue the diary during the period of elimination.

2. When you notice a convincing improvement in your symptoms lasting 48 hours, return the eliminated foods to your diet, one food each day and see if your symptoms return. In this way, you "challenge" the offending food. You may notice a flare up in your symptoms within a few minutes, or they may not occur for several hours or even until the next day.

My Diet Recommendations for the 1990s:

You are unique. And your diet requirements may not be the same as those of your friends or other family members. Yet, in treating my candida patients, I'm certain that diet is important . . . very important. Although I can't provide hard and fast rules that suit every person, here are guidelines that will help you.

• Identify the foods that cause allergic reactions and avoid them.

- Avoid "junk" foods—foods which are refined, overly processed and loaded with sugar, salt, food coloring, additives and hardened (hydrogenated or partially hydrogenated) vegetable oil and other hidden ingredients.
- Especially avoid all sugars, honey, molasses and maple syrup. The candida "Critters" like a baby bird looking for a worm, thrive on sweets. Sugar promotes multiplication of candida organisms, just as it does the tooth decay germs.
- Feature nutritious food obtained from a variety of sources. Eat more vegetables. Also become familiar with the grain alternatives, amaranth, quinoa, buckwheat and teff.
- Avoid all fruits during the first three weeks of your diet. Here's why: As I've already pointed out, although fruits contain complex carbohydrates and furnish many excellent nutrients, they're readily converted into simple sugars in the intestinal tract.
- After you've been on your diet for about 3 weeks, do a fruit challenge. Here's how: Take a small bite of banana, 10 minutes later eat a second bite. If no reaction develops in the next hour, eat the whole banana.
- If you tolerate the banana without developing symptoms, try strawberries, pineapple or apple the next day. If you show no symptoms following these fruit challenges, chances are you can eat fruit in moderate amounts. But feel your way along and *don't overdo it.*
- Diversify or rotate your diet so you'll be eating a variety of foods. Also, rotating your diet may enable you to more easily identify the food that may be disagreeing with you and causing your symptoms.
- If you pass the "yeast challenge" add nuts and seeds into your diet, including especially shelled nuts or nuts and seeds, from a health food store (walnuts, almonds, pecans, cashews, soy, sunflower and pumpkin). Be more cautious on adding peanuts or pistachios especially if you're sensitive to molds of any kind.
- When you follow these recommendations, you should improve. As the weeks and months go by, chances are you'll find that you can "cheat" occasionally without causing problems. Yet, if you throw caution to the wind and load up on sweets and junk foods, your health problems will usually return.

11

The Candida Control Diet Update

During the Early Weeks: Foods You Can Eat Freely...

Vegetables

Most of these vegetables contain lots of fiber and are relatively low in carbohydrates. They can be fresh or frozen, and you can eat them cooked or raw.

Asparagus
Beets
Broccoli
Brussel sprouts
Cabbage
Carrots
Cauliflower
Celery
Cucumbers
Eggplant
Green pepper
Greens:
  Spinach
  Mustard
  Beet
  Collards
  Kale
Lettuce
  all varieties
Okra

Onions
Parsley
Radishes
Soybeans
String beans
Tomatoes, fresh
Turnips

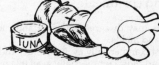

Meats and Eggs

Chicken   Salmon, mackerel, cod, sardines
Turkey   Tuna
Other fresh or frozen fish that is not breaded
Shrimp, lobster, crab & other seafood
Beef, lean cuts
Veal
Pork, lean cuts
Lamb
Wild game
Eggs

Nuts,* Seeds & Oils** (unprocessed)

Almonds	Oils	Butter***
Brazil nuts	Linseed	
Cashews	Safflower	
Filberts	Sunflower	
Pecans	Soy	
Pumpkin seeds	Walnut	
	Corn	

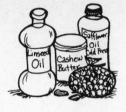

What you can drink. . . .
Water

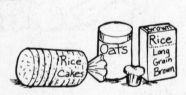

Foods You Can Eat Cautiously

High Carbohydrate Vegetables

Sweet Corn
Lima Beans
English Peas
White Potatoes (baked)
Winter Squash, Acorn,
   or Butternut
Sweet Potatoes
Beans and Peas, dried
   and cooked

Whole Grains

Barley
Corn
Millet
Oats
Rice
Wheat

Breads, Biscuits & Muffins

All breads, biscuits and muffins should be made with baking powder or baking soda as a leavening agent. Do not use yeast unless you pass the yeast challenge. To avoid yeast and to obtain more vitamins and minerals, use whole wheat flour or stone-ground cornmeal.

---

*Nuts may disagree with you and cause symptoms, especially if you're allergic to yeasts and molds.

**Most commercially available nuts and seeds have been processed and contain additives, and most commercially available oils have been heated and processed. So get unprocessed nuts and seeds and unrefined oils from a natural food store.

***Use in moderation.

Foods You Must Avoid

Sugar & Sugar-containing Foods: Sugar & other quick-acting carbohydrates, including sucrose, fructose, maltose, lactose, glycogen, glucose, mannitol, sorbitol, galactose, monosaccharides and polysaccharides. Also avoid honey, molasses, maple syrup, maple sugar, date sugar and turbinado sugar.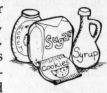

Packaged and Processed Foods: Canned, bottled, boxed and other packaged and processed foods usually contain refined sugar products and other hidden ingredients.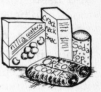

You'll not only need to avoid these sugar-containing foods the early weeks of your diet, *you'll need to avoid them indefinitely.*

Avoid yeasty foods the first 7-10 days of your diet. Then do the yeast challenge as described in Chapter 8. If you're allergic to yeast, you'll need to continue to avoid yeast and mold-containing foods indefinitely. However, if you aren't allergic to yeast, you can rotate yeast-containing foods into your diet and consume them in moderation.

Here's a list of foods that contain yeasts or molds:

Breads, Pastries and other raised bakery goods.

Cheeses: All cheeses (moldy cheeses, such as Roquefort, are the worst). Prepared foods, including Velveeta®, macaroni and cheese, Cheezits® and other cheese-containing snacks. Also buttermilk, sour cream and sour milk products.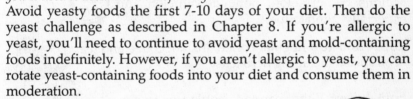

Alcoholic Beverages: Wine, beer, whiskey, brandy, gin, rum, vodka and other fermented liquors and liqueurs. Also, fermented beverages such as cider and root beer.

Condiments, Sauces and Vinegar-containing foods: Mustard, ketchup, Worcestershire®, Accent® (monosodium glutamate); steak, barbecue, chili, shrimp and soy sauces; pickles, pickled vegetables, relishes, green olives, sauerkraut, horseradish, mince meat and tamari. Vinegar and all kinds of vinegar-containing foods such as mayonnaise and salad dressing. (Freshly squeezed lemon juice may be used as a substitute for vinegar in salad dressings prepared with unprocessed vegetable oil.)

Malt Products: Malted milk drinks, cereals and candy. (Malt is sprouted grain that is kiln-dried and used in the preparation of many processed foods and beverages.)

Processed & Smoked Meats: Pickled and smoked meats and fish including sausages, hot dogs, corned beef, pastrami and pickled tongue.

Edible Fungi: All types of mushrooms, morels and truffles.

Melons: Watermelon, honeydew melon and especially cantaloupe.[†]

Coffee and Tea: Regular coffee, instant coffee and teas of all sorts, including herb teas.

Fruit Juices: Either canned, bottled or frozen, including orange juice, grape juice, apple juice, tomato juice, pineapple juice.
Exception: freshly prepared juice.

Dried & Candied Fruits: Raisins, apricots, dates, prunes, figs, pineapple.

Leftovers: Molds grow in leftover food unless it's properly refrigerated. Freezing is better.

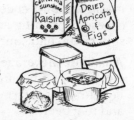

[†]Porous skin of cantaloupe is especially apt to be contaminated with mold. However, careful washing before cutting may enable melons to be tolerated.

[‡]Many individuals tolerate fruit-free, sugar-free, yogurt. For a discussion of *Lactobacillus acidophilus* and other friendly bacteria and their role in controlling candida see Chapter 43, Update.

MEAL SUGGESTIONS

The menus listed and illustrated on the next few pages are all *sugar-free* and *yeast-free* and designed to help you answer that always troublesome question, *"What can my family and I eat?"*

The menus for the early weeks are also *fruit-free* and contain relatively few grains and high carbohydrate vegetables (such as potatoes, yams and lima beans). Depending on your likes and dislikes, using these general guidelines, you can change these menus to suit your tastes and those of other members of your family.

If you pass "the yeast challenge", you can cautiously add cheeses, mushrooms, or other yeast-containing foods to your diet on a rotated basis. *You should also rotate your other foods, especially during the early weeks and months of your treatment program.* Here's why:

Many, and perhaps most, individuals with yeast-connected health problems are allergic to several (and sometimes many) different foods. The more frequently you eat a particular food, the greater are your chances of developing an allergy to that food. Moreover, you tend to become addicted to foods you are allergic to and you crave them, even though they may be contributing to your fatigue, headaches, muscle aches, depression or other symptoms.

When you rotate your diet and eat a food no more frequently than every 4th day, you accomplish two main goals: First, you avoid becoming addicted (allergic) to various foods. Second (and equally important), you are better able to identify foods that could be causing problems.

For a further discussion of food allergies and rotated diets, see Chapter 15 of this book and *The Yeast Connection Cookbook—A Guide to Good Nutrition and Better Health.*

In this book, you'll find over 200 recipes which feature vegetables of all sorts, a variety of grains, plus grain alternatives, amaranth, quinoa, buckwheat and teff. You'll also find information on chemical contaminants in foods and how to avoid them.

The recipes focus on foods most people can eat and enjoy. They're divided into easy-to-follow groups. Even if you're an inexperienced cook, you'll be able to select and prepare foods that will please you and other members of your family.

Meal Suggestions for the Early Weeks*

BREAKFASTS

2/3 cup cooked whole wheat cereal
Butter or linseed oil
Pecans

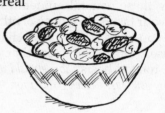

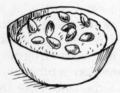

3/4 to 1 cup cooked oatmeal
   with butter
Almonds

3/4 cup cooked brown rice with butter and
   cashew nuts

---

*Recipes for many of the foods recommended in this section can be found in Chapter 12.

Meal Suggestions

BREAKFASTS

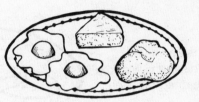

Eggs, any style
3/4 cup cooked grits
   with butter

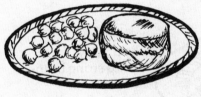

1 or 2 whole wheat biscuits with
   butter
Filberts

Tuna (water packed)
1 or 2 whole wheat popovers with butter

LUNCHES

Chicken salad
2 toasted rice cakes
Steamed broccoli

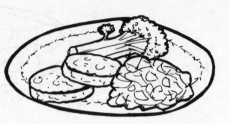

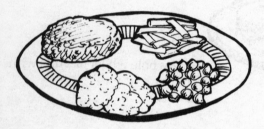

Beef patty
1 cup string beans
Filberts
Steamed cauliflower

Pork chop
Zucchini
Sunflower seeds
Buttered beets

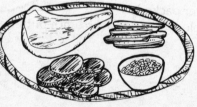

LUNCHES

Tuna fish with lemon & chopped celery
Pecans
Salad with tomato, lettuce, green
  pepper, cucumber, radish
Linseed oil & lemon juice dressing
1 or 2 whole wheat popovers

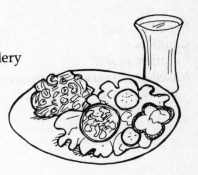

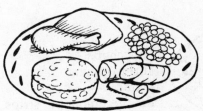

Baked chicken
1/2 to 1 cup peas & carrots
1 or 2 toasted rice cakes

Sliced turkey breast
Steamed asparagus
Almonds
Steamed cabbage

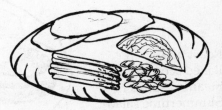

MAIN MEALS

Baked chicken
Cauliflower
Summer squash
Mixed green salad with linseed oil
   and lemon juice dressing
1 piece corn bread

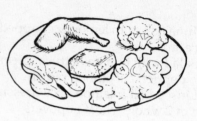

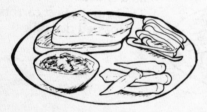

Pork chops
Turnip greens
Okra
Raw green pepper strips

Roast turkey
Baked acorn squash
Steamed spinach
Summertime salad

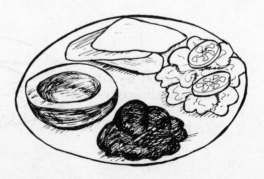

MAIN MEALS

Baked rock Cornish hen
Steamed cabbage
Asparagus
Salad with lettuce,
    pecans

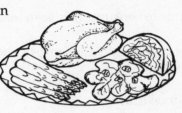

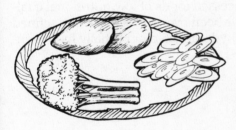

Sauteed liver
Carrots
Raw or steamed broccoli

Steak (or hamburger patty)
Eggplant
Mixed green salad with cucumbers
    and green peppers
Whole wheat popover

After the first several weeks of your diet, you can experiment. And, chances are you can eat freely. . .

All fresh vegetables. . .

All fresh fruits (in moderation) . . .

Whole grains . . .

You can continue to consume fish, lean meat, egg, nuts, seeds and oils . . .

And if you pass the yeast challenge test, you can also include some of the yeast-containing foods.

You must continue to avoid. . . .

Sugar & Sugar-containing Foods: Sugar & other quick-acting carbohydrates, including sucrose, fructose, maltose, lactose, glycogen, glucose, mannitol, sorbitol, galactose, monosaccharides and polysaccharides. Also avoid honey, molasses, maple syrup, maple sugar, date sugar and turbinado sugar.

Most of the packaged and processed foods of low nutritional quality, especially those which have been overly processed and refined and which contain sugar and hydrogenated or partially hydrogenated fats and oils.

Candida Control Diet

Meal Suggestions After the First Few Weeks

BREAKFASTS

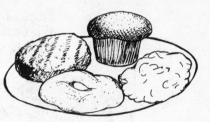

Ground beef patty
Scrambled eggs
Grits with butter
Applesauce muffin

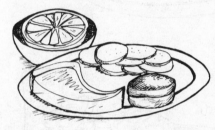

Pork chop
Sliced potatoes
Whole wheat biscuit
Grapefruit

Toasted rice cakes with
    butter
Sliced banana
Cashew nuts

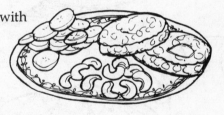

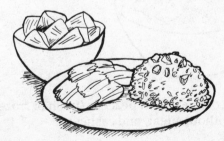

Brown rice with butter
    and chopped almonds
Tuna (water packed)
Fresh pineapple

BREAKFAST

Eggs, any style
Whole wheat pancakes
Freshly squeezed orange juice

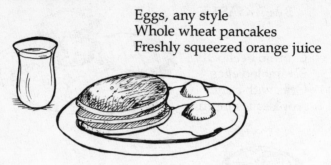

Barley cereal with
  banana and pecans
Milk
Fish (baked or broiled)

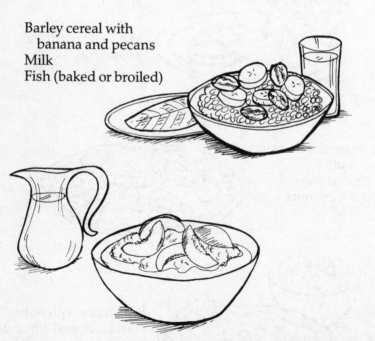

Hot oatmeal with peaches (fresh or frozen),
  without sugar, and cashews
Milk

LUNCHES

Salmon patty
Corn bread
Boiled cabbage
Blackeyed peas
Sliced tomatoes
Orange

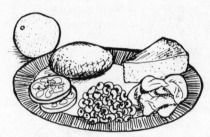

Fish cakes
Steamed cauliflower
Boiled okra
Oat cakes
Strawberries

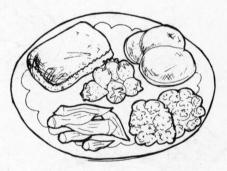

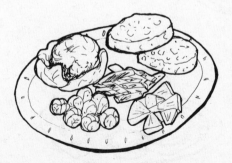

Tuna salad on lettuce
Rice cakes
Steamed green beans
Boiled Brussel sprouts
Fresh pineapple

LUNCHES

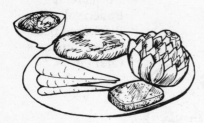

Swiss steak
Steamed artichoke
Turnip greens
Raw carrots
Corn bread

Chicken salad
Rice soup
Spinach
Rice biscuits
Apple

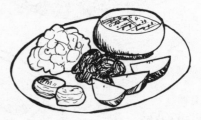

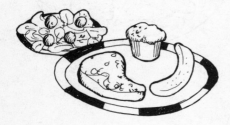

Pork chop
Lettuce & tomato salad
Applesauce muffin
Baked banana

Meat loaf
Barley soup
Celery and carrots
Whole wheat biscuits
Pear

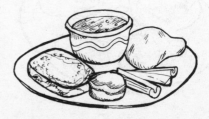

MAIN MEALS

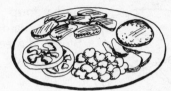

Sauteed liver
Lima beans
Baked acorn squash
Sliced tomato
Banana oat cake

Broiled fish
Cabbage & carrot slaw
Wax beans
Whole wheat popovers
Baked banana

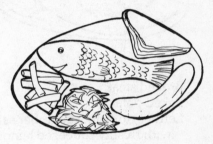

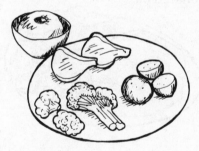

Broiled lamb chops
Steamed cauliflower
Steamed broccoli
Boiled potatoes
Baked apple

Rock Cornish hen
Steamed carrots and peas
Wild rice
Corn bread
Papaya

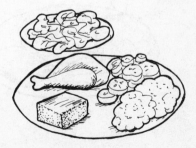

MAIN MEALS

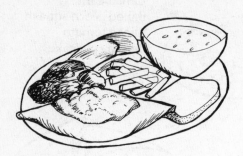

Roast duck
Spinach
Barley soup
Sweet potato
Steamed green beans
Corn bread

Broiled steak
Baked potato
Lettuce, tomato, cucumber salad
   with freshly squeezed lemon
   juice & safflower or linseed oil
   dressing
Lima beans
Spoon bread
Fresh strawberries

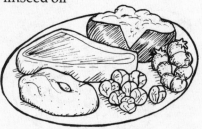

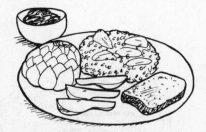

Easy chicken and rice
Steamed artichoke
Turnip greens
Corn bread
Pear

Shopping Tips

1. Feature whole foods.

2. Avoid foods labeled "enriched" if you're allergic to yeast.

3. Since many, and perhaps most canned, packaged and processed foods contain hidden ingredients, including sugar, dextrose and other carbohydrate products, avoid them.

4. If you must use canned or packaged foods, **Read Labels Carefully.**

5. Avoid processed, smoked or cured meats, such as salami, wieners, bacon, sausage, hotdogs, etc., since they often contain sugar, spices, yeast and other additives. Such foods are also loaded with the wrong kind of fat.

6. Use fresh fruits and vegetables. Commercially canned products often contain yeasts and added sugar.

7. Avoid bottled, frozen and canned juices. If you wish juice, buy fresh fruit and prepare your own juice.

8. Most commercially available nuts are roasted in vegetable oil and contain additives. Buy nuts in the shell, or shelled nuts from a natural food store. If you're allergic to yeasts and molds, you may need to avoid peanuts since they're more apt to be contaminated with mold. (And nuts of all kinds, like other foods, may become contaminated with molds.)

9. All commercial breads, cakes and crackers contain yeast. If you wish yeast-free breads, you'll have to obtain them from a special bakery or bake your own. Arden, Chico San or Golden Harvest Rice Cakes contain no sugar or yeast. Most children and adults like them. They're good with nut butters. Also San-Esu Rice Snacks (plain or sesame) and Kame Rice Crackers (usually found at natural food stores.)

10. Use cold pressed vegetable oils (such as sunflower, safflower, linseed and corn). (To make salad dressing, combine the oil with fresh lemon juice.)

11. Buy whole grains (barley, corn, millet, oats, rice and wheat) from a natural food store. Grains can be an important ingredient of a nutritious breakfast. Barley, rice and other grains can also be used in various ways at other meals. Barley or rice casseroles are especially tasty.

Food sources

Rice cakes
Arden Organic
99 Pond Road
Asheville, NC 28806

Vegetable oils, wheat, oats, rye
Arrowhead Mills, Inc.
Hereford, TX 79045

Rice crackers (contain whole brown rice, sesame seeds & salt)
Chico San, Inc.
1144 West First Street
Chico, CA 95926

Puffed corn, rice, wheat, and millet
El Molino Mills
City of Industry, CA 91746

Ener-G Rice Mix®, Ener-G Egg Replacer®, Jolly Joan Soyquick®
Ener-G Foods, Inc.
P.O. Box 24723
Seattle, WA 98124

Sugar-Free Preserves
Judy & Toby's Preserves
Beginnings—Endings—Etc., Inc.
Chatsworth, CA 91311

Vegetable oils, cashew butter, almond butter
Hain Pure Food
 Company, Inc.
Los Angeles, CA 90061

Potato chips (contain potato, safflower oil & salt. No additives)
Health Valley Natural
 Foods, Inc.
700 Union
Montebello, CA 90640

Bottled water, vegetables, nuts, whole grains, flours
Shiloh Farms
Sulphur Springs, AR 72768

Unprocessed nuts
Tropical Nut & Fruit Co.
11517-A Cordage Rd.
P.O. Box 7507
Charlotte, NC 28217

Also check with your local natural food store. They may be able to supply these sugar-free (or yeast-free) foods.

Additional Helpful Suggestions

Many individuals with yeast-connected health problems improve . . . often dramatically . . . when they stop eating foods containing significant amounts of cane sugar, beet sugar, corn syrup, fructose, dextrose or honey. Then if they follow other parts of the candida-control program, after two or three months they may find they can consume small amounts of foods which contain a small amount of sugar. For example, they may eat a low-sugar dry cereal such as Cheerios® without developing symptoms.

Others with candida-related illness, including those who are allergic to yeasts and molds, pay for any dietary infraction. And they may not achieve maximum improvement unless they rigidly avoid all foods which contain sugar, yeasts and molds. So they must stay away from coffee, teas, spices, sprouts, condiments and unfrozen left-over foods (mold quickly grows on any food which isn't eaten as soon as it's prepared).

Still others must carry out food allergy detective work. They must identify and avoid (or otherwise treat) all foods that cause adverse or allergic reactions. Common offenders include milk, egg, wheat, corn and soy. However, any food can be a troublemaker, including beef, pork, lettuce, chicken, apple, tomato, banana, grape and other foods.

When an adverse reaction is caused by a food such as lobster, shrimp or cashew nuts, it can usually be identified with ease. However, when such reactions are caused by foods that are eaten frequently, the relationship of the food to a person's symptoms is rarely suspected.

To identify hidden food allergies requires a carefully designed and appropriately executed elimination diet, as described in my book, *Tracking Down Hidden Food Allergy*[13]. (See also Chapter 15.)

Each person differs from every other person. **YOU ARE UNIQUE.** In following the anti-candida diet, *use a trial and error approach.*

Most of my patients with candida-related illness, as they improve, can follow a less rigid diet, especially if they're following other measures to regain their health. Included are the use of nutritional supplements and exercise, and avoiding exposure to environmental chemicals and mold spores. (See Chapter 17 for a further discussion of these factors.)

Why do sweetened foods and beverages cause symptoms?:

During the past 20 years, I've heard countless patients say,

"When I eat sweets, I feel spaced out, irritable, jittery or depressed."

And many a parent has commented,

"When Johnny eats sugar, he becomes hyperactive and unable to concentrate."

Why do such reactions occur? What is the mechanism? Here are a few possibilities:

1. When you eat refined sugars, you may be feeding yeast germs in your digestive tract and causing them to multiply. As a result toxins are produced which may cause symptoms all over the body.

2. Diets containing large amounts of refined sugar cause your pancreas to put out extra insulin. As a result, rapid up and down fluctuations occur in your blood and brain sugar levels producing nervousness, weakness, irritability, drowsiness and other symptoms of hypoglycemia.

3. If you fill up on sugar-laden foods, chances are you won't consume enough essential nutrients, including calcium and magnesium. Your diet may also be deficient in other essential vitamins and trace minerals, including vitamin B-1, vitamin B-6, chromium, zinc, essential amino acids, essential fatty acids and other nutrients. Such nutrients participate in various body enzyme systems and serve as precursors in the manufacture of hormones and neurotransmitters (chemicals your brain requires to function properly).

4. You may be allergic to sucrose and other sugars derived from a particular botanical source (cane, beet, corn or maple). In my own practice, dozens of my patients have commented, "Cane sugar products cause reactions, yet I can take beet or corn sugar." Or, "Foods sweetened with corn syrup make me irritable and nervous, yet other sweetened foods don't bother me." Other physicians have made similar observations. (For a further discussion of adverse reactions to different sugars, see Chapter 29.)

102

Yeast and mold-containing foods: *Avoiding yeasts and molds in your diet isn't easy*. Molds are everywhere . . . indoors and out-doors. Although dampness and darkness promote mold growth, as do basements and cellars, *molds can grow on any food, including fruits, vegetables, nuts, meats, spices and left-overs.*

Although heating . . . even boiling or processing . . . may kill live molds, mold products may be left behind which may cause prob-lems for some individuals with candida-related disorders. Here are further comments on foods that usually contain yeasts and molds.

Fruit juices: Most fruit juices, including frozen, bottled or canned, are prepared from fruits that have been allowed to stand in bins, barrels and other con-tainers for periods ranging from an hour on up to several days or weeks. Although juice processors discard fruits that are obviously spoiled by mold, most fruits used for juice making contain mold.

Coffee & tea: These popular beverages, including the health food teas, are prepared from plant products. Such products are subject to mold contamination. How much is uncer-tain. If you're allergic to yeasts and feel you can't get along without your coffee or tea, you'll have to experi-ment and see what happens. Some herbal teas have been reported to have therapeutic value. A California physician who has been using Taheebo® tea in treating some of her patients commented,

> "I've found that Taheebo® tea helps. I've been using it since Novem-ber 1982. It seems to help, especially in clearing nasal symptoms."

Alcoholic beverages: Wines, beers and other alcoholic beverages contain high levels of yeast contamination, so if you're allergic to yeast, you'll need to avoid them.

Moreover, I feel you should stay away from alcoholic beverages for another reason: They contain large amounts of quick-acting carbohydrate. If you drink such beverages, you'll be feeding your yeast.

Other beverages:

> "What's a person to drink?"

asked one of my patients.

"You've taken away my beer, my Scotch, my coffee, my tea, my cokes and my juices. That leaves only water. Isn't there something else? How about diet drinks?

Diet drinks have no nutritional value. Moreover, they often contain caffeine, food coloring, phosphates, saccharin and other ingredients which disagree with many individuals. However, since these beverages do not contain mold, individuals with candida-related problems may tolerate them. If you use them, don't go overboard.

Many people with chronic health problems, especially those with chemical sensitivity, require bottled or distilled water to remain symptom-free. Others find they can tolerate tap water if they install a water filter in their home.

In an article in the Summer, 1982 issue of *The Long Island Pediatrician* (published by Chapter 2, District II, American Academy of Pediatrics) entitled, "How Safe is Long Island Drinking Water?", Frances S. Sterrett,[14] Ph.D., Professor of Chemistry, Hofstra University, commented,

> "Several hundred different organic chemical substances have been found in a variety of drinking waters. For this reason, I and many other people on Long Island and in many parts of the country filter our drinking water through an activated carbon water filter . . . Water consumed by infants and small children should be filtered through activated carbon and boiled because cumulative effects of low level contaminants are more critical at such an early age."

(Information on water filters can be found in the book, *Water Fit to Drink,* by Carol Keough, Rodale Press, Inc., Emmaus, PA, 1980, and in the February 1983 issue of *Consumer Reports*).

Left-overs: Such foods provide a rich breeding ground for yeasts and molds. Molds are one of the major micro-organisms causing foods to spoil, and all foods spoil. Although refrigeration retards mold growth, even refrigerated foods develop mold contamination. 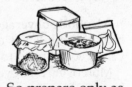 So prepare only as much food as you need and eat it promptly, or freeze left-overs.

At the July 1982 Dallas Candida Conference, Dr. Francis Waickman of Cuyahoga Falls, Ohio commented,

> "Several of my mold sensitive patients must eat foods immediately after they're cooked. Left-overs always cause their symptoms to flare."

Whether or not you can eat left-overs will depend on the severity of your health problems and how sensitive you are to mold. Some individuals can eat left-overs without developing symptoms, while others cannot. It takes trial and error experimenting to find out which foods can cause trouble and which ones do not.

Spices & condiments: These dietary ingredients are usually loaded with mold and should be avoided or approached with caution. Limited quantities of salt and juice from a freshly squeezed lemon are your safest food flavoring agents. And freshly squeezed lemon juice, plus unprocessed vegetable oil, makes a healthy, nutritious salad dressing. Moreover, unprocessed vegetable oils, especially flaxseed or linseed oil, safflower or sunflower oil, are rich in essential fatty acids which are important precursors of substances your body requires for proper functioning. (For further discussion of fatty acids, see Chapters 36, and 43 of the Update.)

Cereal grains: Cereal grains, including oats, wheat, rice, barley, corn and millet, especially those found in natural food stores, are excellent sources of vitamins and minerals. Moreover, such unprocessed grains contain no sugar. However, like other foods, some mold contamination may occur.

Nevertheless, such grains can play an important part in meeting your nutritional needs. If you haven't tried eating a hot cereal that you prepare at home from brown rice, unrefined oats, wheat or barley for breakfast, you're missing a treat. You can add chopped nuts, banana, peaches or strawberries (in season) and enjoy a satisfying nutritious breakfast that will help you start the day right.

How about dry cereals? These cereal grains . . . even the best of them . . . have been processed and subjected to high heat. Accordingly, they're much less desirable than hot cereals you prepare at home made from whole grain. Moreover, most of these cereals contain malt and added yeast-derived B vitamins. So if you're allergic to yeast, you'll need to avoid them.

Several years ago, on the "Today Show", Dr. Art Ulene showed a box of one of the popular cereals advertised for children and said,

> "This 14 ounce box contains 80 teaspoons of sugar. In fact, sugar is the main ingredient. And some two dozen of these cereals contain over 40% sugar."

If, in spite of their limited nutritional value, you decide on a dry cereal, get sugar-free Shredded Wheat®. Cereals which contain less than 6% added sugar include Cheerios®, Puffed Rice®, Wheat Chex®, Puffed Wheat®, Post Toasties®, Product 19®, and Special K®. However, I don't recommend them for anticandida diets as many contain malt and added yeast-derived B vitamins.

Breads: Nearly all commercially-available breads, cakes, crackers and cookies contain yeast or sugar and cause symptoms in patients with candida-related problems. So if you're allergic to yeast, they should be avoided. However, a few yeast-free and sugar-free products may be found in natural food stores and specialty departments of some supermarkets.†

Nuts: Nuts are loaded with good nutrients, especially trace minerals. However, most commercially available nuts on supermarket shelves contain additives of various sorts, including dextrose (corn sugar). So use unprocessed nuts. Ideally, nuts should be freshly shelled, since nuts stored for long periods of time (like fruits and other foods) attract mold growth. Avoid peanuts and peanut products since they're contaminated with mold.

Candies & sweets: Many people crave sugar, especially people with the candida problem. In fact, New York pediatrician, allergist and clinical ecologist Morton Teich commented,

> "Sugar craving is one of the leading symptoms that leads me to suspect candida-related illness in my patients."

What to do about it? Stay away from sugar-containing foods. After your immune system and your health improve, you may be able to cheat occasionally. An alternate: Use bananas and other fruits to prepare cookies, cakes and other sweetened foods. If you'd like a guide to help you prepare such foods, get a copy of the "all-natural, fruit-sweetened cookbook" 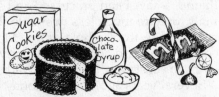 by Karen E. Barkie entitled *Sweet & Sugar Free*, St. Martin's Press, 175 Fifth Ave., New York, New York 10010, 1982.

---

†See Chapter 12 for recipes and suggestions for yeast-free and sugar-free baked products.

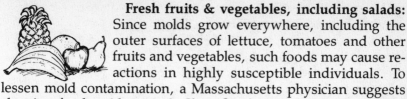**Fresh fruits & vegetables, including salads:** Since molds grow everywhere, including the outer surfaces of lettuce, tomatoes and other fruits and vegetables, such foods may cause reactions in highly susceptible individuals. To lessen mold contamination, a Massachusetts physician suggests cleaning foods with a weak Clorox® solution. (See Chapter 34.) And he said,

> "Although the fumes from Clorox® bother many chemically-sensitive patients, a person can avoid such reactions by using a nose clip while preparing the solution."

Eating out: If you're like most people, you live "on the run" and eat foods away from home. What's the answer? Do the best you can. And during the early weeks and months of your candida-control program, you may need to do a lot of brown-bagging (see Chapter 13). And when you eat out, you'll need to make your selections carefully, so as to avoid foods that trigger your symptoms.

More on Yeast and Mold-Containing Foods

Many patients with yeast-connected disorders develop symptoms when they consume yeast-containing foods. Yet, a number of my patients recently have reported that cheeses, teas, peanuts, mushrooms and other yeast-containing foods do not bother them.

I reported these observations to mold authority John W. Rippon, Ph. D., who commented:

> "Eating a yeast-containing food doesn't make candida organisms multiply. So when your patients develop symptoms from yeasty foods, they do so because they're allergic to yeast products." (See Chapter 10.)

Accordingly, as you improve (if you aren't bothered by mold allergies) you can cautiously try eating some yeast-containing food. But don't go overboard.

12

Sugar-Free, Yeast-Free Recipes

Swiss Steak

2 lbs. round steak, cut into serving
  size pieces

2 tbsp. unrefined vegetable oil

Heat skillet to 370°, add oil, then brown
the meat. Place in casserole and add:

1 medium onion (¹/₂ cup), chopped
¹/₂ cup chopped celery
¹/₄ cup chopped green pepper
1 cup peeled, chopped fresh
  tomatoes
¹/₂ cup carrots
2 cups water

Cover and bake at 300° for 3-4 hours.
Serves 4.

Meat Loaf

2 lbs. ground beef
1 cup oats, uncooked (old fashioned)
1 egg, beaten
¹/₄ cup chopped onion
1 cup water
1 tsp. salt

Combine ingredients. Shape into loaf
and bake in 9 x 5 pan at 350° for about 1
hour. Serves 6.

Sauteed Liver Slivers

¹/₄ cup whole wheat flour
¹/₄ cup cold-pressed veg. oil
1 lb. beef liver cut into slivers
1 onion, chopped
Salt to taste

Roll liver slivers in whole wheat flour.
Heat oil in pan. Saute onions and liver.
Salt and serve.

Fish Cakes

2 cups tuna fish
1 cup cooked brown rice
1 egg
1 small onion, finely chopped
1 tbsp. lemon juice (fresh)
3 tbsp. melted butter or unrefined
  vegetable oil
1 cup finely ground nuts

Beat egg, add tuna, rice, onion, lemon
juice and oil. Blend well and form into
patties. Roll in nut meal and place on
oiled baking sheet. Bake in 350° oven
about 15 minutes or until brown and
bubbly. May substitute any cooked fish
or poultry for tuna. Makes approximately 8 patties. Serves 4.

Pork Chops and Brown Rice

4 pork chops
1 cup brown rice
2½ cups boiling water
½ cup chopped green pepper
¼ cup chopped onion
½ tsp. salt

Soak rice in boiling water for at least 30 min. Brown pork chops. Set aside. In same frying pan, add remaining ingredients. Simmer 10-min. Pour rice mixture into an oiled baking dish. Layer chops on top. Cover. Bake at 350° for 1 hour. Serves 4.

Baked Chicken

Oil bottom of oven-baking dish with a cold-pressed vegetable oil. Lay chicken pieces in pan (skin side down), sprinkle with salt and cover with foil. Bake at 375° for ½ hour. Remove foil, turn pieces, and bake an additional 20 to 30 min., until brown and tender.

Pork Chop Casserole

1-10 oz. package frozen green beans
2 medium onions, sliced
2 or 3 potatoes, peeled and sliced
6 pork chops
Salt

Layer beans, onions, potatoes in an oiled 13 x 9 baking pan or casserole. Sprinkle with a bit of salt. Place pork chops on top, cover and bake at 375° for ¾ hour. Remove cover (or foil) and bake an additional 15 min. until chops are tender and brown. Serves 4.

Chicken Salad

2 cups finely chopped cooked
    chicken
½ cup finely chopped celery
2 to 4 hard cooked, chopped eggs
1 medium onion, chopped

Moisten with blender mayonnaise. Serves 4.

Easy Chicken and Rice

3 lbs. frying chicken pieces
1 cup brown rice
2 cups water
½ tsp. salt
1½ tbsp. butter
3 tbsp. chopped fresh parsley
Optional: Onions, celery, green
    pepper, nuts

Place rice, water, salt, butter and parsley in 4 quart casserole. Stir and bring to a boil. Salt chicken and lay on top of rice. Lower heat to simmer; cover tightly and cook 45 to 60 min. until water is absorbed and chicken is tender.

Barley or Rice Soup

1–3 lbs. chicken, disjointed
8 cups cold water
½ cup onion, chopped
1 tbsp. sea salt
½ cup barley or brown rice
1 cup celery, chopped

Place all ingredients in a large pan and cook over medium heat until done. Or, may be cooked all day in a slow cooker. Serves 4.

Best Barley Soup

1/4 cup whole barley–cooked in 6 cups
of water for 1 hour

Add and cook until tender:

1 cup carrots
1/2 cup celery
1/4 cup onions, chopped
2 cups tomatoes, chopped
1 cup peas–fresh or frozen

Add fresh parsley just before serving.

Salmon Patties

1 lb. salmon with liquid
1/3 cup whole wheat flour
1/4 cup stoneground corn meal
1/4 cup wheat germ
2 eggs, beaten
1/2 cup chopped onion
1/4 cup chopped bell pepper
1 tbsp. lemon juice
1/4 to 1/2 cup unrefined vegetable oil
for frying

Flake salmon, mashing bones well. Mix
all ingredients together. Form into patties. Brown in oil on medium heat for 15
minutes. Serves 4.

Stewed Okra

Okra
Onion
Tomatoes
Corn
Sea Salt

Saute okra and onion in a bit of unrefined vegetable oil. Add fresh tomato,
fresh or frozen corn, a bit of salt and
simmer until tender. May thicken with
stoneground corn meal if desired.

Zucchini and Tomatoes

Zucchini
Onion
Tomato
Fresh Parsley

Saute zucchini and onion until tender.
Add chopped tomato, continue to stir
until cooked. Add parsley and a bit of
sea salt and serve.

Green Beans with Almonds

Fresh or frozen green beans
Onion
Unrefined vegetable oil
Fresh parsley
Slivered blanched almonds

Steam green beans until tender. In separate pan saute onion in vegetable oil
until tender. Add green beans, parsley
and almonds. Sprinkle lightly with salt
and serve.

Summertime Salad

1 cup cucumber, diced
1/4 cup onion, chopped
1 cup tomatoes, diced
1/2 tsp. sea salt (or less)

NO NEED FOR DRESSING
Serves 4.

Acorn Squash

Cut squash in half and remove seeds. In
baking pan place 1 tbsp. unrefined vegetable oil and 1 cup water. Lay halves in
pan cut side down and bake in 370°
oven for 30 minutes. Turn (face up),
brush with oil and sea salt and bake another 20-30 minutes until tender.

Stir Fried Vegetable Scramble

2 tbsp. unrefined vegetable oil or
 butter
2 tbsp. chopped onion
2 tbsp. chopped green pepper
1/2 cup fresh chopped tomato
1/2 to 1 cup cooked vegetables
2 to 4 slightly beaten eggs

Heat skillet, add oil, onions and green peppers. Stir fry until tender. Add tomato and other vegetables. Bring to boil, stirring constantly. Add eggs and cook, stirring gently. Serve immediately.

Wheat Biscuits

2 cups whole wheat flour
4 tsps. baking powder
1/2 tsp. salt
1/3 cup unrefined vegetable oil
3/4 to 1 cup water or milk†

Mix together dry ingredients, add oil and mix well (important). Add enough water to make a soft dough that is not sticky. Mix just enough to moisten dry ingredients. With hands, pat out dough to 3/4" thickness on floured board. Cut with glass, place on oiled baking sheet and bake 20 minutes or until done in a 450° oven. 12 biscuits.

Blender Mayonnaise

2 eggs at room temperature
2 tbsp. fresh squeezed lemon juice
1/4 tsp. sea salt
1 1/4 cup unrefined vegetable oil

Combine all ingredients except oil in blender at high speed for 1 minute. Slowly add oil. Store in glass jar. Refrigerate.

Zucchini Florentine

6 small zucchini-1/4 in. slices
2 tbsp. butter
1 cup water or milk†
3 slightly beaten eggs
1 tsp. salt

Put zucchini in 1 1/2 qt. casserole. Dot with butter. Bake at 400° for 15 minutes.
Combine and pour remaining ingredients over zucchini. Set casserole in shallow pan with one inch hot water. Bake 350° for 40 minutes until knife comes out clean.

Whole Wheat Popovers

3 eggs
1 cup water or milk†
3 tbsp. butter
1 cup whole wheat flour

Beat eggs until foamy. Add water and butter and continue beating. Add flour and blend. Fill greased muffin cups 2/3 full. Bake at 375° for 50 minutes. Makes 12 popovers.

Banana-Oat Cake

2 cups oat flour
1/4 tsp. salt
2 tbsp. unrefined vegetable oil
2 tsp. baking powder
1/2 cup mashed banana
2 eggs
3 tbsp. cold water

Mix dry ingredients. Beat eggs. Add water, oil and mashed banana. Blend with dry ingredients. Bake in 8" x 8" pan at 350° for 25 to 30 minutes. Cut in 9 pieces.

†Milk may be used if tolerated.

Better Butter

1 stick (1/2 cup) butter, room
   temperature
1/2 cup linseed oil

Blend until light and fluffy. Store in glass container. Use as you would regular butter or margarine.

Corn Bread

1 3/4 cups stoneground corn meal
1/3 cup whole wheat flour
3 tsp. baking powder
1 tsp. sea salt
1 egg lightly beaten
3 tbsp. cold pressed vegetable oil
1 1/2 cups water or milk†

Combine dry ingredients, beat egg, add oil and water and blend all together. Bake in oiled 8" square pan 425°, 20 to 25 minutes. Cut 9 pieces.

Spoon Bread

1 1/2 cups water or milk†
3/4 cup stoneground cornmeal
3/4 tsp. sea salt
3 eggs, separated
3 tbsp. cold pressed vegetable oil

Bring water to boil. Pour in cornmeal and stir constantly and cook until thickened. Add salt and lightly beaten egg yolks and oil. Remove from heat and cool slightly. Fold in stiffly beaten egg whites. Bake in greased 8" square baking dish at 375°, 35 to 40 minutes. Cut in 9 squares.

Rice-Oat Pancakes

1/2 cup rice flour
3/4 cup Old Fashioned oats-blend in
   blender until fine
1 tbsp. baking powder
1/4 tsp. baking soda
2 tbsp. unrefined vegetable oil
1/2 tsp. sea salt
3 tbsp. apricot puree (or egg)
1/2 cup Soyquick

Mix all ingredients together and drop tablespoonsful onto oiled skillet.

Sunflower Crackers

1 cup whole wheat flour
3 tbsp. sunflower seed butter (blend
   seeds in food processor)
2 tbsp. cold pressed vegetable oil
3 tbsp. water
1/4 tsp. sea salt

Combine flour, sunflower seed butter and oil. Gradually add water, adding just enough to form a soft dough. Add salt. Knead and roll on floured surface to 1/8" thickness. Cut in shapes, prick with a fork and bake at 350° for 10 minutes or until browned. Cool.

Oat Griddle Cakes

3/4 cup cooked Old Fashioned oats
1 1/4 to 1 1/2 cup milk or water
1 egg
2 tbsp. pressed oil
3/4 cup oat flour
1 tsp. baking powder
1/2 tsp. salt

Mix all ingredients together and spoon onto greased skillet.

†Milk may be used if tolerated.

Potato Pancakes

3 cups potatoes, grated raw
1 cup onion, grated
3 eggs, beaten
1/2 tsp. sea salt
2 tbsp. whole wheat flour
2 tbsp. unrefined vegetable oil

Drop by tablespoonsful on hot oiled skillet. Lower heat slightly and brown, turn and brown other side. Makes 12 pancakes.

Rice Muffins

1 1/2 cups rice flour
1/2 tsp. sea salt
2 tsp. baking powder
1/4 tsp. baking soda
4 tbsp. unrefined vegetable oil
3 tbsp. apricot puree
1 cup water or Soyquick

Mix and spoon into greased muffin tins and bake at 350° for 15 to 20 minutes. Makes 12 muffins.

Pancakes

1 1/2 to 2 cups water or milk†
2 eggs
2 tbsp. unrefined vegetable oil
3 tsp. salt
2 cups whole wheat flour
2 tsp. baking powder

Beat eggs, add water and oil and blend. Add dry ingredients and blend well. Bake on hot, oiled griddle. Makes about 2 dozen 4″ cakes.

†Milk may be used if tolerated.

Corn Muffins

1 1/4 cup whole wheat flour
3/4 cup stoneground corn meal
4 1/2 tsp. baking powder
1 tsp. sea salt (optional)
1 egg
2/3 cup water or milk†
1/3 cup unrefined vegetable oil

Sift dry ingredients together. In separate bowl blend egg, water and oil; add to dry mixture and stir with a spoon just enough to dampen all ingredients. Place in 12 greased muffin tins and bake in 425° oven 25 to 30 minutes. Serves 12.

Applesauce Muffins

1 large egg
2 tbsp. unrefined vegetable oil
1 1/2 cups unsweetened applesauce
2 cups whole wheat flour
3/4 tsp. baking soda
2 tsp. baking powder
1/4 tsp. sea salt

Beat together egg, oil and applesauce. Add flour, soda, baking powder and salt; beat well. Spoon into oiled and floured muffin tins. Bake at 375° for 20 to 25 minutes until firm to touch and browned. Makes 12 muffins.

Wheat-Nut Snack

3 cups shredded wheat bits
3 cups pecans
1/4 cup butter, melted

Melt butter in baking pan in 250° oven. Add wheat bits and nuts; mix well and bake 30 to 40 minutes.

13

Ideas For Breakfast And Eating On The Run

"Since you *have* to get up, you might as well fix a cheerful breakfast. Not overbearingly cheerful, please! And nothing that requires intricate measuring, sifting, blending or beating . . ."

In her continuing discussion, Janet Lorimer said,

"Experts tell us that breakfast is the most essential meal of the day. It should be nutritious *and* quick-and-easy *and* well-balanced *and* appealing to the tastebuds. Studies confirm that children and adults learn and work better when they've eaten breakfast. Unfortunately, breakfast is the most maligned meal of all! Everyone is rushing about in seventeen different directions, and eating seems to be *one* thing no one wants to spend time doing. So, how can you possibly make breakfast your favorite meal against those odds?

"Plan ahead! Spend a few moments the night before planning tomorrow's first meal. Who likes to think about breakfast at 10:30 at night? But it beats staggering into the kitchen the next morning totally unprepared."

Janet's article gives many other suggestions, including making a list of menu ideas, glamorizing the table setting, making your own mixes and freezing for the future.

In discussing these, she commented,

"Never underestimate the power of your freezer to work breakfast miracles. If all you have in your freezer is frozen pizza and two bags of ice cubes, you're not using a valuable ally!"

"When fruit goes on sale, buy in bulk and freeze, following the proper freezing instructions in your cookbook! Frozen fruits lose their crispness when they're thawed, but they make a delicious hot com-

---

†Adapted from the article "How to Make Breakfast Your Favorite Meal," by Janet Lorimer which was published in the March 1983 issue of *Bestways Magazine*. Used with permission.

pote. There's nothing quite so much fun as eating summer fruit in the dead of winter."

Although all of the "goodies" Janet talks about can't be used on your diet, special yeast free breads can be baked ahead of time and frozen. When you want to use them just reheat in a moderate oven.

For snacks, lunch or eating on the run, you can fill a "brown bag" with hard boiled eggs, raw vegetables and fruits, nuts, rice cakes or meat and bread from your freezer.

More on Breakfast:

In our recipe section of *The Yeast Connection Cookbook*, my collaborator and co-author, Marge Jones, commented,

> *"What can I eat for breakfast?* Time and time I hear this and it's a valid concern for people who are on a diet to control candida."
> If you strip breakfast of yeast, you eliminate toast, French toast, bagels, sweet rolls, even sourdough bread. If you also omit wheat, milk, corn, sugar, soy and egg—you end up with a gaping void in your menus where breakfast used to be."

Marge then gives you lots of breakfast suggestions. These include pancakes or flatbread that you can make a few days ahead, package and freeze. Then when you're ready, you can put them in your toaster oven.

> "Eat these versatile little treasures with your fingers, like dainty pieces of toast. Or top them with your favorite filling or bean dip for open faced mini-sandwiches. They go brown bagging easily and travel well on trips too."

Marge is a real authority on the non-grain alternatives, amaranth, buckwheat, quinoa and teff. These nutritious foods are rich in carbohydrates and help fill you up. They're especially useful in people who are sensitive to wheat and corn.

She also tells you how to fix breakfast "pudding." Ingredients in this recipe include foods that you may not think of as breakfast foods, such as sweet potato (and/or other vegetables), and chopped nuts.

14

If Sugar Is A "No-No," What Can I Use?

If candida plays a role in causing your health problems, avoid sugar, because sugar seems to feed the yeast germ and hundreds of my patients have reported,

"When I eat sugar, my symptoms flare up."

Sugar may also trigger symptoms in individuals who do not have candida-related illness.

Yet, because sweetened foods taste good, I'm sure you'd like to know other ways that you can safely sweeten your foods and beverages. Here are comments on sweeteners you may have considered, including some you can use and others which aren't recommended:

Aspartame: In July 1981, the Food and Drug Administration finally gave its approval for use of a new low calorie sweetener. This product is 200 times sweeter than sugar, but contains only 1/8th the calories found in sugar. The product tastes like sugar, but contains no saccharin or other artificial sweetener.

Aspartame can be found on supermarket shelves across the country under the brand name Equal® or Nutra-Sweet®.

Aspartame was discovered in 1965 when a chemist wet his fingers to pick up a piece of paper and noticed a sweet taste. The two compounds he was working with were aspartic acid and the amino acid, phenylalanine (found in proteins). Although neither of these compounds alone taste sweet, combined they're very sweet.

Since the discovery of this product, more than 100 scientific tests for its safety have been conducted during the last 15 years. In addition, scientists at Searle Consumer Products (which markets Equal®) have conducted many formal and impromptu consumer taste tests with men, women and children. These results show that aspartame could be widely accepted as a sugar substitute.

How about safety? Most scientists feel aspartame is safe, since it's made of two normal food ingredients (amino acids) which have been joined together. So when it goes into your body, it's like a tiny bit of food, rather than a synthetic chemical.[†]

One packet of Equal®[††] has the sweetness of two teaspoons of sugar, but supplies only 4 calories. It costs about 4 cents per packet, so it's much more expensive than saccharin.[††] Also, it can't be used in baking because high heat for long periods of time cause chemical changes in the amino acids, eliminating the sweet taste.

Saccharin: Foods and beverages containing saccharin must be labeled with the following warning:

> "Use of this product may be hazardous to your health. This product contains saccharin which has been determined to cause cancer in laboratory animals."

In spite of this label, I prefer saccharin to sugar, and when used in limited quantities, I feel it is relatively safe. Moreover, a study in a leading medical journal comparing patients with bladder cancer to a similar group who had no cancer, showed no evidence that the cancer patients had consumed more saccharin than those who did not have cancer.

Fruits: Some of my patients with yeast-connected illness tolerate complex carbohydrates, including apples, bananas and pineapple. If you are such a person, Karen Barkie's cookbook, *Sweet and Sugar Free*, (St. Martin's Press, New York, N.Y.) should interest you. It's full of recipes for sugar-free, fruit-sweetened foods.

Other of my patients develop symptoms when they eat fruits. For example, Ted F., a patient with MS who was doing well, was in for a follow-up visit on April 22, 1983. Ted commented,

> "I'm doing great. No symptoms unless I eat yeast-breads or sugar. These foods trigger numbness and weakness, and a large banana will do the same thing.

---

†R. J. Wurtman recently reported that undesirable effects may occur if large amounts of aspartame are ingested. (*New England Journal of Medicine*, August 18, 1983)

††Since the packets of powdered, artificial sweeteners contain cane and/or corn sugar, I do not recommend them. If you must sweeten a food artificially, use liquid saccharin. (For a further discussion, see Chapter 44, Update).

And 39-year-old Lynn, a patient with fatigue, depression and abdominal symptoms, commented,

"Grains and fruits of all kinds make my symptoms worse."

Because fruits promote yeast growth, I now tell my patients to avoid them—especially during the first three weeks of their treatment program.

Honey: Many people like honey. And honey is sweeter than sugar. Moreover, over the years, many parents of hyperactive children have reported,

"Sugar makes my child hyperactive, yet he can take honey."

Nevertheless, if your illness is related to candida, stay away from honey . . . at least until your health problems are well controlled. Here's why: Honey resembles sugar in many ways and tends to feed the yeast organism.

Fructose or High Fructose Corn Syrup: This substance has received a great deal of publicity. It's sweeter than cane and beet sugar in cold liquids and is now used in many commercially sweetened foods.

Is it better or safer for you than ordinary table sugar? No, because it feeds the yeast germ just as much as ordinary sugar. Also, it's a lot more expensive.

15

Food Allergies

Reactions to foods have been recognized by numerous observers for many centuries. For example, over 2,000 years ago, Lucretius commented,

> "What is food to one may be fierce poison to others."

And perhaps the first report of the use of an elimination diet can be found in the Bible in the first chapter of the Book of Daniel (1:12—15). Hippocrates[15] also commented,

> " . . . There are certain persons who cannot readily change their diet with impunity; and if they make any alteration in it for one day, or even for a part of a day, are greatly injured thereby. Such persons, provided they take dinner when it is not their wont, immediately become heavy and inactive, both in body and mind, and are weighed down with yawning, slumbering, and thirst; . . . to many this has been the commencement of a serious disease, when they have merely taken twice in a day the same food which they have been in the custom of taking once."

Although scattered references can be found on the relationship of food and food odors to physical symptoms during the past several centuries, it wasn't until about 100 years ago that physicians began to pay attention to what was then called "food idiosyncrasy."

During the current century, thousands of physicians have made clinical observations on the relationship of foods to a wide variety of clinical syndromes and several hundred reports of such food-related reactions can be found in the medical literature.

In spite of these numerous reports, many allergists ignore food-induced reactions and say in effect, "If you can't establish an immunologic mechanism you can't term such reactions allergy." But growing numbers of individuals, including physicians in practice as well as in academic centers, are now recognizing that food-related reactions are common. And one academician commented,

"It will be a long time before we understand all aspects of food allergy; certainly it will not happen in our lifetime."

Obvious Food Allergies: Such allergies are usually caused by uncommonly eaten foods such as shrimp, lobster, cashew nuts or strawberries. However, they can also be caused by peanuts, eggs and other common foods. Individuals with obvious food allergies will show positive reactions to various immunological tests, including the scratch or prick test and the RAST test. By contrast, such tests are usually negative in individuals with hidden food allergies.

Hidden Food Allergies: During the past 27 years, I've found that food-induced reactions have caused health problems in thousands of my patients. And because the foods causing the patients' symptoms are rarely suspected, I've termed these reactions "hidden food allergies."

Such allergies are caused by foods a person eats every day, including especially milk, corn, wheat, sugar, chocolate, citrus and food colors, flavors and additives. They usually develop gradually over a period of weeks, months and years. A person tends to become "addicted" to the foods causing his symptoms. So he's apt to crave them. Symptoms caused by hidden food allergies include fatigue, nasal congestions, dark shadows under the eyes (allergic "shiners"), headache, abdominal pain, muscle and joint pains, bladder symptoms and nervous system symptoms of all types.

Experiences of Other Physicians: Hundreds of other physicians, including Dr. Elmer Cranton of Trout Dale, Virginia, Dr. Harold Hedges of Little Rock, Arkansas, and Dr. Doris Rapp of Buffalo, New York, have also found that hidden allergies to common foods often cause chronic and often disabling symptoms in their patients. And Dr. Cranton commented,

"In addition to prescribing nystatin, I nearly always prescribe Elimination Diet A in your book, *Tracking Down Hidden Food Allergy.*[13] This enables me to identify trouble-making foods and remove them from the diet. And by decreasing the patient's allergy load, my overall treatment program is more apt to be successful."

In carrying out Elimination Diet A, the patient avoids milk, egg, wheat, corn, sugar, chocolate, citrus fruits, along with the food colors, dyes and most of the packaged and processed foods. The elimination phase of the diet usually lasts about a week or until there is convincing improvement in symptoms which continues for 48 hours. Then foods are returned to the diet, one food per day, and reactions are noted. By using this diet, I'm able to identify troublemaking foods and remove them from the diet.

And in a Letter to the Editor in the January 1982 issue of *The Journal of the Arkansas State Medical Association*, Dr. Harold Hedges commented,

> "The longer I practice medicine, the more I'm convinced that many illnesses are caused by what we eat, drink and breathe.
>
> "Since 1963, I've treated many patients with diseases and disorders which I could neither see with the naked eye nor help. Included among these that I label in good faith are patients with tension headache, chronic fatigue, chronic ear problems, sinusitis, irritable colon, depression, anxiety, hyperactivity, nervous stomach and hypochrondriasis. And when I couldn't find another cause, I'd even lay the blame on the poor lowly virus . . . I thank God for viruses, even if I couldn't prove it, the patient couldn't prove me wrong."

Dr. Hedges has found similar success in using elimination diets. And in a recent conversation with me, he said,

> "I usually use the 'cave man diet' from your book, *Tracking Down Hidden Food Allergy*[13], in working with my adult patients. And this more comprehensive diagnostic diet has enabled me to identify sensitivity to beef, pork, chicken, soy and other foods usually recommended for candida patients. And by identifying these foods and eliminating them, my treatment results are significantly improved."

Rotated Diets: In spite of the gaps which remain in our understanding of food-related problems, countless observers, dating from the time of Hippocrates, have noted that variety or diversity in selecting one's foods lessens a person's chances of developing food-induced reactions. And dur-

Rotated Diets

Day	1	2	3	4	5
Meats	Beef	Chicken	Shrimp	Pork	Trout
Fruits	Orange	Banana	Pineapple	Grape	Apple
Vegetables	White potato	Sweet potato	Carrot	Squash	Peas, beans or other legumes
Grains	Wheat	Oats	Rice	Barley	Corn

ing the past decade, many individuals, including physicians (and other professionals) and allergy sufferers, have found they can tolerate trouble-making foods and experience fewer symptoms if they rotate their diet.

Karen Dilatush commented,

> "I began having severe problems from eating the same *good* foods over and over. I improved as soon as I began *rotating* my diet.

In *rotating* your diet, you eat a food only once every 4 to 7 days. For example, in rotating fruits, you'd eat oranges on Monday, bananas on Tuesday, apples on Wednesday and pineapple on Thursday. Then on Friday you could start over again with oranges. The same system can be used with other food groups, including meats, vegetables and grains.

Further information about rotated diets can be found in a number of reference books, including "If This Is Tuesday, It Must Be Chicken", by Natalie Golos (available from *Dickey Enterprises*, 635 Gregory Road, Fort Collins, Colorado 80524), the "Cookbook/ Guide to Eating for Allergy", by Virginia Nichols (available from 3350 Fair Oaks Drive, Xenia, Ohio 45385), and the *Allergy Self-Help Cookbook*, by Marjorie Hurt Jones (published by Rodale Press, Emmaus, Pennsylvania.)

Section
C

**Keeping Candida
under control requires
more than medication
and a special diet.**

A number of concepts, drawings and charts in this section have been adapted and modified from material published by Sidney M. Baker, M.D.

16

Introduction

My grandfather was a country doctor who started practicing medicine in West Tennessee over 100 years ago. My father followed in his footsteps and joined him in practice around 1900. They were both "people doctors" who tried to help their patients with the limited resources available to them at the time. No x-rays; no antibiotics; no polio vaccine; no corticosteroids; no birth control pills; no endoscopic examination; no CAT scans; no cataract or open heart surgery and no hip replacements. No renal dialyses or exchange transfusions; no heart or kidney transplants.

In medicine, just as in transportation, communication and every other area of our lives, changes have been amazing, fantastic and breath-taking. And because of these advances in medicine, many lives have been saved and much suffering relieved.

When my oldest daughter was 4 years old, she developed severe peritonitis following a ruptured appendix. Antibiotics saved her life. And my mother-in-law, who had a total hip replacement when she was 80, kept driving her car and walking a mile a day until she was 90.

Countless numbers of my patients enjoy healthy, productive lives because medical science provided new answers and new therapies.

To cope with the explosion in medical knowledge during the past several decades, medicine has become more highly specialized. Not long ago I visited John Lingo, a medical school classmate. John, an ophthalmologist, practices with a group of nine eye specialists in Mobile, Alabama. As we toured his clinic, Dr. Lingo commented,

"Dr. A. specializes in blepharoplasty (taking tucks in eyelids of people who want to look younger). Dr. B. specializes in diseases of the cornea; Dr. C. specializes in the retina, and Dr. D. specializes in the parts in between!"

Similar specialization has taken place in internal medicine, pediatrics, surgery and other areas of medicine. And during the last 10 years, all sorts of new specialists and subspecialists have entered practice in my town and in communities across the country. Many doctors specialize in treating only one part of the body or only one type of disease. Some specialize in treating arthritis or thyroid disease while others specialize in diseases of the digestive tract. Still others specialize in treating headaches, psoriasis, hyperactivity or multiple sclerosis.

With the great increase in medical knowledge, medical education has increasingly stressed the importance of correct diagnosis. Accordingly, great emphasis has been placed on the naming of diseases. Then once a disease is identified and labeled, a treatment plan is established which usually includes drugs or surgery. Without question, such diagnosis and treatment is effective in coping with many contemporary health problems, ranging from acute bacterial meningitis to gallstones.

But is this a perfect answer for every medical problem? Suppose you "feel like the devil" and you undergo a variety of medical examinations and learn that you don't have a "disease"? No brain tumor; no diabetes; no tuberculosis; no gallstones; no appendicitis; no anemia; no "nothing." What then?

This was Marilyn's problem. Marilyn, a 38-year-old professional, enjoyed a happy marriage and a successful career. Moreover, her two youngsters were bright and healthy and added to the happiness of her family. *Her only problem: She rarely felt good.*

Because of premenstrual tension, abdominal pain and menstrual irregularities, Marilyn usually went to her gynecologist for medical care. However, when her headaches became almost incapacitating, she was referred to a neurologist who carried out a variety of tests, including EEG studies and brain scans. Both were said to be "normal."

Then because of recurrent abdominal pain, bloating and other digestive symptoms, Marilyn was referred to a gastroenterologist. After upper and lower GI x-rays, gallbladder x-rays and endoscopic examinations, she was told, "All of your studies are normal." But because of continued abdominal pain and occasional urinary tract infections, she was cystoscoped and kidney x-rays were carried out. These studies were also normal.

Finally, because no "disease" could be identified and she continued to feel tired and depressed, Marilyn's gynecologist suggested that she talk to clinical psychologist, Cheryl Robley, Ph.D. After two visits, Cheryl called me saying,

> "I'd like for you to see Marilyn and see if you can help her with her fatigue and depression. She has no significant psychological hangups and I feel her symptoms are yeast connected."

After taking nystatin and changing her diet, Marilyn improved. She improved even more when she really worked on her diet and avoided all junk foods and began taking yeast-free vitamins and minerals. Further improvement followed the banning of odorous colognes and perfumes, insecticides, bathroom chemicals and other chemical pollutants from her home. Marilyn and her husband, John, have also been taking out more time for exercise, rest and relaxation and Marilyn feels that taking essential fatty acids in the form of linseed oil helps her get rid of her premenstrual tension.

In talking to the patients who come to see me seeking help for yeast-connected illness, here's what I tell them:

1. I possess no "quick fix." No magic pill. Yet, I'll do my best to help you get rid of your symptoms and regain your health.
2. Each person differs from every other person. And I do not think of the "yeast problem" as a disease. Instead, it's only one factor which plays a role in causing your health problems. Other important factors include the quality of the food you eat, the air you breathe, the water you drink and the relationship you enjoy with your family and friends.

So to overcome yeast-connected health problems, we have to take a comprehensive approach. This means you need to understand the many factors that play a role in making you sick and take control of them. Then you can help your own immune system conquer them.

17

To Overcome Candida And Enjoy Good Physical, Mental And Emotional Health:

You Must Seek These Vital Nutrients

Good food provides calories and many other essential substances your body needs to function properly. Proteins, carbohydrates (starches) and fats or oils provide the calories. When they're obtained from good sources, they also furnish your body with essential "micronutrients," including vitamins and minerals.

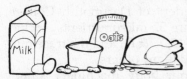

Proteins: Found in meat, fish, eggs, dairy products, nuts & seeds, whole grains, peas and beans (& other vegetables to a lesser extent). Proteins are made up of substances called "amino acids." There are 22 of these and many of them are essential. You increase your chances of good health if you obtain your proteins from a wide variety of sources.

Carbohydrates or starches: There are two types of these; the *"complex" carbohydrates* (found in a wide variety of vegetables, fruits and whole grains), and the *"refined" carbohydrates* found especially in refined sugar and white flour. Although both types of carbohydrates furnish energy, only the complex carbohydrates provide the vitamins and minerals needed for their proper utilization.

Fats & oils: Limited amounts of these nutrients are an important part of your diet. Yet, there are "good" fats and "bad" fats. The good fats are the *essential fatty acids* ("EFA's"), including linoleic acid and linolenic acid (obtained especially from unprocessed vegetable oils, including linseed, sunflower, safflower, corn and primrose oils). They play an important role in many of your body's biochemical processes, including the manufacture of prostaglandins and the strengthening of your immune system.

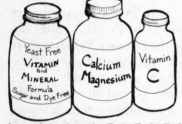

The bad fats include hydrogenated or partially hydrogenated vegetable oils and fats obtained from animal products. Although such fats provide calories, they appear to play a role in plugging up your arteries, leading to the premature development of degenerative disorders.

Other nutrients include iron, calcium and magnesium which are necessary for many vital body functions, including the prevention of anemia, the promotion of strong teeth and bones, a sound heart and a properly functioning nervous system.

You also need other *"micronutrients"* (*micro* means very small), including both vitamins and minerals. According to the late Dr. Henry Schroeder[16] of Dartmouth College, there are 37 micronutrients, including vitamins A, B-1, B-2, B-3, B-6, B-12, C & D, and the trace minerals, zinc, selenium, chromium, and many others.

Without these micronutrients, your body machinery simply doesn't work well. For example, a zinc deficiency interferes with normal taste, growth and resistance to infection. If you don't get enough chromium, you cannot properly metabolize carbohydrates. Without sufficient vitamin B-6, prostaglandin synthesis is impaired and calcium deficiency renders the white blood cells incapable of making substances they need to kill candida. These are only a few of the hundreds (or even thousands) of important interactions in the body which require micronutrients.

Iron appears to be especially important to people with yeast-related illness. Studies by Higgs & Wells[17] and others suggest that some individuals, even those who aren't anemic, may require iron supplements. Calcium and magnesium supplements are particularly important in young women, especially those of slender build who do not consume dairy products. Without an adequate calcium intake, bones lose their minerals and women, especially those past the menopause, develop osteoporosis.[181a-b-c] This condition weakens the bones, leading to collapsed vertebrae, pinched nerves, broken hips and other disabling health problems.

and you must avoid

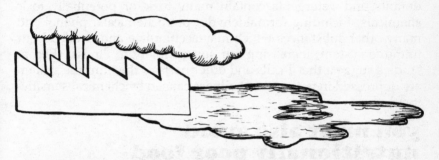

poisons and pollutants of all kinds including those which contaminate the air, soil and water.

Toxic or poisonous substances: Lead from many sources, including leaded gasoline, is polluting our planet. Evidence of such lead pollution can be found in the North Polar ice cap which contains much more lead than the South Pole, the difference being fewer automobiles in the Southern Hemisphere.

Other toxic minerals include cadmium and mercury. There's also growing evidence that we're ingesting aluminum in many processed foods as well as in foods wrapped in aluminum foil, aluminum in drinking water, aluminum cans and cooking utensils. Although aluminum doesn't appear to be a major environmental poison, it would appear prudent to lessen your exposure to it.

Insecticides and weed killers: These chemicals, sprayed on our fields and farms and in our homes, get into the water supply and into the food chain. And all of us now have DDT and similar poisons in our bodies.

Other chemicals: A variety of other industrial chemicals have been introduced into our environment which are causing health problems in many persons. Substances such as PCB's (polychlorinated biphenyls) have gotten into our soil and water and into the food chain, and have made their way into our bodies. Moreover, human breast milk contains these toxins and pollutants to a degree that concerns many people.

Home chemicals: Our clothing, homes, cosmetics, soaps, deodorants and detergents contain many toxic or potentially toxic chemicals, including formaldehyde, petrochemicals, phenol and many other substances which may accumulate and overload our immune system, increasing our susceptibility to illness. (Recent studies suggest that T-cells and other parts of the immune system are depressed in patients with illness caused by chemical sensitivity.)

you must also avoid nutritionally poor food especially sugar, white flour and hardened vegetable oil

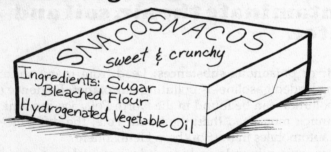

You are what you eat. And if you load up on poor quality foods, including especially foods containing sugar, white flour and hardened vegetable oil, you won't enjoy good health.

Studies by Cheraskin[19] of the University of Alabama indicate that diets high in refined sugar impair the function of the body's phagocytes (germ-eating white blood cells) which play an important role in resisting bacterial infection.

Studies by Schroeder[16] (and many others) clearly indicate that when whole wheat flour is refined, many essential nutrients are removed, including vitamins and minerals. Included among these are B-vitamins, magnesium, zinc and selenium. Moreover, even when white flour is "enriched" by the addition of a few nutrients, it still lacks other nutrients which are equally essential.

Research by Horrobin and Rudin[20-a-b-c-d] shows that diets containing hardened vegetable oil found in many processed and packaged foods may be deficient in essential fatty acids. Such diets may interfere with the formation of prostaglandins E-1 (PGE-1). This, in turn, depresses T-lymphocytes which (as previously mentioned) play an important role in resisting allergies and infections.

Their research also suggests that diets deficient in essential vitamins, trace minerals, essential fatty acids and other nutrients lessen the integrity of the immune system.

you must be treated for . . . allergies caused by inhalants and foods

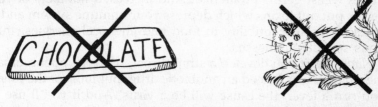

and infections caused by harmful microorganisms

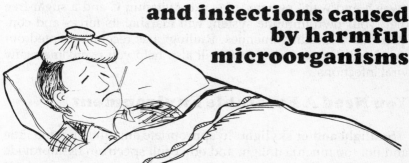

Allergies: Many people are troubled by adverse or allergic reactions to substances which do not appear to bother the average person. Such substances include pollens, molds, dust, animal danders, and foods. A number of observers now feel that individuals who react to substances in their diet or environment experience such reactions because their immune system is depressed by poor nutrition and an overload of environmental chemicals.

Many of my patients with food and chemical sensitivities improve and their allergies lessen when they take nystatin and follow a comprehensive program of management. Yet others, especially patients with inhalant allergy, may require allergy testing, followed by the use of allergy extracts, in order to achieve maximum improvement.

Infections caused by harmful micro-organisms, including bacteria, viruses and yeasts (and invasion by parasites). The healthy body with its marvelous immune system and other protective forces, both known and unknown, is usually able to resist or overcome invasion by many such organisms. Yet, when we pollute our environment or eat a poor diet, or upset our body balance with prolonged courses of drugs (including antibiotics and birth control pills), our immune system becomes depressed and these organisms can enter.

For example, when you take a diet high in refined carbohydrates, yeast germs proliferate. And increased numbers of yeast germs put out toxins which depress your immune system and increase your susceptibility to food and chemical allergies, infections, and other illnesses.

Naturally, if you develop a strep throat, bacterial pneumonia or meningitis, you'll need an antibiotic drug. But most of the time, if you run a fever, the cause will be a virus. And if you'll use the "watch and wait" system, plus extra vitamin C and a sugar-free diet, your own immune system will marshal its forces and conquer many invading enemies. Pauling[21] has recently pointed out that large doses of vitamin C will also help you overcome many viral infections.

You Need A Favorable Environment

Sunlight and/or skylight: In appropriate amounts (not too little and not too much) sunlight and other full spectrum light provide vitamin D and other essentials needed for proper growth of plants, animals and humans. (Further information on the importance of full spectrum light can be found in the writings of John Ott. See chapter 47, Update for reference.)

Fresh air. You must have fresh air (including oxygen) in order to live.

Pure water. Without water, you cannot survive. And the purer and less polluted the water, the better it is for you.

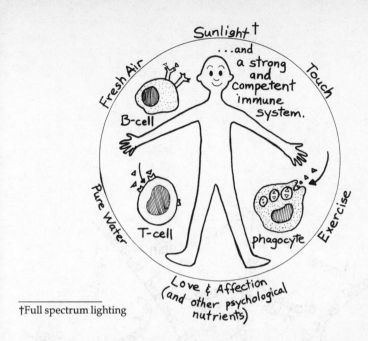

Sunlight †
...and a strong and competent immune system.
Fresh Air
B-cell
Touch
Pure Water
T-cell
phagocyte
Exercise
Love & Affection
(and other psychological nutrients)

†Full spectrum lighting

Exercise. Absolutely essential for proper function of your body, including not only your bones and muscles, but also your heart, lungs, brain, and immune system.

Love & Affection. All human beings require affection from the moment of birth throughout life. You must feel accepted, loved, respected and valued for what you are. Without love and affection, you cannot thrive.

Touch. Many recent scientific studies show that touch stimulates the production of hormones and body chemicals, including endorphins which play an important role in your overall health.

A competent and properly functioning immune system: Your immune system resembles your army, navy and marines. It protects you from foreign invaders, including bacteria, viruses, yeasts and chemicals. Some of your defenders are called phagocytes (phago = to eat; cyte = cell). These cells gobble up strep germs, pneumonia germs and other threatening invaders and help you overcome an infection.

Other defenders in your immune system include B-cells and T-cells. These make immunoglobulins of several types which block or neutralize invaders and help the phagocytes and other body defenders protect you. (See, also, chapter 24.)

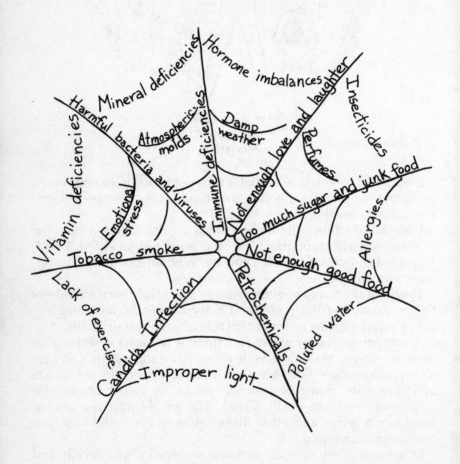

18
The Causes Of Illness Resemble A Web

When you don't feel well, there's always a reason (or many reasons). Some of these are obvious; yet others may be hard to find. Moreover, when you become ill, *your illness is nearly always caused by a web of interacting factors*, rather than a single cause. Although *Candida albicans* may play an important role in making you sick, to get well and stay well you'll need to pay attention to other factors.

In so doing, you must eat good food, stay away from junk, and make your environment a favorable one. So you'll need fresh air, appropriate lighting (indoors and outdoors) and pure water. You must also avoid or limit your exposure to the many chemicals which are polluting our environment.

Finally, you must receive liberal quantities of "psychological vitamins," including an affectionate, caring relationship with those with whom you live and work.

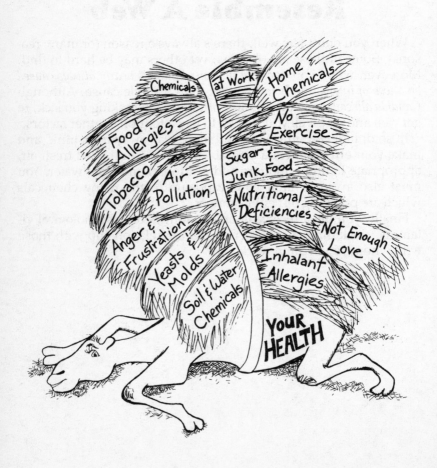

19
Is Your Camel's Load Too Heavy?

Suppose a stray bullet pierced your body or a tornado caused your roof to fall in on you. In such a distressing situation, it would be easy for your doctor to see how and why you'd be unable to work and/or take care of your family. But, if your symptoms have bothered you for years and affect many parts of your body, there's almost never such a single cause.

If your health problems are yeast connected, a special diet and antifungal medication will usually start you on the road to recovery. Yet, such therapy is rarely a "quick fix" or a "magic bullet."

If you're like most people with candidiasis, you resemble an overburdened camel. To regain your health—to look good, feel good, and enjoy life, you'll need to unload many "bundles of straw". This may take months—even a year or two. But then, your camel will be off and running!

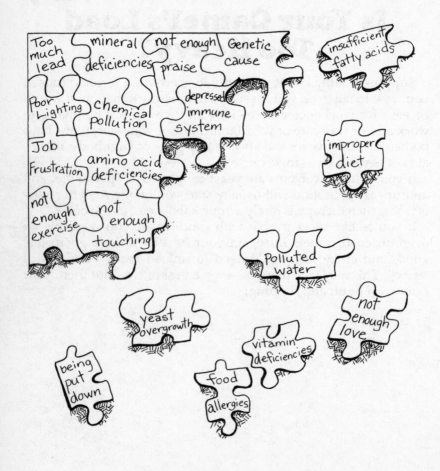

Adapted from Carl Pfeiffer, Ph.D., M.D. Used with permission.

20

The Puzzle
Of Chronic Illness

During the past seven years, I've treated over 1000 patients with chronic health problems related to "the yeast connection." And although nystatin and diet played an important role in helping most of these patients, many did not improve until other pieces of the puzzle were appropriately treated. Examples:

A 40-year-old school teacher felt much worse on damp, muggy days. A room dehumidifier and ionizer helped her symptoms. Control of mold growth in the home played an important role in contributing to the improvement of many other patients.

A 34-year-old mother of four, with candida-related health problems, was improving slowly. When blood studies showed a low blood vitamin A level, she was given digestive enzymes and additional vitamin A. Within a short time, she began to show more rapid improvement.

A 16-year-old with severe systemic and nervous system symptoms, including peculiar "seizures," was found to be sensitive to a number of common foods he was eating every day. Eliminating these foods and carrying out other parts of a comprehensive program of management resulted in significant improvement.

A 42-year-old secretary suffered from chronic hives, fatigue, depression and mental confusion. Her hives and mental confusion disappeared on treatment with diet and nystatin. A series of vitamin B-12 injections helped relieve her fatigue.

A 4-year-old with recurrent rhinitis, ear problems and irritability improved on diet, nystatin and nutritional supplements. Yet, rhinitis continued until a foam rubber pillow and rubber-stuffed dolls were removed from the child's bed.

Many of my patients continued to be bothered by headaches,

rhinitis, cough, burning eyes and other symptoms until tobacco smoke, insecticides, furniture polishes, colognes and other odorous or "outgassing chemicals" were removed from their homes. Other patients improved when they began drinking filtered water.

Improvement in many patients occurred when essential fatty acids in the form of linseed oil or primrose oil were added to their treatment programs. Still others improved when their inhalant and food allergies were treated with allergy vaccines and extracts.

21
Chemicals May Play A Role In Making You Sick

Margaret, a 58-year-old housewife, came to my office in January 1983. Here are excerpts from a letter she sent in before her visit:

"In my thirties, I developed post nasal drainage which irritated my throat. The doctors blamed it on 'sinus' and gave me antibiotics which didn't help. Later I read about allergies and experimented with my diet. My symptoms improved when I left off milk.

"At age 39, I gave birth to my fourth child and developed inner ear trouble with dizziness, nausea and vomiting. I was treated by a head specialist with various medications, including antibiotics. I was allergic to all of them. Through further experimentation, I learned I felt better, with less dizziness and heart palpitations, when I left off corn, sweets, dairy products and eggs.

"At the age of 53, I developed stiff and aching joints and began to notice that tobacco smoke, cosmetics, cleaners, paints, dyes and printing ink would bother me. More recently, I've developed reactions to polyester and had to quit crocheting and quilting because I coughed so much when I worked with them."

Margaret was put on a comprehensive treatment program, including nystatin and a yeast-free, sugar-free diet. She was also tested for a number of foods and given food extracts.

On February 18, 1983, Margaret wrote,

"I feel so much better; it's like I died and went to heaven. I'm still sensitive to chemical fumes and odors so I decided to stay away from church and public places for a while to avoid these reactions."

On March 22, 1983, Margaret reported,

"I'm still improving, although slowly in some ways. My chemical sensitivity is still bad. It seems I find more things in my house each day that bother me. I'm trying to get rid of them but it seems to be an endless task.

"I'm continuing my rotating diet, along with vitamins and primrose oil. My dry skin has improved tremendously and my feelings of depression and uneasiness are also much improved. I'm able to sleep most nights without problems. I'm grateful to you for helping me. Thank you so much."

Like Margaret, many of my patients with yeast-connected health problems develop symptoms when they're exposed to diesel fumes, colognes, perfumes, formaldehyde, insecticides, laundry detergents, polyester clothing and other chemicals. *If you suffer from a yeast-related illness, learn as much as you can about chemicals and how to avoid them.*

Some chemicals are normally present in your body, including sodium chloride (salt), potassium, calcium and magnesium. They're "normal chemicals" and aren't the ones you need to worry about. Instead, pay attention to "foreign chemicals," especially those derived from petroleum and related sources. These include:

Gasoline	Coal burning stoves	Inks
Natural gas	Brass, metal or shoe polish	Carbon paper
Diesel fumes	Floor waxes	Typewriter stencils
Garage fumes	Wax candles	Clothing dyes
Cleaning fluids	Car roofs & roads	Cosmetics
Nail polish	Asphalt pavements	Disinfectants
Formaldehyde	Furniture polishes	Marking pencils

Others include:

Phenol derivatives (carbolic acid or Lysol®), alcohols, defoliants, and household detergents.

Rubber, including sponge rubber, foam rubber pillows, typewriter pads, rubber-base paints, rubber tires, automobile accessories.

Plastics, including plastic upholstery, pillow covers, shoe bags, handbags, plastic folding doors, plastic cement, adhesive tapes.

Synthetic textiles, including dacron, orlon, polyester, rayon, etc.

Paints, varnishes, shellacs, window cleaning fluids, banana oil, ammonia fumes, moth balls, insect repellants, termite exterminating materials, insecticides (chlordane, lindane, parathion).

Chlorinated water, chlorox, bleaches.

Sulfur dioxide, cedar-scented furniture polish, pine odors from knotty pine interiors and pine-scented household deodorants, bath oils, turpentine-containing paints.

In addition, many drugs contain chemicals, including aspirin, tranquilizers, sedatives and antibiotics.

Cosmetics nearly always contain chemicals, including toilet soaps, shampoos, hand lotions, antiseptic preparations, face powders, lipsticks, nail polish, mascara, hair sprays, perfumes, colognes, shaving lotions, hair dressings, scented toilet paper and douches.

Foods may be chemically contaminated in a number of different ways, including coloring added to hot dogs and to the rinds of fruits and vegetables (orange to make citrus fruit look more orange; red coloring to make apples look redder, etc.) Fruit and vegetables may also be waxed, or contaminated by insecticides or by wrappings derived from petrochemical sources.

Finally, tobacco pollutes the environment of many people.

Your level of chemical tolerance: If phosgene, chlorine and other poisonous gases are released, everyone who breathes them will be poisoned. Illness from such chemicals is called "toxicity." By contrast, indoor and outdoor pollution from chemicals including formaldehyde, insecticides, weed killers, diesel fumes and other industrial odors, may make some individuals sick; while others seem to remain well.

Whether or not you'll be made ill by exposure to chemicals appears to depend on several variables, including:

1. Your inherited tendency.
2. The load of chemicals you're exposed to.
3. Your load of other allergy troublemakers (foods, pollens, molds, etc.).
4. The integrity of your immune system (see, also, chapter 24).

Managing chemical sensitivities: If you show symptoms from any chemicals, you're apt to develop sensitivity to other chemicals . . . especially if you're exposed to them in quantity over a prolonged period of time. *So one of the best ways to treat chemical sensitivity is to lighten your chemical load at home and at work.*

Since we're polluting our planet with automobile exhaust, industrial wastes, insecticides, weed killers, perfumes and other chemicals, keeping your chemical load low poses difficult problems. Yet, by learning about chemicals and by planning your life so as to avoid them, you'll increase your chances of remaining well.

Your understanding of chemical sensitivity will be made clearer if you understand the term, "outgassing." This term refers to the volatility of a material . . . its tendency to discharge molecules into the air.

As a rule, hard materials outgas less than soft materials. And natural substances outgas less than synthetics. Marble and stone are the least outgassing substances. And, of the man-made materials, ceramic tile is the least volatile. Soft plastics and polyurethane foam rank among the strongest outgassing substances. Other offenders include smokes, perfumes and sprays.

Here's a list of materials in your home which may cause problems:

Your Bedroom:

Foam rubber pillows or pillows made of other synthetic materials.

Mattresses covered with plastic and other synthetic material. Even cotton mattresses may be treated with fungicides and insecticides.

Sheets made of polyester.

Blankets . . . wool blankets may be treated with chemicals to make them less flammable or to keep moths away.

Pajamas & nightgowns may be made of polyester or other synthetics. (Use, instead, those made of cotton or silk.)

Floors . . . most floors today are covered with carpets which are made of chemicals. Moreover, carpet pads often are made of rubber or other outgassing materials. Some of the glues are even worse. Ideally, floors should be of ceramic tile, hardwood or stone with cotton scatter rugs. (Of the carpets, nylon with jute backing is best.)

Chairs & furniture. Many of these outgas, especially naughahyde, stuffed furniture containing foam rubber padding, or even cotton padding treated with insecticides.

Other chemical contaminants in your bedroom include perfumes and other cosmetics, hair sprays, tobacco smoke, synthetic curtains, floor waxes, television sets (put out an odor of phenol), and clothing.

Living room, family room and other rooms in your house:
Many of these rooms contain the same carpet as your bedroom. They also contain sofas, chairs and other materials that may outgas and cause trouble. Tobacco smoke is a common problem in many homes, either from the occupants or from visitors.

Kitchen:
Your kitchen is often loaded with outgassing substances, including a gas stove, soft vinyl flooring, soaps, detergents, insecticides and cleaning substances. Plastic dishes and Teflon® skillets may cause trouble in highly susceptible individuals.

Bathroom:
Your bathroom is often loaded with chemical odors, including cosmetics, soaps and deodorants. And even the chlorine odor from water causes trouble in some people. Plastic shower curtains may also offend.

Garage & Yard:
Gasoline and especially diesel odors cause problems in many people. This is especially true if the garage is connected to the house, and more especially if the garage has closed doors and lies under the house. Weed killers, bug killers and other chemicals stored in the garage may also cause trouble.

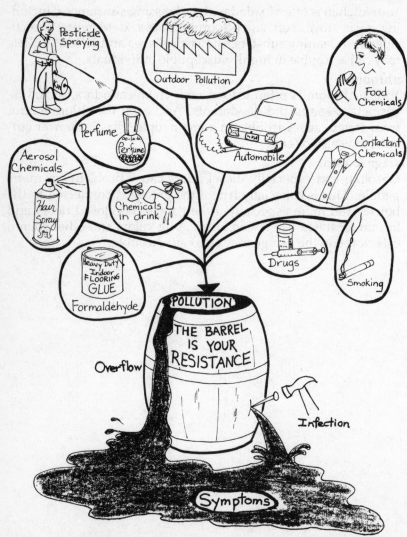

Adapted from William Rea M.D. Used with permission.

22

How Chemicals Make You Sick

You may be able to drive in traffic without experiencing symptoms; and chlorine and other chemicals in your drinking water may not bother you. You may also tolerate laundry detergents, furniture polishes, bathroom chemicals, perfumes and colognes. And you may tolerate foods containing coloring and additives or foods which are wrapped or stored in plastic.

You may also be able to go to a party or attend a conference in a room filled with tobacco smoke.

Yet, if you suffer from an immune system disorder and your health problems are yeast connected, you're apt to be bothered by chemicals. And you may develop burning eyes, stuffy nose, itching, tingling, headache, muscle and joint pains, and all sorts of strange mental and nervous symptoms when you're exposed to outgassing chemicals.

Studies by Dr. William Rea[24] and others[25a-b] show that chemical exposure adversely affects many parts of the immune system. And the more chemicals you're exposed to, the greater the adverse effects.

If you're troubled by allergies and chemical exposures of any type, the "barrel concept" of Dr. Rea may help you understand how chemicals affect you.

Chemicals you're exposed to resemble pipes draining into a rain barrel. The barrel represents your resistance. If heavy chemical exposure continues, the barrel overflows and you develop symptoms. Also, infection often precipitates a "leak in your barrel," even when the barrel isn't full.

If you develop symptoms when exposed to chemicals, reading these books will help you:

Dickey, L: CLINICAL ECOLOGY, Springfield, IL, Charles C. Thomas, 1975.

Golos, N., & Golbitz F., COPING WITH YOUR ALLERGIES (paperback), New York, Simon & Schuster, 1986.

Mackarness, R: CHEMICAL VICTIMS, London, Pan Books, 1980.

Mackarness, R: LIVING SAFELY IN A POLLUTED WORLD, New York, Stein & Day, 1981.

Pfeiffer, Guy O., & Nikel, Casimere, (Edited by) THE HOUSE-HOLD ENVIRONMENT & CHRONIC ILLNESS, Springfield, IL, Charles C. Thomas, 1980.

Randolph, T. G.: HUMAN ECOLOGY AND SUSCEPTIBILITY TO THE CHEMICAL ENVIRONMENT, Springfield, IL, Charles C. Thomas, 1962.

Saifer, P. & Zellerbach, M.: DETOX, New York, Ballantine, 1986.

Small, B & B: SUNNYHILL, Goodwood, Ontario, Canada, Small Associates, 1980.

Zamm, A. V. with Gannon, R.: WHY YOUR HOUSE MAY EN-DANGER YOUR HEALTH, New York, Simon & Schuster, 1980.

These books are available in some stores and from Dickey Enter-prises, 635 Gregory Road, Fort Collins, CO 80524.

23

When Candida Is Treated, Your Chemical Sensitivity Will Often Improve

In September, 1982, 27-year-old Mary Ann wrote:

"My general health has been reasonably good, although I've taken Keflex® and other antibiotics a couple of times a year for sore throat. Also, while on birth control pills several years ago, I was bothered by severe depression and irritability.

"Several months ago, while driving, I developed a strange sensation in my head and blacked out. It was a terrifying experience and I feared for my life. Three weeks later I had a trance-like experience along with a funny taste in my mouth. Soon thereafter, my symptoms went wild. I developed strange sensations in my head off and on all day, with one or two blackouts a day, extreme fever, nausea, difficulty in breathing, sinus problems, heart irregularities and emotional instability. My headaches were severe.

"I consulted a neurologist who hospitalized me for a complete workup, including CAT scans and brain wave tests which were said to be 'just slightly irregular'. And because of questionable findings on the CAT scan, an arteriogram was carried out.

"Meanwhile, I had been put on Dilantin®. When the arteriogram showed no problem in my brain, my medicine was changed to phenobarbital.

"I was exhausted all the time and I felt awful trying to run a business and carry on as a wife and mother. My headaches persisted and I was so dopey I couldn't function well at all. My doctor and his nurse seemed to feel I was 'making much out of nothing' and wouldn't return my calls. So I found another doctor. By the way, the first doctor diagnosed me as epileptic and would not let me drive.

"The new neurologist said he couldn't fit me neatly into any category, such as epilepsy or brain tumor and that it was perhaps just 'nerves'. But to make sure, he would do another CAT scan, EEG, EKG and lumbar puncture. However, he told me to slowly wean myself off the phenobarbital which is where I am now. Yet my symptoms are recurring.

"Then last week I remembered developing an extreme reaction . . . dizziness, headaches, coughing . . . when we had cabinets built in the shop I was remodeling. This happened last March. The cabinets were built of pressed wood (containing formaldehyde) and I sat beside them daily. Also, I personalized gifts all day using enamel paints, paint thinners and turpentine. Moreover, the building I work in is poorly ventilated because my electric heat and air conditioning do not draw in outside air. The building is also very old and the back rooms are dusty. I also receive merchandise packed in straw which has been treated with formaldehyde.

"After reading recently about chemical sensitivity, I'm relieved to think that this might be my problem. Yet I'm desperate for help."

Because Mary Ann lived in another state and found it impossible to come to my office for a visit, after reviewing her history and because of her chemical sensitivity, I sent her personal physician information about yeast-connected illness. I suggested a therapeutic trial of nystatin, diet and nutritional supplements and changes in Mary Ann's work place so as to lessen chemical exposures. Six months later, in March, 1983, Mary Ann came in with the following report:

"I've improved to some degree, even though my physician decided not to prescribe nystatin. Yet, I'm still sensitive to many chemicals I come in contact with in the car and elsewhere."

After re-reviewing Mary Ann's history, I prescribed a therapeutic trial of nystatin, diet and nutritional supplements.

In a follow-up report in July, 1983, Mary Ann wrote:

"My improvement has been amazing . . . more than I expected. I've been on all-day car trips with no problems. The greatest thing that has happened is the nervousness, grouchiness and irritability that I thought was 'just me' has gone. The first two weeks on nystatin were terrible, but then I began to improve amazingly. My 4-year-old daughter recently commented, 'Mommie, you don't fuss like you used to'.

"For a while I wasn't able to cheat on my diet without experiencing depression, but now I can eat anything although I still adhere to the diet most of the time.

"My monthly period is no longer a time I consider commiting myself to a mental hospital. I feel great even then . . . and I certainly wasn't expecting this.

"I've never had so many compliments on how good I look . . . it all shows doesn't it? My husband lost 14 pounds on the diet and he feels beautiful, too.

"I have to admit now that I was very skeptical when I first came looking for help. Now I'm a real believer and it's such a wonderful relief to know I'm not just naturally an old grouch.

"I know now my problems began when I started taking birth control

154

pills 13 years ago which contributed to my nervous breakdown. It's truly an answer to my prayers to find relief for so many of my physical and mental problems."

John Smith, M.D. (name changed), a 40-year-old physician lived in the suburbs of a large city. John was bothered by many health problems, including severe chemical sensitivity. In searching for help he underwent many different tests and therapies, including hospitalization in an environmental unit. Yet, his chemical sensitivity continued.

Dr. Smith commented,

"I had to live like a hermit. I moved to a rural area, ate organically grown foods, drank spring water and avoided all petrochemicals and synthetic products, including those found in clothing and housing. Any break in my routine triggered symptoms.

"Then two years ago, I learned of the work of Dr. Truss and began taking nystatin and a low carbohydrate diet, plus nutritional supplements including garlic. Gradually my immune system improved and my chemical sensitivity lessened. More recently I've found that other anticandida therapies have helped, including inhaling amphotericin B powder and using the herb tea from the South American LaPacho tree.

"Although it's been a long struggle, I'm excited to report that I'm able to travel, eat in restaurants and I no longer have to follow my diet as closely as I once did. I've been able to rejoin the human race! Anticandida therapy has certainly played a major role in helping me and my immune system recover from severe chemical sensitivity."

The stories of Mary Ann and John clearly illustrate a number of important points that I've talked about in various parts of this book, including:

1. Each person with yeast-connected illness differs from every other person. Yet, common threads run through the histories of many patients.

2. Birth control pills (while tolerated by many women) have triggered severe and complex illnesses in many of my patients.

3. Antibiotics, especially "broad spectrum" drugs (while they save lives and relieve suffering) are a "two-edged sword." By encouraging yeast growth, their use often leads to other chronic health problems.

4. When the immune system is adversely affected, symptoms involving every part of the body often develop. The endocrine, digestive and nervous systems are especially affected.

5. Intolerance to environmental chemicals is found in many pa-

tients with yeast-connected illness. Such chemical sensitivity usually lessens following anticandida therapy.

6. Although such therapy increases a person's tolerance for chemicals, reducing the chemical load remains a sound part of therapy.

7. Nystatin and diet rank at the top of the list of treatment measures used in helping individuals with yeast-connected health disorders. However, in my experience, other measures are important in strengthening the immune system and speeding recovery. Included especially are vitamins, minerals, garlic, linseed and primrose oils and sugar-free yogurt. For a more comprehensive discussion, see Section D.

8. Still other patients are helped by additional therapies, many of which are discussed in Sections E and F of this book.

24

About Your Immune System And How It Protects You[†]

All around you are harmful substances that can "do you in" . . . bacteria, viruses and chemicals.

Yet, you survive. Here's why: You possess "the most stunning, effective protection the world has ever seen . . . your immune system." Like the army, navy, marines and air force, your immune system is composed of a number of defenders with different capabilities.

These defenders hold harmful organisms in check and retard their growth. Occasionally, they even kill a few. *However, in the end, it is your body itself which must destroy the harmful organisms.* Your body must clean up the battlefield, seek out and destroy each germ. No matter where these germs hide, it is your body that must do the killing. Among your body's defenders are several types of white blood cells. And one group of these cells (called *granulocytes*) chase germs and gobble them up.

If you put these white blood cells in a small dish of salt water, they'll move around randomly in a tranquil manner. Yet, all you have to do is add one bacterium to the dish . . . just one . . . and the whole scene changes. The granulocytes, like a cat stalking its prey, creep relentlessly toward the bacterium. Then they attack. Later, they back off and let a different army of germ-fighting cells called *macrophages* take over.

Under the microscope you can see these different white blood

[†]Excerpted and adapted from *The Body is the Hero* by Ronald T. Glasser, M.D., Random House, 1976.

cells *fighting for your life.* You can actually see them grab bacteria and hold them while they empty their granules on them; you can see the microbes twist and turn and finally break apart.

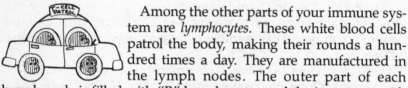

The second part of your immune system . . . your *antibodies* . . . are special proteins circulating in your blood stream. A protein, as you may know, is made of linked-together *amino acids.* And they can be made to fit around almost any "foreign" structure. In so doing, they help you conquer your enemies.

How do the antibodies work? They clump microbes together and slow them down a bit, making it easier for granulocytes to eat them. They also unlock a series of physical events which lead to the microbes' death.

In addition to white blood cells and antibodies, the third and perhaps the most important part of your immune system is a group of nine separate proteins made in the liver called *"complement."* When activated, these complement components unite and help destroy the bacteria.

Among the other parts of your immune system are *lymphocytes.* These white blood cells patrol the body, making their rounds a hundred times a day. They are manufactured in the lymph nodes. The outer part of each lymph node is filled with "B" lymphocytes and the inner part with "T" cells or "T" lymphocytes. *These lymphocytes comprise the master mind of your immune system.* They'll attack bacteria, even ones you don't have antibodies against.

All parts of your immune system are needed to keep you healthy. In his book, *The Body is the Hero,* (see Reading List, chapter 47, Update) Dr. Ronald J. Glasser commented,

> *"To cure a disease, not just to treat it, you must help the body to do it itself.* It is the body that is the hero, not science, not antibodies, not machines or new devices. It is the body making antibodies against the swallowed polio vaccine, not the iron lung, that cures polio. It is the body, not radiation or drugs, that must destroy cancer cells if the patient is to survive."

There is growing evidence that if you're troubled with allergies, chemical sensitivity, chronic and recurring infection, including candida, with symptoms which involve just about any and every part of your body, it is your body which must be strengthened. And for your body to resist the harmful substances around it which are making you ill, your body's immune system must be on the job and functioning well.

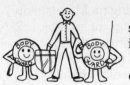

Many different factors play a role in strengthening (or weakening) your body's immune system. These include:

1. The presence of excessive numbers of candida organisms in your intestinal tract and other parts of the body. And large numbers of candida organisms appear to put out a toxin which weaken your immune system.

2. Molds in your environment.

3. Chemicals you eat, breathe and touch.

4. Your nutritional status. A diet loaded with *sugar* interferes with the function of your granulocytes[6]. Similarly, a diet loaded with hardened fat, white flour, sugar, and other processed food lacks many essential nutrients your body needs to function properly.

These nutrients include essential amino acids (from proteins), complex carbohydrates (found in vegetables, fruits and whole grains), essential fatty acids (found in unprocessed vegetable oil), and a variety of vitamins and minerals.

Moreover, as pointed out by Roger Williams,[26] Ph.D. of the University of Texas, and Sidney Baker, M.D.[27a-b], head of the Gesell Institute in New Haven, Connecticut, *each person is biochemically unique.* And some individuals require much more of a particular vitamin . . . such as vitamin C or vitamin B-6 . . . than do others.

Minerals are still another story. And according to the late Henry Schroeder, M.D., Ph.D.[28] of Dartmouth College, *your mineral needs are even more important than your vitamin needs, since your body cannot make minerals.* You not only need the minerals found in large quantities in your body (such as magnesium and calcium), you also need many *trace minerals* including zinc, chromium and selenium.

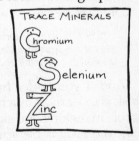

These trace minerals are essential for taste, appetite, growth and for the proper functioning of your immune system and for many of the other metabolic and biochemical processes which keep your body strong and disease-free.

Studies by Pauling[29] and others indicate that vitamin C strengthens the immune system. Other studies show similar results. For example, in 1980, Anah and associates[30] told of a double-blind study on 41 Nigerian asthmatics who had noted increased asthmatic symptoms during the rainy season (suggesting mold sensitivity).

Twenty-two individuals were given 1000 mgs. of ascorbic acid (vitamin C) daily, while 19 other patients were treated with a placebo (dummy pill) for the 14-week duration of the rainy season. The group of patients who received no supplemental vitamin C experienced 35 asthmatic attacks, while the vitamin C group suffered only 9 such attacks. Subsequently, vitamin C was withheld from the individuals in group A and "the asthma attack rate increased remarkably."

Psychological factors are important. The late Dr. William Osler of Johns Hopkins pointed out that people who develop severe tuberculosis are often unhappy people. More recently, experiments in biofeedback show that you can speed up your heart or slow it down, or even regulate your blood pressure. And psychological factors may determine whether or not a person recovers from cancer.

A fascinating story about the role of psychological factors in curing a severe chronic illness can be found in Norman Cousins' book *Anatomy of an Illness*[31]. Cousins, a former editor of the *Saturday Review of Literature*, developed a severe, crippling and supposedly incurable illness. Yet he got well. And he attributed his recovery to large doses of vitamin C, plus measures designed to make him laugh, along with a positive attitude and an intense desire to get well.

In his book, *The Body is the Hero*, Dr. Glasser commented,

> "The idea that an individual can control his immune system doesn't seem so far fetched anymore." And he suggested that we could use our minds to "will our white cells into a more efficient attack against infection."

Dr. Glasser continued,

> "The task of the physician today is what it has always been, to help the body do what it has learned so well to do on its own during the unending struggle for survival . . . to heal itself."

And if you suffer from yeast-connected health problems, your task is to learn as much as you can about the many things that play a role in making you sick, and do your best to cope with them. *After all, your body is the hero, and your body will recover if you'll give it a chance.*

25

Labeling Diseases Isn't The Way We Should Go†

In a paper some 10 years ago, E. Cheraskin, M.D., D.M.D.[22], then Chairman of the Department of Oral Medicine at the University of Alabama, said in effect,

> "We physicians are taught to diagnose, classify and label 'diseases'. And most of us feel if we can put a diagnostic label on each patient who comes to us, we've done our duty. Then we feel we can relax because our task becomes easy. All we have to do then is to go to our procedure book, medical library, Physicians Desk Reference® or computer and find the recommended treatment. Then we prescribe drugs, surgery or psychotherapy."

Cheraskin emphasized,

> "There's a better way."

And in his numerous publications, including his book, *Predictive Medicine*[23], he pointed out that many disabling health disorders could be prevented by recognizing early signs and symptoms and helping patients make appropriate changes in their life styles and, more especially, in their diets.

In his book, *The Missing Diagnosis*[5], Dr. Orian Truss commented,

> "I would like to call attention once again to the pitfall inherent in dividing human illness into 'diseases'. The organs and systems of the body are so integrated, with each playing its specialized role in the maintenance of good health and efficient function, that to speak of disease of an individual organ is to suggest an autonomy that is undeserved. If one organ malfunctions, it is likely that there will be repercussions in most other systems."

---

†Illustrations adapted from Sidney Baker, M.D., and used with permission.

And recently Dr. Sidney Baker commented, saying in effect,

> "Labeling diseases isn't the way we should go. And in working with people with the yeast problem, we need to take a new look at illness in terms of the differences between people. This is the important thing, rather than using so much of our time and energy trying to put labels on diseases, whether it be psoriasis, multiple sclerosis or Crohn's disease."

I agree. Although labeling disorders such as migraine, ulcerative colitis, asthma, the attention-deficit disorder, multiple sclerosis, or systemic lupus erythematosus serves a useful purpose, new scientific data suggest that many of these diseases are interrelated and result from environmental, nutritional, biochemical and other influences that affect the immune system. By recognizing these causes, and taking steps to alter them, physicians may be able to help many of their patients without resorting to hospitalization, surgery or drugs.

As physicians, we're taught to label diseases and divide them into separate and seemingly unrelated compartments. Some diseases are considered to be "mental" and to have mainly psychological causes, while others are categorized as being "physical."

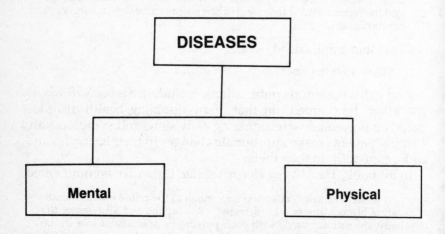

The mental diseases are usually divided into the following categories:
1. *Psychotic* ("crazy", disoriented, out of touch, paranoid). Treatment of such patients often includes custodial care.
2. *Neurotic & nervous*, ("can't cope," hypochondriacal).

Psychological explanations are usually furnished (rejection, inadequate personality, sexual or religious worries, etc.).
3. *Childhood disorders.* Applied to those whose symptoms began early in life.
4. *Organic.* Caused by infection, trauma, poisoning or hardening of the arteries.

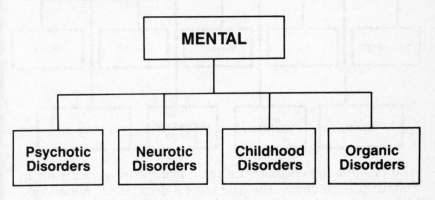

The physical diseases are also split up. Some are handled by medical doctors and others by surgeons.

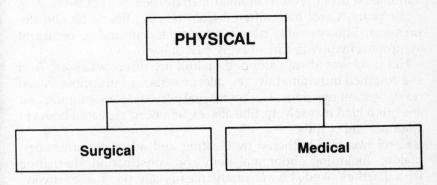

Then they are subdivided into organs or systems.

If you suffer from yeast-connected illness, you'll usually show symptoms involving your brain, your gastrointestinal tract and your reproductive organs. Yet you may also be bothered by symptoms in your bones and joints, your skin, your respiratory tract, urinary tract or other parts of your body.

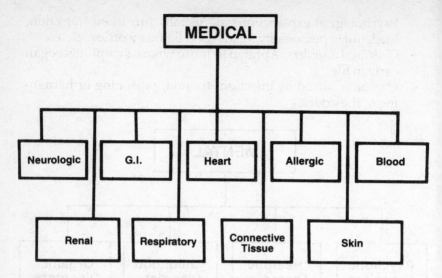

```
                    ┌─────────────┐
                    │   MEDICAL   │
                    └─────────────┘
```

MEDICAL

Neurologic · G.I. · Heart · Allergic · Blood

Renal · Respiratory · Connective Tissue · Skin

I'd like to acknowledge once again that the advances made by medical science during the past several decades are remarkable. Moreover, suffering is often relieved and health care costs are lessened by appropriate diagnostic and treatment procedures carried out by contemporary specialists and subspecialists. But there is "another side of the coin" as illustrated by the story of Carol.

For years, Carol had suffered from fatigue, headache and depression. She was also troubled by persistent and/or recurrent symptoms involving almost every part of her body.

Her nose was always stopped up and her throat was sore. And she coughed intermittently. Yet, allergy tests for inhalants showed no significant reactions. Her menstrual periods were irregular and she often bled excessively. She also experienced repeated bouts of vaginitis and cystitis.

Carol was also bothered by bloating and other digestive complaints, including abdominal pain and constipation alternating with diarrhea. And she was rarely free of scaly skin rashes involving her hands and feet.

In talking about her health problems, Carol commented:

> "During the past ten years my medical and hospital expenses have been more than $100,000. I've consulted internists, neurologists, dermatologists and psychiatrists. Every orifice of my body has been looked into and x-rays of every type have been made. My tonsils, uterus and one ovary have been removed and my bladder outlet has been dilated repeatedly."

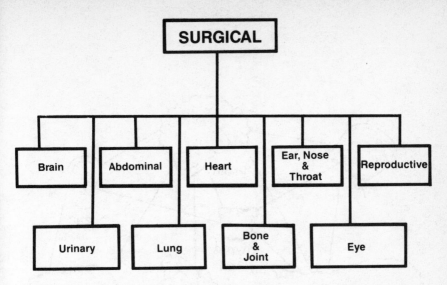

I first saw Carol early in 1982 and on the Candida Questionnaire (see chapter 6), she scored over 300.

On a program of diet and nystatin (with intermittent courses of Nizoral®), vitamins, minerals, linseed oil, garlic, yogurt, exercise and immunotherapy with yeast and mold extracts, Carol improved remarkably. Love and understanding from her family and a lay-support group also helped.

In January 1984, Carol commented:

> "I've improved in every way and many of my symptoms have disappeared. However, on damp, muggy days I don't feel as 'with it' as I do on clear, crisp days. Tobacco smoke and perfume still stuff up my nose and give me a headache. Also, if I really cheat on my diet, I pay for it. But compared to the way I felt and looked two years ago, I'm a 'new woman'."

Patients like Carol are being helped by a small but growing number of physicians all over the country. And as I pointed out in the Preface, "I sincerely feel that recognition and appropriate management of yeast-connected illness . . . will help physicians and their co-workers relieve much unnecessary suffering (and) . . . save patients, the government, business and industry (including the health insurance industry) billions of dollars."

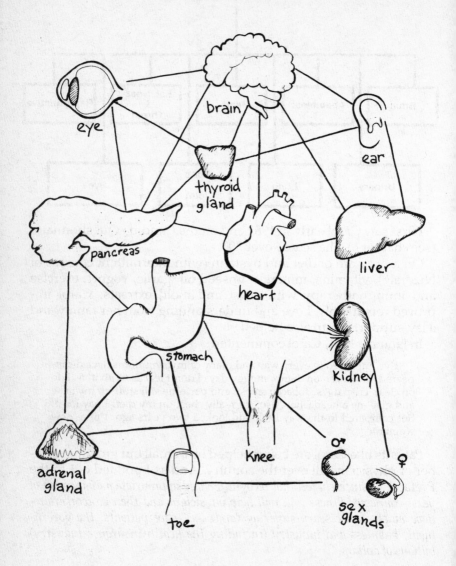

eye

brain

ear

thyroid
gland

pancreas

heart

liver

stomach

kidney

adrenal
gland

Knee

♂

♀

toe

sex
glands

26

Every Part Of Your Body Is Connected To Every Other Part

Obviously (although we often forget it), every part of your body is connected to every other part. Moreover, this interrelationship was clearly pointed out in the old spiritual song "Dry Bones" which went something like this. "Your foot bone is connected to your ankle bone and your ankle bone is connected to your knee bone" . . . and so on.

In my practice every day, I see many examples of these interrelationships. Here are two of them:

1. John, a 55-year-old business man, had been troubled with bloating and digestive problems for many years. He also was bothered by headache, buzzing in his ears and persistent athlete's foot. On the anticandida treatment program, his symptoms subsided rapidly. Interestingly enough, John did not come to me as a patient originally; he only came along to give his wife emotional support. Then when he saw his wife improving, he said, "Can I go on the program, too?" He did, and he improved even more than his wife.

2. Louise, a 29-year-old school teacher was bothered by recurrent episodes of rhinitis and wheezing. Her problems were severe enough to require hospitalization. She also was troubled with premenstrual tension, fatigue, depression and menstrual irregularity. Her respiratory symptoms persisted even though she took allergy extracts for several years. Helping Louise hasn't been easy. Yet, after following a compre-

hensive program of management for a year, many of her health problems have improved.

Among the more important and recently recognized connections are those between the *immune system,* the *endocrine system* and the *brain. And since candida toxins affect each of these systems and one system affects the other, the yeast connection can cause all sorts of symptoms.*

Here are examples:

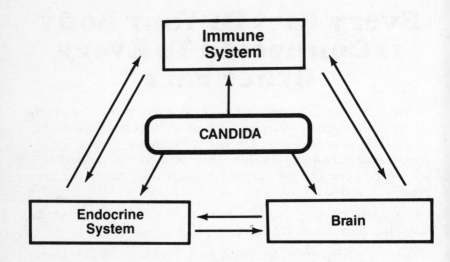

1. 33-year-old Barbara commented,

   "Candida-related health problems made me tired, gave me headaches, irritability, menstrual problems and cystitis. And after the birth of my last baby, I lost all sexual feeling. Now, following three months of treatment with nystatin, diet, vitamins and minerals, it's just like it used to be. My husband and I are both grateful."

2. One of my patients, 27-year-old Anne commented,

   "My nervous system wasn't working right. I was clumsy, uncoordinated and spaced out. My memory was terrible . . . worse than my 80-year-old grandmother's. At times my hands would be numb and would tingle. Following treatment, I feel better all over and my nervous system symptoms have disappeared."

3. Eleanor, a 25-year-old patient with headache, fatigue, constipation and recurrent vaginitis improved on diet and nystatin.

However, she continued to be bothered by morning fatigue. And, at times, she would complain of feeling chilly. Thyroid and other tests were normal. However, her underarm thermometer reading in the mornings was usually 96° to 97°. Following thyroid supplementation, she improved more rapidly.

4. A gynecologist commented,

"I've seen several hundred young women with symptoms related to hormone dysfunction. These same patients were also experiencing candida-related health problems. I've noted that by treating their yeast problems, premenstrual tension, menstrual cramps and other problems related to hormonal dysfunction improve . . . often dramatically."

Section
D

Manifestations
of
yeast-connected
illness

Premenstrual
Syndrome

Vaginal
Problems

Menstrual
Difficulties

Small
Breasts

Skin
Problems

Painful
Intercourse

Pelvic
Pain

Headache

Fatigue

Depression

Irritability

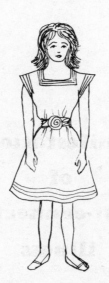

Infertility

27

Health Problems Of Women

Health problems of women are often yeast-connected. A young woman (I'll call her Sherry) went to her physician complaining of fatigue, menstrual irregularities and severe migraine headaches. Sherry was also worried about her poor breast development and remarked,

> "I dread going to the beach and putting on a bathing suit."

Following treatment with diet and nystatin, Sherry's headaches, fatigue, constipation, premenstrual tension and abdominal pain improved. And her breasts enlarged significantly.

Recently, John Curlin, M.D., a Jackson, Tennessee gynecologist who has developed an interest in yeast-connected health problems commented,

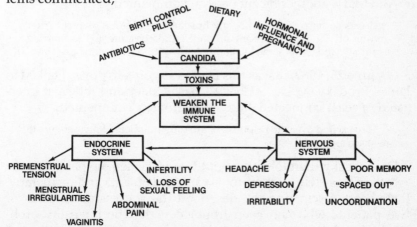

"Since entering practice, I've seen thousands of patients with symptoms related to hormone dysfunction. Their complaints have included pelvic pain, menstrual irregularities, PMS (premenstrual syndrome), infertility, nausea and vomiting of pregnancy, endometriosis, vaginitis, painful intercourse and absence of normal sexual interest and responsiveness.

"Three years ago I learned of the observations of Joseph Miller[42] and Richard Mabray[43] who noted that women who experienced painful menstruation, premenstrual syndrome and other symptoms of hormone dysfunction often responded to tiny doses of progesterone. I began to use this method of therapy in patients in my own practice and found that many of them improved, often dramatically.

"Then two years ago I learned about yeast-related illness and began to use diet, nystatin and candida extracts in treating these patients. Although this program doesn't relieve all of the symptoms caused by hormone dysfunction, the response in most of my patients has been gratifying. In addition to the 'typical' gynecological problems that have responded, many patients with other health problems, including arthritis, colitis and other auto-immune disorders, have also improved."

Even though I was trained as a pediatrician, most of my new patients are adults . . . especially young women burdened with dozens of complaints involving especially their reproductive organs and nervous system. The response in many of these patients have been phenomenal . . . and exciting. Some of them give a history of marital discord and many have been divorced. A recent patient (I'll call her Laura) commented,

"I was sexually unresponsive, depressed and irritable. I acted like a real bitch. No wonder my marriage failed."

And Mary, another recent patient, commented,

"I was so hard to live with, my husband and I got a divorce. After getting off the pill and receiving anticandida treatment, I'm married again . . . and to the same husband. And we're getting along just fine."

On June 25, 1983, just as this book was going to press, I talked to James Brodsky, M.D., a Chevy Chase, Maryland internist interested in yeast-connected illness. Dr. Brodsky commented,

"I'm excited over the response of growing numbers of my patients to nystatin and diet."

Dr. Brodsky then told me about two of his female patients with "restless legs" whose symptoms vanished on anticandida therapy. Even more fascinating, he described the successful outcome of two patients who had been troubled with "the infertility problem." One patient had been trying to conceive for 7 months and the other for over 10 months. On diet and nystatin, one woman became pregnant in 30 days and the other in 60 days.[†]

I don't claim that an anticandida treatment program will increase the brassiere size, banish infertility, cut the divorce rate in half or cure all the health problems of young women. Yet, it can work wonders in helping many women . . . and their spouses, too. What's more, women of all ages with chronic health disorders respond. Here are more detailed reports on some of my female patients:

I first saw Sara in 1951, a few hours after she was born. During the ensuing years, she came to see me dozens of times for routine checkups and for the treatment of colds and ear infections. During the 50's, she received many antibiotic drugs, including the tetracyclines. When Sara was 7 or 8, she began to sneeze and cough when she picked up a cat. About the same time, her mother commented,

> "When Sara drinks chocolate milk she feels tired and develops dark circles under her eyes. On one occasion, she wheezed after playing in a wheat field."

Through her early and mid-teen years, Sara enjoyed reasonably good health. Yet she often complained of feeling tired. She came in for a checkup at the age of 16 with the complaint of "falling asleep in study hall." She also was bothered by menstrual cramps, premenstrual tension and occasional episodes of vaginal yeast infection.

I didn't see Sara again as a patient until she was 27 when she came back to me saying,

> I'm wondering if my allergies have anything to do with my health problems."

In going over her history, I found that she had continued to experience extreme fatigue accompanied by many other nervous symptoms.

Sara commented,

> "I fall asleep anywhere and if I don't eat at frequent intervals I become weak. I'm also bothered by mood swings, frequent frontal head-

---

[†]In September, 1983, a 34-year-old patient from Memphis came to see me with an infertility problem. She and her husband had been trying to have a baby for six years. Four weeks after starting diet and nystatin, she became pregnant. And an 8 lb., 9 oz. healthy son was born on July 8, 1984!

aches and severe menstrual cramps. And during the past 6 to 8 years, I've been treated repeatedly for vaginal yeast infections and cystitis."

Her records forwarded to me by her internist included two glucose tolerance tests. Both revealed elevations of her blood sugar level one-half hour after glucose was administered. On one occasion it went to 212 and on another it went to 221. Sugar also appeared in her urine. Then at the third and fourth hours, her blood sugar dropped rapidly; on one occasion it went to 41.

In talking further to Sara she said,

> "I feel dizzy on getting up and at times I feel 'real spaced out' like I'm not on this planet. My memory has been poor during recent years and at times I can't remember the names of people I know well. I feel uncoordinated, I stumble and drop things. My arms and legs ache."

Because of the complexity of her problems, I referred Sara to an endocrinologist for further study and treatment. She was hospitalized and, after a comprehensive work-up, her physician recorded this diagnosis in her chart: "Reactive hypoglycemia, symptomatic, with associated narcolepsy." Her treatment program included a high protein diet, supplemental vitamins, avoidance of food allergens, including wheat, chocolate and milk.

On this program, Sara improved; yet she continued to be troubled by severe vaginal yeast infections and bouts of fatigue and lethargy.

She came to see me again in the summer of 1980, saying,

> "I wonder if I need further allergy testing."

As I reviewed her history, I said,

"Sara, since you last came to see me, I've learned of the work of Dr. Orian Truss of Birmingham who feels that *Candida albicans*, the common yeast germ which causes vaginitis, plays an important role in causing health problems similar to those you've experienced over the years."

I prescribed nystatin, a yeast free diet and nutritional supplements. Although Sara has experienced a few ups and downs, she has improved remarkably. When I last saw her in January, 1983, she said,

> "I feel great. No headaches, no spaced out feelings, lots of energy, only occasional mild premenstrual cramps. Life is full and exciting."

Was candida "the cause" of Sara's multiple and complex health problems? No. Many other factors were involved, including food and inhalant allergies, hormonal dysfunction and metabolic problems. But based on her response to anticandida treatment, plus my experiences in hundreds of other patients . . . especially young women . . . I feel Sara's illnesses were due to a weakened immune system and that the anticandida treatment program has played a major role in enabling her to regain her health.

Now I'd like to tell about Cindy who was born in 1963. Although I saw Cindy on one or two occasions during infancy and childhood, she was usually seen by one of my pediatric associates. Over the years, Cindy (like other members of her family), was troubled by allergies of all sorts, including rhinitis, otitis and bronchitis. However, Cindy's main complaints were more widespread. When she was 10, her physician commented,

> "Cindy complains of headaches, abdominal pain . . . she aches everywhere!"

Cindy came in for a checkup at the age of 14 with the complaint of "not feeling well for a long time." Her symptoms included shortness of breath, substernal discomfort, headache, nervousness and anxiety. Although her mother had noted that milk and corn contributed to her symptoms, she never felt well. Treatment of spring and fall hayfever with allergy extracts and medication helped a little; yet she continued to experience multiple symptoms.

At the age of 15, Cindy came to me as an allergy patient. Her mother commented,

> "Cindy has been through the mill. She's been seen by numerous doctors and although some of her treatments have helped, she never really feels good."

On a program of allergy testing and treatment with food and inhalant extracts, Cindy improved. Yet she continued to be a difficult and complex patient who experienced all sorts of ups and downs.

In an effort to obtain help, she consulted many other physicians, including gynecologists and urologists. She was hospitalized for study on several occasions. Because of severe menstrual cramps, she was placed on birth control pills and antibiotic drugs were prescribed for her bladder and respiratory infections.

In July 1982, after an absence of three years, Cindy (age 19) came in with many of her same complaints. These included severe premenstrual tension, menstrual cramps and recurrent bladder infections (she had been treated with Keflex®), recurrent vaginitis and abdominal pain. I commented,

"Cindy, I've learned a lot since I last saw you. And I feel most of your problems are yeast related. Let's start over again and see if we can help you get well."

I sent Cindy to a gynecologist (who was interested in yeast-connected health problems) for a checkup. He prescribed a diet and nystatin. Cindy returned to my office in May 1983 and commented,

"I feel much better. Although I'm occasionally bothered by burning on urination, muscle aching and headache, I feel better than I've felt in years. Nystatin and diet have enabled me to conquer my unbearable menstrual cramps, fatigue and many of the other problems which had plagued me. Avoiding milk, corn, chocolate and other troublemaking foods helps. So do my allergy vaccines and nutritional supplements. *But the most important factor in helping me really feel better and look forward to college is my treatment with nystatin and diet."*

Here's the story of a patient whose health problems began over 25 years before I saw her on May 24, 1983. Margie was born in 1940 and came in complaining of recurrent vaginitis, abdominal pain, asthma and severe sensitivity to chemical fumes and tobacco. Other symptoms included sugar craving, headache, itching, muscle aches, numbness, tingling, depression, poor memory and fatigue. Here are excerpts from the letter she wrote me:

"As a child I was sick all the time with a runny nose and cough. I had pneumonia several times. During my teen years, I moved to another state for six years and my health improved. Then when I moved back home, I again began coughing and had further bouts of pneumonia. After I went to work in a flower shop, I started having asthma attacks. My doctor sent me to an allergist who ran tests. I took shots and quit smoking and I got better.

"Then after taking birth control pills for five years, I started having vaginitis. I stopped the pill and my vaginitis cleared. But then I began having asthma at work from colognes, perfumes, soaps and cleaning products. I improved a little after being retested and started on shots for dust, pollens and tobacco. And my lungs were better until I painted the inside of my house. Finally, I had to quit work because I was sensitive to the perfumes the people I worked with were wearing.

"At some point, because of vaginitis, abdominal pain and persistent menstrual difficulties, I had a hysterectomy and bladder repair. Before surgery, I had so many bladder problems I was given all sorts of drugs including Terramycin®, Keflex® and Ceclor®.

"After taking these drugs, my vaginitis came back and has been one of my worst problems during the past three years. In August of last year, I had pneumonia which developed after I polished my floors using an odorous floor wax. I was treated with Keflex®, Erythromycin® and cortisone.

"My home doctor saw me in April of this year and said, 'I think yeast allergies are a big part of your problem.' So he put me on a yeast-free diet, nystatin, and sent me to see you. The nystatin caused 'die-off' reactions and my vaginitis is driving me crazy. So here I am."

Just as this book went to press, Margie wrote me and said,

"I've been on treatment for a month. I'm somewhat better. I'm really sticking to my diet for the first time. I can now tolerate the nystatin and it's helping. So are digestive enzymes and linseed oil. The congestion in my head and lungs is definitely better, but my vaginitis continues. But now that I know why I've been sick so much and so long, I believe I can get well."

Here's the story of a more recent patient, Linda, who came in with severe premenstrual syndrome (PMS). This young woman first came to see me on May 3, 1983 on referral from psychologist Cheryl Robley, Ph.D.:

Linda complained of anxiety, fatigue and many other mental and nervous system symptoms. Here are excerpts from her medical history written in her own words:

"I've been married for 12 years, have two sons . . . ages 7 and 3 . . . and a very loving, understanding husband. I've been a happy person who never complained. I've loved my role as a wife, housewife and mother. Like everyone else, I'd occasionally be upset or moody, but this was never a real problem. Gradually, over the past few years, my moodiness increased to a point where, within minutes, it could change either way, from depression to anxiety and then back again. I could feel it coming on, but I had no control over it. *I found that mood swings were especially severe during the five or six days before my monthly period.*

"Increasingly, I began to have 'attacks' where I would get so upset I would clinch my fists, grit my teeth, wring my hands and tense every muscle in my body. I'd feel like screaming. I wouldn't be able to sit down or lie down. I would usually end up getting in the car and driving until I calmed down. I would feel as though I'm MAD. During these times I would feel completely irrational; I could not calm down or talk to anyone. Thoughts would race through my mind and become exaggerated.

"Even when I wasn't having attacks, I found I could not cope without getting upset with any situation, such as a washer or dryer going out or my husband forgetting to call me and tell me he'd be late in coming home after work.

"I resented my duties as a housewife, cleaning, washing, cooking, going shopping. At times, I didn't even want to get up off the couch and tuck my two children in bed . . . that's awful!

"Until the birth of my second son, the only symptoms I can remember were severe tension headaches and pains in my left shoulder blade and shoulder joint which developed after I sat at the telephone and typewriter for hours at a time. After my son was born in 1979, I developed bladder infections and had to take a lot of antibiotics. Soon afterward, I began to notice nausea, stomachache and occasional diarrhea.

"In the last few years, insomnia has taken over. I don't fight the bed, I just lie awake . . . sometimes for 3 hours or more. I cry at anything. I've gotten to the point of not feeling loved . . . not trusting my husband, not feeling secure. My self-confidence has begun to diminish.

"The episode that sent me to Dr. Robley was provoked by my husband not calling me to say he'd play cards one evening. He didn't come home until late. By that time, I was a 'raving maniac.' (*This was four days before my period was due to start.*) I tried to talk to him but ended up screaming insults. When I got no response, I started hitting him. It scared me so bad that I got in my car at 1 AM and drove around until 3 AM. I prayed out loud that God would give me an answer. I was tired of battling this thing. Finally, I called my gynecologist who referred me to the psychologist who sent me to see you.

"I'm tired of feeling this way, I want to feel happy again and be able to cope day to day . . . enjoy life, my husband and my two boys.

"During the many years of our marriage, my husband and I have been through many emotional stresses, including job changes, financial problems and all sorts of other things. Yet I was able to cope until the last several years."

I put Linda on "the anticandida program," including a yeast-free diet and nystatin. At a recheck visit on May 24, 1983, Linda said,

"I'm better. However, the acid test will be this week, since my period is due to start in 7 days."

Linda came back again on June 20, 1983.

"I'm much better! For the first time in three years, my premenstrual period wasn't hell. I got through it without any blowups. Although I still have a little vaginal discharge and some of my old emotional symptoms pop up occasionally, I can deal with them."

A Special Word About PMS†
(Premenstrual Syndrome)

In a comprehensive article in the June 1983 issue of *Hospital Practice*, Doctors Robert M. Rose and Judith M. Abplanalp of the University of Texas Medical Branch at Galveston commented,

"This syndrome has become a popular scape-goat for behavioral aberrations ranging from malaise to murder . . . Largely as a consequence of media attention (it has changed) over the past few years from a relatively obscure clinical entity to a household word."

---

†For a further discussion of PMS, including a report on scientific studies, see Chapter 42, Update.

What is PMS? It is a group of physical and psychological symptoms which occur or are accentuated during the week or so preceding menstruation, and are relieved when the period starts. Physical complaints often include painful or swollen breasts, bloating, abdominal pain, headache and backache. Even more striking are the mental and nervous system symptoms, including especially depression, anxiety, irritability and behavioral changes.

What causes PMS and how should it be treated? It depends on who you ask. British gynecologist Katharina Dalton feels that women with PMS suffer from a relative deficiency of progesterone during the week before menstruation. She has found that relief can often be obtained through the use of progesterone vaginal suppositories.

Other physicians studying and treating PMS have emphasized the role of emotional factors; still others feel deficiencies of vitamins A and B-6, magnesium and other nutrients are at fault. Other viewpoints include prostaglandin excess, progesterone allergy and immune and endocrine system disorders related to *Candida albicans.*

C. Orian Truss, in his writings, has repeatedly emphasized the role of yeasts in causing health problems in women, including PMS.[51-52] More recently, a number of gynecologists have confirmed Truss' observations and are successfully treating many of their PMS patients with an anticandida program.

Gynecologist Richard Mabray of Victoria, Texas recently commented,

> "A large percentage of phone calls and visits to gynecologists are related to vaginal yeast infections. At best, they're a nuisance to the patients; they're costly; they cause pain and often interfere with normal sexual relations. Of even greater importance is the effect of yeast toxins on the whole person. *I'm increasingly impressed with the role of candida in causing a whole host of health disorders in women, including depression, irritability and the premenstrual syndrome.*
>
> "The most exciting thing I'm involved in now is a new association of PMS clinics in Texas, Arizona, Colorado and Utah. We'll be studying patients using clinical, psychological and laboratory studies and we'll put our findings on computers. It'll take a while to generate the data we need but we should have a lot to report in another year or two."

Gynecologist A. Stephens Orr of Atlanta had this to say,

> Today, January, 1984, the first thing I think about when I see a patient with severe PMS syndrome is the association of this disorder with chronic candidiasis. I look for a yeast-connected PMS, especially in

women who give a history of receiving repeated antibiotics, feeling worse on damp days, chemical hypersensitivity, intolerance to birth control pills and recurrent vaginitis.

"In patients with such a history, I prescribe nystatin and a low carbohydrate diet. I'm very happy with the response, so are the patients, including some who have been referred by psychiatrists and psychologists. Candida isn't the only cause of PMS and some patients don't improve until they've been on treatment for 3 to 6 months. Nevertheless, anticandida therapy is an important addition to successful PMS management."

My observations in my own patients resemble those of Doctors Truss, Mabray and Orr. Candida certainly isn't "the cause" of PMS. *Yet I feel that in the patient with the characteristic history suggesting yeast-connected illness, a trial of anticandida therapy is warranted.* I've observed that diet, nystatin and nutritional supplements, including primrose and linseed oils (which are rich in essential fatty acids), zinc and vitamins B-6 and E, often work dramatically in relieving PMS and a wide variety of other health problems of young women (see also chapter 43, Update). Included among these are recurrent vaginitis, pelvic pain, headache, fatigue, irritability, depression, infertility and other complaints related to poor hormone functioning (small breasts, lack of sexual interest and response, and painful intercourse).

Moreover, other health problems which do not involve the reproductive organs and other parts of the endocrine system may also improve, including rhinitis, bronchitis, arthritis, bursitis. Since "everything is connected to everything else," what helps a woman's reproductive organs and endocrine system helps every part of her body.

Why Yeast-Connected Illness Occurs More In Women, Especially Young Women

Many women with yeast-connected illness are tired, depressed and feel bad all over. They tend to complain of aches and pains in almost every part of their bodies. The typical young woman with these symptoms has consulted many different physicians, including gynecologists, internists, urologists, otolaryngologists and neurologists. And because their complaints continue and no apparent explanation is found, they may be told, "You'll just have to learn to live with these symptoms." If they continue to complain, their families, friends and physicians will usually label them as "hypochondriacs." And if their symptoms are severe and disabl-

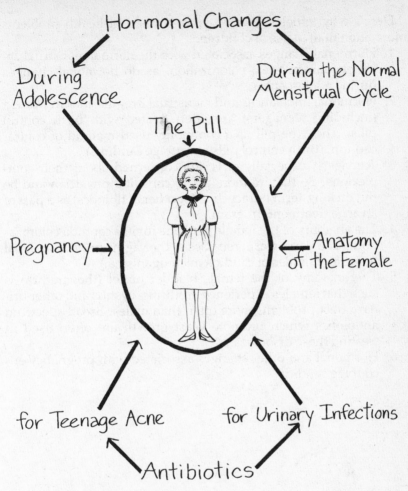

Hormonal Changes

During Adolescence

During the Normal Menstrual Cycle

The Pill

Pregnancy →

← Anatomy of the Female

for Teenage Acne

for Urinary Infections

Antibiotics

ing, their physicians are apt to say, "I think you should discuss your problems with a psychiatrist."[†]

[†]On October 25, 1984, John Espy, Ph.D., Director, Character Disorders Treatment Institute, 4130 Linden Ave., Dayton, Ohio 45432, reported the exciting responses of some of his patients to anticandida therapy.

Dr. Espy had this to say, "These patients were all female and were diagnosed 'borderline personality disorder' (with a score of 8 or greater on the Gunderson Diagnostic Interview). Most had received repeated broad spectrum antibiotics.

All patients reported states of *unrealness, self-mutilation* and *severe depression.* Symptoms were especially acute during the 3 or 4 days prior to menstruation.

"These patients were placed on nystatin and a yeast-free, sugar-free special diet. Symptoms were exacerbated initially; thereafter improvement was dramatic."

Here's why females develop yeast-connected health problems more often than males or children:

1. Hormonal changes associated with the normal menstrual cycle encourage yeast colonization, as do hormonal changes during adolescence.

2. Hormonal imbalances and menstrual irregularities in women (including teenagers) are often treated with birth control pills. And "the pill' is a commonly used method of contraception. (Birth control pills encourage candida.)

3. Teenagers, especially girls, are concerned about their complexions. So they're more apt to consult a physician and be put on long-term tetracycline (or other antibiotics) as a part of an acne treatment program.

4. The anatomy of the female genitalia invites candida colonization. (The dark, warm recesses of the vagina provide an ideal home for families of candida microorganisms.)

5. The anatomy of the female bladder outlet (the urethra) is such that females experience urethritis, cystitis and other urinary tract problems more often than males. Broad spectrum antibiotics which promote yeast growth are often used in treating these disorders.

6. Hormonal and other changes associated with pregnancy encourage candida.

28

Men, Too, Develop Yeast-Connected Health Problems†

Jim, a 36-year-old engineer, came to see me on February 23, 1982. His main complaint . . . "athlete's foot for 20 years." For four years, Jim had also been troubled by other rashes involving especially his hands.

Jim commented,

> "I've been bothered with abdominal pain and sinus trouble off and on for many years. My energy supply is low and I experience a lot more fatigue than I feel is normal for a person my age. During the last 6 months, I frequently develop inappropriate drowsiness and trouble in concentrating. And at times I feel 'spaced out' and 'not with it'. These mental and nervous symptoms became worse when I went to work at an aluminum plant."

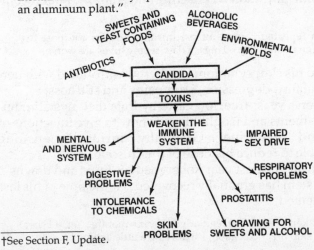

On examination, Jim showed what appeared to be a chronic fungous infection of his toenails plus a rash involving his fingers and hands. Following a blood test (the "liver panel"), I prescribed Nizoral® which Jim took for a year. In addition, I treated him with yeast and mold extracts which he took sublingually (under-the-tongue). He began to improve within a few weeks and at a checkup in February 1983, Jim commented,

> "My rashes have disappeared and my nails are 95% well. My fatigue, nasal congestion, headaches and other symptoms are better, and my tolerance for environmental chemicals has improved."

Robert, a 31-year-old refrigeration technician, came to see me on December 30, 1982 with severe hives and swelling. He was frightened and said,

> "I feel my throat is swelling and I have a lump in my stomach."

I gave Robert a shot of Adrenalin® which provided partial relief. In 30 minutes, I repeated the Adrenalin® injection.

In reviewing Robert's history, I found he had taken many antibiotics as a child. Then, while serving in the army, he developed a peculiar form of encephalitis or meningitis which was treated for several weeks with antibiotics, including tetracycline.

In 1979, Robert was again given a prolonged course of antibiotics because of "prostate infection." In 1981, he broke out in hives which persisted for a week. The rash returned in June 1982 and recurred daily during the next 6 months. Medication included repeated Adrenalin® injections, Periactin® and Atarax®. Robert commented,

> "I've taken repeated courses of prednisone, and for the past two weeks I've been taking 30 to 60 mgs. a day. Yet my hives are worse."

In addition to his skin symptoms, Robert was troubled with nervousness, irritability, depression, joint pains and stiffness.

I put Robert on a yeast-free, low carbohydrate diet, nystatin, nutritional supplements and taught his wife how to give injections of Adrenalin® and Susphrine®. Gradually, during the ensuing weeks, I was able to reduce his dose of prednisone.

Although during the past year Robert had his "ups and downs", his immune system has gradually recovered. At the time of his last visit, he commented,

> "I haven't taken prednisone regularly for over 6 months. Yet, if I cheat on my diet or skip my medication, I'll develop a little itching."

George, a 36-year-old banker, came to see me on March 25, 1983. Here are excerpts from his letter:

"I've been bothered by sinus problems and sore throats all of my life. The severity varies and I've taken many antibiotics. For the past several months, I've felt light-headed and dizzy. I feel drained and 'zapped' most of the time and extremely anxious. In addition, I have spring and fall hayfever. I thought that my mental and nervous symptoms were caused by stress, but during a prolonged rainy period several weeks ago, I could tell I felt considerably worse. My sister, who has been helped by diet and nystatin, talked me into coming to see you."

Following allergy testing and a treatment program which included immunotherapy, diet, nystatin and nutrition supplements, George commented,

"All of my problems aren't solved, but I have more energy, feel less depressed and am enjoying life once more."

Paul, a 43-year-old factory worker wrote to me in February 1983. Here are excerpts from his letter.

"As a child I was bothered by persistent colds and sinus congestion and during my early teens I took lots of antibiotics. Finally, when I was 16, my tonsils were removed and I got better. But by 18, I noticed that deodorants, colognes and perfumes gave me a headache and irritated my nose and throat.

"Soon afterward, I started working in a factory and my nose irritation, drainage, headaches and sore throats became worse. I took daily decongestants for several years and tried to stay away from perfumed soaps and deodorants.

"When I was 30, I bought an older home to remodel and began to work with panelling. About that time, I noticed more problems with my head, nose and throat. Then 4 or 5 years ago, my symptoms got worse and I began to have stomach trouble as well as head and throat trouble. A gastroenterologist made x-rays and used an instrument to look in my stomach. It showed only 'gastritis.'

"What really bothers me now is tobacco smoke at my work place. It sent me to the doctor three times in the last six months. Two minutes of smoke inhalation causes headache, tingling in my chest, dizziness, runny nose, burning eyes and mental confusion."

At the time of Paul's first visit on March 22, 1983, I put him on a comprehensive program of management, including nystatin, a yeast-free, sugar-free diet, extra vitamin C (2,000 to 3,000 milligrams a day) and nutritional supplements.

Paul steadily improved and at a followup visit on June 3, 1983, he said,

"I'm much better. Now my bad days are as good as my good days were before I started treatment. My stomach no longer hurts; I don't need to take Tagamet® and my tolerance to tobacco and other chemicals has improved."

(Paul's wife, Betty, had been troubled with recurrent abdominal pain, respiratory problems and menstrual irregularity for years. Her stomach was x-rayed three times and a diagnosis of "nervous stomach and spastic colon" had been made. In May 1982, her gynecologist prescribed nystatin and diet. Betty commented, "I feel better than I can remember feeling in a long time.")

In my practice over ¾ of my patients with yeast-connected health problems are women. *Yet, men, too, develop yeast-connected health problems.** I particularly suspect such problems in men . . .

1. Who are troubled by food and inhalant allergies.
2. Who have been bothered by persistent "jock itch," athlete's foot, or fungous infection of the nails.
3. Who have taken repeated courses of antibiotics for acne, prostatitis, sinusitis or other infections.
4. Who consume lots of beer, breads and sweets.
5. Who crave alcohol.
6. Whose wives or children are bothered by yeast-connected illness.
7. Who feel bad on damp days or on exposure to chemicals and/or tobacco.
8. Whose sex drive is impaired.
9. Who are troubled by fatigue, depression and other peculiar nervous system symptoms.
10. Who are bothered by recurrent digestive problems, including constipation, bloating, diarrhea and abdominal pain.

---

*Even if men do not appear to have a yeast-related health disorder if their wives or sexual partners are experiencing such problems, they too may need treatment (see chapter 42, Update).

29

Health Problems Of Children

Although children differ from adults in many respects, many of the same factors which lead to candida colonization and a weakened immune system in adults also affect children. These include prolonged or repeated courses of antibiotic drugs and the consumption of diets with a high sugar and yeast content.

Yeast-connected illness should also be suspected in children whose parents have been bothered by similar problems. It is also more apt to occur in children who give a history of thrush and persistent diaper rashes.

In the summer of 1980, I was discussing the "American epidemic" of recurrent ear problems in children with another physician interested in yeast-connected illness. We both agreed that these problems seemed to be getting worse, rather than better. And in spite of polyethylene tubes and repeated or long-term antibiotics, ear problems were continuing to recur.

Since these drugs had encouraged candida and depressed the immune system in many of my adult patients, it seemed logical to prescribe nystatin for children who required an antibiotic for their ear infections. However, because I had limited my practice to allergy, I saw only an occasional child with ear problems. Accordingly, I had little opportunity to note the effectiveness of an anti-yeast program in children.

Then in January 1982 I saw Rusty, a 5½ year old child with multiple health problems. He had been troubled with colic, recurrent colds, ear infections and hyperactivity during his first year of life. According to his mother,

"The doctor changed Rusty's formula several times. He was hyperactive, even as an infant, but he was a smart baby who learned quickly.

> "Rusty's constant colds continued and he averaged one ear infection a month. His developmental milestones were normal . . . sitting alone at 6 months, standing alone at 8 months, walking across the room at 11 months. His speech developed normally and by one year he could say 20 words. But then his progression seemed to cease. Around the age of 2 he became worse with increasing hyperactivity. Mild autistic symptoms began to appear and communication became an increasing problem; speech was broken and very fast."

Also, at age 2, the family moved into a new home which subsequently was found to be contaminated with formaldehyde. Rusty also ate lots of junk food. His recurrent ear infections continued and he always had dark circles under his eyes and a runny nose. Studies at a university medical center resulted in a diagnosis of "pervasive developmental disorder, with symptoms of autism."

At the time of his first visit to me, Rusty was put on the "cave man diet", a basic elimination diet[†] which avoided any and every food he ate more than once a week. After following this diet for a week, his mother reported,

> "Rusty showed a dramatic improvement. He became more responsive and began to cooperate."

After challenging Rusty with mushrooms, his mother reported,

> "Rusty became hyper, wild . . . aggressive, ill, crying, throwing things. Pupils dilated. Yeast caused a similar reaction."

Other foods, including wheat, corn and raisins also caused reactions . . . some of which were severe. For example, Rusty's mother reported,

> "Thirty minutes after eating wheat, his pupils dilated and he stared into space more. Within a few hours he showed more autistic behavior."

The history of recurrent ear troubles treated with multiple antibiotic drugs, plus the sharp flareup in symptoms on challenge with yeast and mushrooms, made me feel that this child's problem was related, in part at least, to candida. Accordingly, as a part of his treatment program, Rusty was put on nystatin and a yeast and sugar-free diet. After 3 months of therapy, Rusty's teachers reported "dramatic improvement in his behavior and readiness for learning." And on April 6, 1982 Rusty's mother sent me this report:

> "Rusty continues to improve. He is now writing more of his ABC's and can write the alphabet in order down to H. He is using more language and putting words together, such as 'cook cookies', 'want to go'.

---

†*Tracking Down Hidden Food Allergy,* chapter 34.

His understanding of language is still improving, although speech is still fast. He is dressing himself and is awakening to the world!"

In the next six months, Rusty's autistic behavior[†] and related developmental problems continued to improve. However, there were ups and downs. Exposure to chemical fumes caused a relapse; also, his family noted that larger doses of B vitamins, especially B-6, were essential for optimal functioning. Rusty still requires special education, yet his family is pleased.

Early in 1982, while I was working with Rusty, Truss' third article, "The Role of Candida Albicans in Human Illness," was published in the *Journal of Orthomolecular Psychiatry*. (This report was first presented at the Huxley Institute Symposium in September 1981). Although it dealt mainly with the role of *Candida albicans* in health problems in adults, Truss summarized,

---

[†]In December, 1983, I learned of another child with severe developmental problems, including autistic behavior, who improved on anticandida therapy. The story of this child (Duffy Mayo) was described in the September 25, 1983 issue of the *Los Angeles Times* by Don Campbell and was featured on Charles Kuralt's "American Parade" (CBS).

I called Duffy's physician, Dr. Alan Levin, to get more information. Here's what Dr. Levin told me: "During Duffy's first 18 months, his development was superior. Then because of recurrent ear infections, he received lots of antibiotics. Soon he began to slip backward and develop autistic-type behavior. He stopped talking, lost his vigor, and began withdrawing. He'd go from acting depressed and stuporous to 'climbing the walls'.

"When Duffy was about 3½, Dr. Phyllis Saifer and I began to study and treat Duffy using anti-allergy therapy. He began to improve. Subsequently, because of the history of antibiotic drugs, I prescribed nystatin and for a while he improved even more. Then another colleague, Dr. Cecil A. Bradley, put Duffy on Nizoral® in a dose of one tablet a day. He later increased the dose to two tablets and then to three tablets a day. Duffy improved dramatically and has maintained this improvement. Although he still shows some fine motor and comprehension problems, he's reading ahead of his milestones. I'm pleased and so is his family."

Was Duffy, like Charlie Swaart (see chapter 32), actually drunk? According to Dr. Levin, no blood alcohol studies were carried out. Yet, before his anticandida therapy, Duffy would stagger, giggle and break into silly laughs and act drunk. The research of Kazuo Iwata, M.D. of Japan shows that many candida species put out toxins. So regardless of whether it was alcohol or toxins affecting Duffy Mayo's nervous system, the trial of an anticandida treatment program helped.

Recently, Bernard Rimland, Ph.D. of San Diego, California told me of other autistic children who had improved following anticandida therapy. And in October, 1984, at a Chicago medical conference, Dr. Bradley described his finding in 13 additional autistic children. "All had an inordinate number of bacterial infections with the use of broad-spectrum antibiotics preceding the onset. Most improved on a diet eliminating cow's milk, wheat and other starches. Skin testing for candida (and other fungi) revealed a high degree of sensitivity."

During 1984, I've treated two other autistic children who resembled Rusty and Duffy in many ways. Both were sensitive to wheat, sugar and other foods, and both improved significantly on nystatin and/or Nizoral® and a special diet.

". . . the categories of illness [in which he felt] the relationship to yeast is well established, those in which the evidence is strongly suggestive and those I believe deserve careful study with respect to the possibility of such a relationship.

"Infants and children with frequent infections and much antibiotic. Bowel disturbances, oral thrush, diaper rash, and respiratory allergy are common. Chronic irritability and hyperactivity, and even one case of stuttering, have been seen in children, many of whom carry the diagnosis of 'learning disabled'."

Truss also briefly discussed the manifestations of candidiasis in early adolescence,

". . . often with devastating effect on mood and on intellectual functions."

My interest in yeast-connected illness was further stimulated by the presentations at the Dallas Candida Conference on July 9-11, 1982. In the discussion period, several pediatricians told of their experiences in treating children with an anticandida program:

Dr. Aubrey Worrell:

"Over the years, I've seen kids who are sick one week out of a month and each time they seem to require antibiotics. A year and a half ago, I began to use small doses of nystatin three times a day for 4 to 6 weeks. My patients seemed to do better. I think it works."

Dr. Morton Teich:

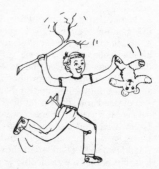

"I've treated quite a number of hyperactive children and have done quite well with them, using the anticandida approach. One of our most significant findings in studying hyperactive patients was the history of sugar craving. This relationship is so striking that I've come to feel if a patient doesn't have some form of sugar and yeast craving, I tend to question the diagnosis."

Dr. Francis Waickman:

"Sixty percent of the illnesses which take children to doctors are viral. Yet, many of these viral illnesses are treated with antibiotics. In my opinion, stopping the overuse of antibiotic drugs in children is the number one way to lessen candida colonization. Most children with recurrent infections receive excessive amounts of sugar. And cutting down on sugar is the next most important thing physicians can do. I've had better results by paying attention to these factors than by giving nystatin."

Another pediatrician commented,

> "Until recently, I had not developed a clear and consistent policy in dealing with this problem. But I'm now tending more and more to put my regular pediatric patients (who are given ampicillin or other broad-spectrum drugs for treatment of otitis media) on prophylactic nystatin. However, I feel that curbing the use of antibiotics is really the key."

In my general pediatric and allergy practice during the past 10 years, I've found that sugar is the *number one cause* of hyperactivity. Accordingly, the observations of Rusty's mother, along with those of the physicians at the Dallas Candida Conference, turned a light on in my "computer." And I easily recalled dozens of hyperactive children I'd seen whose mothers commented,

> "Johnny's addicted to sugar. He'll cheat, lie or steal to get it. I have to watch him like a hawk."

I began to ask myself, *"Is it possible that my sugar-craving children who show hyperative behavior when they eat sweets are developing these nervous system symptoms because sugar feeds their candida? And is this the answer rather than sugar allergy?"*

Perhaps, it is, yet I realize candida isn't the whole story. Here's why: Several years ago, I carried out a clinical study on 10 of my hyperactive patients whose parents had reported,

> "When my child eats sugar, he becomes hyperactive."

Here's what I did.

I bought 50 pounds of cane sugar and 50 pounds of beet sugar. I gave a 2-pound sack of both types of sugar to the parents of each of these hyperactive youngsters. And I outlined a special plan for giving them the sugar.

I won't review this study in detail. However, I was fascinated to find that *some children reacted to cane sugar who did not react to beet sugar, and some reacted to beet who did not react to cane. Some reacted to both sugars and some reacted to neither.* I've also observed on many occasions that foods containing corn sugar cause reactions in some patients. Yet, such patients may be able to take equivalent amounts of carbohydrates from other sources, including cane and beet. Also, many patients who react to cane, corn and beet may be able to take honey or maple syrup.

My brief study, along with my clinical observations, confirmed the findings of pioneer food allergist Theron Randolph[32] of Chicago who, many years ago, noted that *sensitivity to sugar depends, in part at least, on the botanical source of the sugar. Accordingly, I feel that some sugar reactions are allergic or allergic-like, even though the mechanisms causing these reactions remain obscure.*

But now that I've become aware of candida-related illness, I feel some hyperactive children, especially those who have taken repeated courses of antibiotics, react to sugar because the sugar triggers candida.

During the past year, I've seen additional children in whom candida appeared to be a major thread in the "web" of their health problems. And I feel I now possess sufficient clinical evidence to change the way I treat children with ear infections, urinary tract infections, hyperactivity, behavior and learning problems and acne.

More specifically, when I treat a respiratory or urinary tract infection with amoxicillin, Ceclor,® Septra,® Bactrim,® Keflex,® or other broad-spectrum antibiotic drugs, I also prescribe nystatin during the time the child is receiving the drug. And if the child has taken antibiotics repeatedly over a prolonged period of time, I feel more prolonged courses of nystatin are indicated. In addition, I recommend a diet which eliminates yeast and refined carbohydrates, especially sugar and corn syrup.

In treating bacterial respiratory infections in children, I prefer penicillin V or penicillin G. Here's why: These drugs help mainly in eradicating the families of bacteria which cause respiratory tract infection and they do not wipe out the normal bacteria found in the intestinal tract. By contrast, the broad-spectrum drugs just referred to not only eradicate the harmful germs causing respiratory tract infections, they also wipe out many of the friendly germs found in the intestinal tract. And when these friendly germs are knocked out, *Candida albicans* moves in.

In treating urinary tract infections in children, I prefer Furadantin® or Macrodantin® since these drugs are usually effective and are less apt to encourage the growth of candida.

According to Dennis B. Worthen,[33] Ph.D., Chief, Information Services of Norwich Eaton Pharmaceuticals, Inc.:

> ". . . Nitrofurantoin drugs, Furadantin® and Macrodantin®, have less effect on intestinal flora than do systemic antibiotics such as ampicillin, tetracycline, Bactrim® and Septra®. Since nitrofurantoin is effective only in urinary tract infections, concentrations in the gastrointestinal tract are not sufficiently high to significantly alter the normal flora. Consequently, the problems that would normally occur due to an altered flora/fauna balance are not normally observed."

In my experience, the causes of hyperactivity resemble a jigsaw puzzle. And to help the hyperactive child, many pieces need to be put into place, including attention to food allergies, nutritional needs, avoidance of lead and other toxic metals, appropriate light, good teaching, and so on. *However, if a hyperactive, learning disabled child gives a history of recurrent ear and other infections, and if his hyperactive behavior is triggered by sugar, I feel the anticandida program should be a part of his overall management.*

Here are further clinical reports indicating that the yeast connection plays a role in causing health problems in children, including ear problems and related behavior and learning problems:

In his book, *The Missing Diagnosis*,[52] Truss in his chapter on "Infants and Children," comments,

> "The problem of chronic candidiasis in infants and children is especially important, not alone as it related to their health at this period of their lives, but also as it may relate to problems with yeast later in life."

Truss points out that antibiotics are frequently given to children and that . . .

> "after the use of antibiotic has been discontinued, the previous state of health may not return . . . Restlessness, discontent and irritability often accompany 'the runny nose'."

He also discusses other health problems in children, including learning disabilities and depression. He said,

> "At any age, but particulary in young children experiencing difficulty with school, this condition (meaning candidiasis) is one worth considering."

Allan Lieberman, M.D., a South Carolina pediatrician†, commented:

> "I treat almost every patient I see, including children with hyperactivity, behavior and learning problems, using a therapeutic trial of the anticandida program. The dramatic results I've obtained in so many encourage me to continue this approach. I've found that young children with recurrent respiratory and ear infections seem to really benefit. So do children, especially teenagers, with chronic depression."

---

†Here are other observations on the relationship of antibiotics to health problems in children: Gary Oberg, M.D., a Crystal Lake, Illinois pediatrician (who specializes in allergy and environmental medicine) commented, "Children with behavior and learning problems are usually allergic. Helping them requires a comprehensive program of management. Recently, I've observed that some of these children, *especially those who have received repeated broad-spectrum antibiotics, improve when nystatin is added to their treatment program.*"

195

Tennessee gynecologist John Curlin had this to say:

> "My 13-year-old daughter is a well-coordinated gymnast. However, since infancy, she had shown periods of moodiness, depression and fatigue. And during the past year or so, she has noticed periodic changes in her ability to concentrate and coordinate her movements.
>
> "During the past year, we've learned that she *does extremely well if she maintains her diet and nystatin therapy.* If she does not, her moodiness and marked fatigue will return. And, interestingly, she'll show a lack of physical coordination in her gymnastics.
>
> "Our youngest son, now 14 months of age, was fed only breast milk during his first six months of life and continued on breast milk plus other foods until the age of one year. Nevertheless, he was constantly irritable and suffered from a chronic rhinitis.
>
> "*Almost within 24 hours after I began giving him small doses of nystatin powder, his rhinitis cleared and he showed a noticeable change in personality. His irritability subsided and he became much more pleasant.*
>
> "This is so impressive that family members can recognize when his daily doses of nystatin have been forgotten by the sudden changes in his behavior. Then when he receives his nystatin, he settles down."

Dr. Curlin's comments about his young son led me to speculate about some of the hundreds of crabby, irritable and colicky infants I've seen. Many of these babies experienced persistent abdominal pain and discomfort, regardless of formula changes or other treatment measures I prescribed. Moreover, I've seen many colicky or crabby infants who were totally breast fed.

Would a therapeutic trial of nystatin be appropriate for such infants? And would it be safe?

Again my answer is "Yes."

Abdominal discomfort and other digestive symptoms occur so commonly in adults with candida-connected health problems it seems reasonable to anticipate that similar abdominal symptoms also trouble infants. Candida-related colic[†] should especially be suspected in infants who have been troubled by persistent diaper rashes, and/or thrush, or whose mothers have experienced candida-related health problems.

Ear Problems In Children . . . Isn't There A Better Answer?

In my opinion, which is shared by thousands of physicians and untold numbers of parents, recurrent ear problems in infants and

---

†Obviously, candida isn't "the cause" of colic in all babies. If you need further suggestions for coping with an uncomfortable, unhappy baby, get a copy of Sandy Jones' new book, "Crying Baby, Sleepless Nights" (See *Reading List*, chapter 47).

young children are one of the most perplexing dilemmas of the 1980s. One mother commented,

> "My two sons and just about all of my friends' children have had ear tubes. Isn't there a better answer?"

At a meeting of the Society for Clinical Ecology and Environmental Medicine, held concurrently with the annual meeting of the American Academy of Pediatrics (New York, October 24, 1982), Dr. George Shambaugh, Professor Emeritus of Otolaryngology at Northwestern University and a former President of the American Academy of Otolaryngology, gave an address entitled,

> "Serous Otitis: Are Tubes the Answer?"

In this address, Dr. Shambaugh commented,

> "Serous otitis . . . *is the largest single cause of hearing loss in children.* And the operation of inserting a ventilating tube through the tympanic membrane (ear drum) to restore hearing has become the most frequent hospital surgical procedure with anesthesia today.
> "Removal of enlarged adenoids and tonsils in children, most of them with OME (otitis media with effusion) and with tube insertion, is the second most frequent operation. Together, these operations, along with treatment of acute otitis media in children, is estimated by Dr. Charles D. Bluestone of Pittsburgh (in an article in the *New England Journal of Medicine*) to cost two billion dollars a year. The estimated cost of one operation for adenoidectomy and tube insertion . . . for the anesthesia, operating room, surgical fee, two nights in the hospital . . . is $1,000 or more. I think mostly more."

In his continuing discussion, Dr. Shambaugh said, in effect,

> "There's no questions of the usefulness of ventilating tubes for OME to equalize the air pressure on both sides of the tympanic membrane, thus allowing the fluid to resolve or to be expelled by ciliary action to the eustachian tube.
> "Yet, tubes alone aren't the answer for parents who are struggling to cope . . . often unsuccessfully . . . with the management of recurrent ear problems in their children. Neither are they an answer for their pediatricians, family physicians and otolaryngologists who are trying to help them."

Dr. Shambaugh urged pediatricians, otolaryngologists, allergists, clinical ecologists and other physicians to take a look at the allergic aspects of ear problems in children. And he commented,

> "Although allergies in children are often hard to identify by the usual allergy scratch tests, I've found that a program of allergic management with attention to hidden or delayed-in-onset food allergy helps me manage recurrent ear problems in children. Moreover, my results with

allergy management are far better than those obtained by putting children on prolonged courses of antibiotics and relying on tubes to clear up the condition."

Are Recurrent Ear Problems in Children Related to Candida? I don't know. Yet, based on my experiences in treating hundreds of adults who developed yeast-connected illness following prolonged or repeated courses of antibiotic drugs, such a relationship seems possible or even probable. Moreover, my own experiences in using nystatin and a special diet in a limited number of children with recurrent ear problems make me feel that an anticandida treatment program in these children is appropriate.

Here's a report on Wesley, a 4-year-old youngster I saw for a follow-up visit a few days before I finished the manuscript for this book and sent it to the publisher:

Wesley was born May 4, 1979 and had been seen regularly by his pediatricians. Here are items I excerpted from the medical record which was sent to me:

Treated for thrush and monilia diaper rash with oral Mycostatin® and Mycostatin Cream® to his diaper area at the age of 2 months. At 2½ months, thrush was still bothering him and gentian violet was prescribed.

At age 3 months, still having thrush; gentian violet treatment again prescribed. Ear infection noted at age 5 months, antibiotics prescribed. Began to have recurrent ear problems which responded poorly to antibiotics which he received on many occasions between the ages of 6 and 13 months.

Beginning June 1, 1980, more antibiotics were prescribed, including Pediazole®. Noted to be crying and irritable, was changed to Cyclopen® on June 9th. On June 17th, put on Ceclor® because of "persistent otitis media."

On July 1, 1980, Ceclor® was continued and on July 12 ears were noted to be 'finally looking better'. Put on Gantrisin® "suppression" . . . two 1-pint bottles prescribed, to be given 1 teaspoon twice daily.

On September 11, 1980 . . . irritable, picking at ears. Ears dull but not infected. Put on Septra®, 1 teaspoon twice daily.

January 31, 1981 . . . bilateral otitis. Amoxicillin prescribed.

February 14, 1981 . . . put on Cyclopen® for 10 days.

March 11, 1981 . . . In for checkup because of earache and hyperactivity. The child's mother commented,

"Wesley periodically goes stark raving mad . . . wild . . . climbing the walls . . . chocolate and corn seem to provoke these symptoms. Chemicals, including colognes and after shave lotions, do the same."

Cyclopen® prescribed for otitis. Mother phoned that Cyclopen® made his hyperactivity worse. Medication changed to Septra.®

April 4, 1981 . . . ears noted to be clear.

May 18, 1981 . . . respiratory infection, ears dull and red. Amoxicillin prescribed.

July 5, 1981 . . . viral infection, "ears look good without evidence of infection."

August 25, 1981 . . . in for checkup because of hyperactivity.

"Having temper tantrums, beats his head and carries on for at least an hour. Bites his sister. Nothing seems to help. Attacks not brought on by frustration or being upset. Sleeps poorly, mother worn out."

Because of sleep problems, hyperactivity and prolonged 'fits' . . . much worse than routine temper tantrums, referred to a clinical psychologist.

December 28, 1981 . . . In with fever of 104° to 105°. Ears 'sharp and clear'. Exudative pharyngitis. White blood count 20,800. Treatment . . . bicillin.

February 11, 1982 . . . left otitis media, given amoxicillin.

February 23, 1982 . . . ears still dull, 10 more days of amoxicillin prescribed.

March 20, 1982 . . . otitis media, amoxicillin prescribed.

April 9, 1982 . . . ears clear.

August 17, 1982 . . . age 3 years, 3 months. Referred to me for consultation. Review of history showed that Wesley reacted to sweets of any kind. Corn said to be a major troublemaker. The child also experienced episodes characterized by nasal congestion, swelling of the mouth and bags under his eyes associated with hyperactivity. Anti-yeast program prescribed, including yeast-free, sugar-free diet and nystatin. Supplemental nutrients also prescribed, including linseed oil and vitamins.

September 17, 1982 . . . much, much better. 'Like an entirely different child.' Challenged with 'junk food' . . . caused hyperactivity and irritability.

October 15, 1982 . . . doing well. Sugar in any amount triggers symptoms. So do apples. Nystatin being continued.

April 1, 1983 . . . in for recheck. Has been continued on diet and nystatin, but taking only small 'dots' of nystatin two or three times a day. Symptoms still recur on eating sweets.

Recommendations: Tighten up on diet. Give 1/16 teaspoon of nystatin four times a day.

Follow up visit, May 1, 1983 . . . Comments by mother:

> "Wesley has had a great month as far as his hyperactivity is concerned. He's been on the nystatin in full force and a sugar-free, yeast-free diet. We only had one outbreak of the hyperactivity . . . this past Sunday . . . at a wedding anniversary celebration. He got some cake and punch. That night he was in terrible shape."

In her notes Wesley's mother commented,

> "I'm very sure that nystatin helps. Taking it on a regular basis four times a day has made a real difference as compared to taking it now and then. We've had a great month. Wesley is so much better. He sits down and looks at books, he can be taken places without tearing the place apart. He's very cooperative and things are running so smoothly. As I said before, I really believe in the nystatin."

In his book, *The Missing Diagnosis*,[52] Truss describes in detail

> "a 16-month-old baby boy (who) was seen because of almost constant health problems that began at 2½ months of age."

At that age, because of cough and fever, the child received an antibiotic (Erythromycin®). One week later, Keflex® was prescribed. Although the child temporarily improved, he was seen at least once a month with recurrent respiratory problems, including ear infections. At 10 months, tubes were put in both ears. Health problems, including recurrent otitis, constant irritability and difficulty sleeping continued.

At the time of his first visit with Truss, the child was given a prescription for oral nystatin, 200,000 units four times a day as a liquid suspension. After one week of nystatin his mother reported he

> "feels excellent—running around, clapping his hands. Just feels better all over."

After three weeks of nystatin, the medication was discontinued and the child's symptoms returned. Nystatin was again prescribed and continued for four months. The child remained well through the entire ensuring winter.

In commenting on this child, Truss noted,

> "In my opinion, this is not an isolated problem. In fact, it probably is very common. Antibiotics save countless lives, but as with most forms of medical treatment some individuals are left with residual problems related to their use . . .
>
> Perhaps the single most fascinating potentially important aspect of

200

this case was the abrupt cessation of the ear infections. This suggests that *Candida albicans* was actually causing this problem and makes one wonder about the possible relationship of this yeast to what seems almost a national epidemic of otitis and tubes in the ears."

The response of Rusty, Wesley and other of my pediatric patients, along with the reports from other physicians, including Doctors Teich, Curlin and Truss, make me feel that *it is urgent for pediatricians, family practitioners, otolaryngologists and other physicians to know about "the yeast connection."* Moreover, I hope these anecdotal reports will stimulate physicians, both in practice and in the academic centers, to carry out studies to document the relationship of candida to a wide variety of health problems which are troubling children and perplexing parents and physicians.

For example, one group of young children with ear problems could be given "the routine treatment"; a second group could be put on a special diet and 1/16 to 1/8 teaspoon of nystatin four times a day.

Candida isn't "the cause" of recurrent ear disorders. And like all health problems, such disorders are related to many different factors which combine to lessen the child's resistance. Yet, if the response of the children given nystatin and a special diet resembled that shown by Rusty or Wesley, much suffering and expense could be avoided.

Suggestions for Managing the Infant and Young Child with Persistent or Recurring Respiratory Disorders, Including Ear Problems:
1. Milk-Free, Chocolate/Cola-Free, Corn-Free, Sugar-Free, Citrus-Free, Egg-Free, Yeast-Free Diet.

Pediatricians and allergists continue to argue about food allergy and its incidence in infants and young children. Yet, many observers,[34a-b-c-d-e-f-g-h-i] including Deamer, Gerrard and Speer, feel that hidden or delayed-onset food allergy, especially cow's milk allergy, is a common cause of health problems in children. And they commented recently, "Far too many children have tubes put in their ears before allergy is even considered."

They also pointed out that "milk allergy is difficult to diagnose by the usual immunologic tests, including skin tests and RAST tests. Ogle and Bullock[35] made similar observations and urged physicians to use elimination diets in working with their young patients.

And in a study of 1000 patients with food allergy, Speer[36] found that milk, chocolate/cola, corn, citrus and egg were at the top of his list of "most common food allergens." Milk allergy was especially common in children under two.

Other observers[37a-b] have described the relationship of cow's milk to persistent rhinitis and other health problems in children. The Price-Pottenger Foundation[38] has also documented the relationship of cow's milk, especially heat-treated cow's milk, to respiratory problems in kittens.

And the studies of Cheraskin and Ringsdorf[19] suggest that sugar and other refined carbohydrates lessen the ability of a person's phagocytes (germ eating white blood cells) to gobble up attacking germs.

So it seems possible that traditional sugar or corn syrup-containing cow's milk formulas in infants may play a role in causing health problems.

Putting all of these factors together, I've devised a feeding program for my infant patients with persistent or recurrent rhinitis and otitis. In addition, I suggest that foods be rotated to the extent possible to lessen the chances of other food allergies developing. (See, also, chapter 15.) Admittedly, this diet won't help every infant, and some 25% of milk-sensitive babies develop soy allergy. So Nutramigen® or goat's milk or other breast milk substitutes must be sought if human breast milk isn't available.

Here are the ingredients of this diet:

a. A special carbohydrate-free soy formula, RCF (Ross Laboratories). This formula is available in 13-ounce cans at most pharmacies, and contains a balanced amount of protein, fat, vitamins and minerals.

b. Carbohydrates are obtained from fruits, vegetables and whole grain cereals rather than from corn syrup or cane sugar. (A baby who takes a can of RCF per day needs 45 to 60 grams of carbohydrate.)

Sugar-Free Baby Food	Amount	Carbohydrate Content
Sweet potato	4¾ oz. (1 jar)	21 grams
Spinach	4¾ oz. (1 jar)	8 grams
Squash	4½ oz. (1 jar)	7 grams
Carrots	4½ oz. (1 jar)	7 grams
Beets	4½ oz. (1 jar)	7 grams

Peas, green	4½ oz. (1 jar)	8 grams
Pears	4½ oz. (1 jar)	14 grams
Applesauce	4½ oz. (1 jar)	15 grams
Fresh banana	½ small	11 grams
Apple-grape juice	4 oz.	16 grams
Apple juice	4 oz.	15 grams
Apple-plum	4 oz.	18 grams
Orange-apple	4 oz.	16 grams

Sugar-Free Baby Food	**Amount**	**Carbohydrate Content**
Rice baby cereal	6 tbsp.	11 grams
Oatmeal baby cereal	6 tbsp.	10 grams
Barley baby cereal	6 tbsp.	10 grams

Example: 1 jar of sweet potatoes, 1 jar of applesauce, 1 jar of pears, and 6 tbsp. of oatmeal cereal contains 60 grams of carbohydrate. Equivalent amounts of home-prepared food may also be used. Here are representative foods and their carbohydrate contents:

Baked potato	2 ½″ diameter	21 grams
Black-eyed peas	½ cup	18 grams
Cream of wheat	½ cup	14 grams
Rice cake	1 cake	7 grams

I also recommend the following treatment measures:

1. Nystatin, 100,000 to 300,000 units (1 to 4 ml) four times a day for two to three months or longer (nystatin oral suspension—Squibb or Lederle), or nystatin powder, 1/32 to 1/8 teaspoon four times a day. (Nystatin powder can be obtained by any pharmacist from the American Cyanamid Company. See, also, chapter 8).

2. Clean up the chemicals in the child's environment, including tobacco smoke, perfume, formaldehyde, floor waxes, bathroom cleaners and laundry detergents (see chapter 21.) These substances irritate the lining of the child's nose and throat and adversely affect the immune system and make the child more susceptible to infections and allergies. Other environmental control measures should also be instituted so as to lessen exposure to house dust, molds and animal danders.

3. Additional vitamin C, 100 to 250 milligrams three or four

times a day. Recent research, reported in the Abstract Section of the *Journal of Allergy and Clinical Immunology*,[30] suggests that larger than usual doses of vitamin C may strengthen the immune system in allergic individuals.

If a child experiences persistent or repeated ear problems, ventilating tubes may become necessary. Yet, this treatment program may strengthen his immune system and enable him to overcome his ear problems without surgery or the repeated use of antibiotics.

30

Physical And Mental Problems Of Teenagers

According to an article on May 26, 1983 by Mary Reed, Features Editor of my hometown paper, *The Jackson Sun,*

> "A once carefree teenager, Chris Avrett, would spend some days sitting in one spot, depressed and oblivious to the world. At times he would be so disoriented he couldn't tie his shoe or get food to his mouth. After trips to physicians in Memphis, Jackson and Nashville, several hospital stays and $30,000 in medical bills, his parents still didn't have the answer to the cause or treatment for his problem."

Chris was referred to me on January 26, 1983 by Dr. Cheryl Robley, a clinical psychologist, who felt his problems could be related to candida. Chris gave a history of asthma and other allergies during his early years of life. Tubes were put in his ears when he was in the second grade and again in the fourth. He also had taken

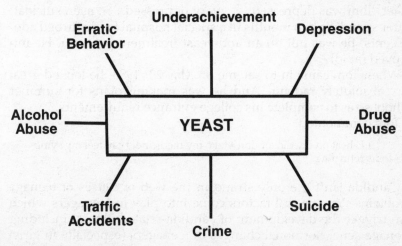

many antibiotics (especially the "broad spectrum" drugs which wipe out good germs along with the bad).

Like most youngsters, Chris loved sweets. Beginning at age 13, he changed from a happy boy who made good grades into a youngster with problems involving especially his nervous system . . . headache, anxiety, nervous twitching, short attention span and depression.

Continuing with Mary Reed's report,

> "Peggy Avrett, Chris' mother, says that within a week of starting the diet and nystatin her son was much better. You wouldn't believe he was the same child, like daylight to dark. On the anti-yeast treatment his mother 'watched him go from being a helpless baby to his old self again'."

How many teenagers like Chris are "out there?" Could there be a yeast-connection to under-achievement in school? Or mental and nervous system disorders ranging from nervous tics to severe depression? And how about alcoholism and other substance abuse, traffic accidents, crime and suicide? Could these perplexing disorders with multi-factoral causes also have a yeast connection?

I don't know, but my experiences during the past couple of years make me answer "Yes."

Tom (not his real name), a 17-year-old youngster enjoyed many economic, educational and cultural advantages. His parents were "super." They cared a lot. Tom was handsome, talented and smart.

Yet, Tom was depressed . . . very depressed . . . even suicidal. After spending two months in a special hospital for disturbed adolescents, he was put on an anti-yeast treatment program. He improved rapidly.

When Tom came in to see me on May 23, 1983, he looked great . . . absolutely radiant. And he was making plans for summer school so as to complete his college entrance requirements.

Tom commented,

> "If I cheat on my diet or don't take my medicine, I can feel my symptoms returning."

Candida isn't the only strand in the web of causes of teenage problems. Yet, several factors come into play in teenagers which can trigger the development of candida-related illness, including teenage acne, hormonal changes in teenagers (especially in girls) and ingestion of large amounts of sugar and yeast-containing foods.

Teenage Acne: Due to hormonal and other changes as the youngster matures, the oil glands of his face, chest and back become more active. And according to one report, 90% of all teenagers will show evidences of acne. Although most teenage acne will respond to soap and water and simple dietary changes, the "routine" treatment of more extensive teenage acne during the past two or three decades has included the use of antibiotics, especially the tetracycline group of drugs, including Sumycin,® Panmycin,® Vibramycin® and Minocin.®

Recently I've seen a number of patients with severe candida-related problems who gave a history of long-term tetracycline treatment for acne and I submitted a clinical report on one such patient recently.[39]

I now feel that routine use of tetracycline in managing teenage acne should be discontinued. And if, for any reason, tetracycline is prescribed for acne (or for any other condition), the Squibb preparation Mysteclin F® should be used, since it contains the anticandida drug, amphotericin B in combination with tetracycline.

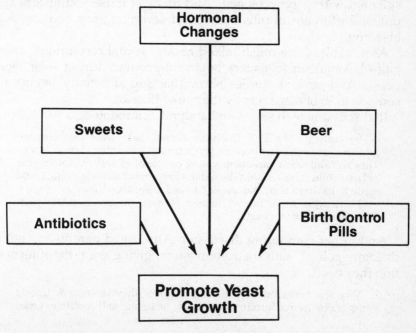

Admittedly, acne troubles many teenagers and the condition is often difficult to manage. Yet, the risks of long-term tetracycline treatment are greater than the possible benefits. Moreover, if a teenager will eat a good diet and seek out the factors which promote good health, and avoid those factors which interfere with it, he'll usually be able to control and overcome his acne without resorting to potentially dangerous drugs.

Hormonal Changes and "The Pill": When your child enters his teen years, all sorts of interrelated hormonal changes occur. His pituitary gland, like Rip Van Winkle, "wakes up." And it sends messages to other endocrine glands, including the thyroid, the adrenals and the sex glands (testicles or ovaries). These various glands also interact with each other.

These hormonal changes help turn your child into an adult. Yet, sometimes, the process isn't easy. Hormonal imbalances especially cause problems in the maturing female; and many girls are troubled by premenstrual tension, cramps, irregular periods, abdominal pain, headache, fatigue and other problems related to the menstrual cycle.

In some girls, these problems are severe enough to warrant consultation with a gynecologist. And many of these youngsters are put on birth control pills because of severe cramps or excessive bleeding.

As a result of the much talked about "sexual revolution", over half of American teenagers begin intercourse during their teen years. And several studies show that sexual activity begins in some $1/4$ to $1/3$ of teenagers by the age of 15 or 16.

In discussing teen sex, Ann Landers[40] commented,

> "Recently on the Phil Donahue Show, there were two teenage mothers, one who had become pregnant at 13 and the other at 14 . . . They were attractive, articulate young people of 15 and 19. The 19 year old (her child is now 4) said she did not know what she was doing could result in having a baby. No one had talked to her about sex . . .
>
> "There were more than 1 million teenage pregnancies last year. Something is not working."

And in her continuing discussion Ann urged parents to "get a dialogue going" with their youngsters, giving them the information they need.

> "Very few teenagers stop having sex once they've started. Unless yours is one in five hundred thousand, he or she will continue. Once

you have the knowledge that your child is sexually active, you must do what you can to protect him or her."

Helping and guiding teenagers (especially those who are sexually active) isn't easy for parents, and you or your physician may feel "the pill" is appropriate therapy for treating menstrual problems or for pregnancy prevention. However, since the pill stimulates candida, it's a two-edged sword which involves significant risks. So, in my opinion, alternate methods of pregnancy prevention should be sought.

Teenage Diet: As your youngsters grow up, you'll be astounded at how much they can eat . . . boys especially. They'll consume tremendous numbers of calories because they're growing so rapidly. I've seen teenage boys grow 6 inches and gain 30 pounds in a year. Many teenagers will eat anything that doesn't bite them first! Foods and beverages they like include pizza, candies, cakes, soft drinks and beer. All of these items are loaded with yeast and sugar.

Although many youngsters who consume these foods and beverages do not develop candida-related illness, such diets, especially when combined with hormonal changes, antibiotics, birth control pills and other anti-nutrient factors, lead to the development of candida-related health problems.

Although you may find it impossible to control your youngster's diet when he's away from home, offer him good foods when he is at home. What's more, good foods will contribute to the health of your entire family.

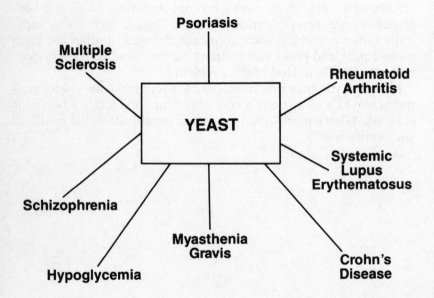

Psoriasis

Multiple
Sclerosis

Rheumatoid
Arthritis

YEAST

Systemic
Lupus
Erythematosus

Schizophrenia

Myasthenia
Gravis

Crohn's
Disease

Hypoglycemia

31

Does Candida Cause Multiple Sclerosis, Psoriasis, Arthritis Or Schizophrenia?

No—Candida isn't THE cause of these and other often devastating disorders including Crohn's disease (inflammation of the intestine), myasthenia gravis, systemic lupus erythematosus and some forms of hypoglycemia—but . . . there's growing evidence based on exciting clinical experiences of many physicians that there is a yeast connection.

And by treating the candida strand in the "Spider web" many individuals with these other disorders will start on the road to recovery.

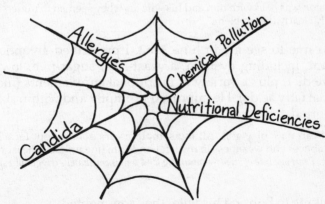

Bob, a 42-year-old soft drink executive, began to have twinges of pain in his left hand in March 1982. It was worse if he struck his hand against an object during his daily routines. Gradually, the pain, with associated numbness, involved his entire left arm. He than developed numbness and tingling in his left leg. Soon his left arm and leg became weak and he needed a cane for support.

Bob commented,

> "I have trouble knowing where my left arm and my leg are. And, at times, I've noticed tingling in my right buttock and thigh."

During the next few weeks his symptoms progressed and he was examined by a number of specialists in our town. In May, he was referred to a world famous clinic in the upper midwest for further observation and study. Here are excerpts from the medical report of the consultant who examined Bob:

> "Neurological exam revealed an ataxic, broad based, jerky gait. His deep tendon reflexes were brisk in both legs, more so on the left than the right . . . His reflexes in the left upper arm . . . were reduced . . . His muscle testing revealed mild left facial weakness and moderate weakness of the left upper extremities and mild weakness of the left lower extremity and right upper extremity. Muscle tone was increased in the left arm and both legs in a spastic fashion. There was some impairment of vibratory and joint sense in both the upper and lower extremities.
>
> *"It is our feeling that he has some type of demyelinating CNS disease. Whether this represents an acute episode of acute disseminating encephalomyelitis or a disease which will have recurrent episodes and be progressive cannot be determined at this time.* We told him that only further observation would confirm the diagnosis and that, in the case of acute flareups in the future, a short course of corticosteroids might be indicated. A long discussion was held with him and his wife and they seemed to understand fairly clearly the problem."

Bob came to see me in June 1982. I prescribed an anticandida program, including nystatin, a yeast-free, sugar-free, low carbohydrate diet, plus a variety of nutritional supplements (including essential fatty acids). He improved promptly and within six weeks he reported,

> "I can now play golf. All my symptoms are gone except for a little numbness and weakness in my left hand. I'm fine unless I cheat on my diet. *Even one bite of sugar-containing food will immediately trigger my symptoms.*"

In talking to Bob and his wife, they commented,

> "The doctors told us that Bob did indeed have multiple sclerosis and that the course was uncertain."

Bob comes in to see me at regular intervals and continues on his diet, nystatin, linseed oil and other nutritional supplements. In June 1983 he commented, "I'm doing great."

Has Bob's severe neurological disease improved through coincidence, or has anticandida treatment helped?

Multiple sclerosis is a disease that waxes and wanes, regardless of the sort of treatment used. Nevertheless, I feel the anticandida treatment has definitely helped Bob. Although I can't prove it, neither Bob nor his wife want to take a chance on discontinuing the anticandida program.

A similar patient, Ted, first came to me on October 1, 1982. Ted, a truck driver, had enjoyed general good health during his childhood, although he said,

> "I had a number of ear and throat infections and took a lot of antibiotics."

Then five years ago, he was involved in a serious accident and suffered extensive injuries. Treatment included insertion of an acrylic plate in his skull, plus lots of antibiotics.

Ted began to notice numbness, tingling and weakness in both of his feet and legs in December 1981. He also experienced back pain and a loss of coordination. He was checked by a neurologist in March 1982. The diagnosis: *multiple sclerosis*. Ted was checked at the same famous midwestern clinic in April 1982. Here are excerpts from the report of his neurological examination:

> "His gait was slightly wide-based with circumduction of the right lower limb; there was mild tandem ataxia; there was mild static tremor in the hands bilaterally; coordination was slightly impaired in the left upper limb and alternate motion rate was minimally impaired in the left foot.
> "Mr. F. has demyelinating disease or multiple sclerosis. In view of the diagnosis, I suggest he strongly consider other types of work . . . I do not feel he should try to continue as a truck driver in view of the nature of his disease and the uncertain prognosis."

I prescribed a comprehensive program of management for Ted, including nystatin, a yeast-free diet containing, initially, 100 grams of carbohydrates, essential fatty acid and vitamin/mineral supplements.

When I checked Ted one month later, he said,

> "I'm significantly better. The numbness, tingling and weakness are less intense. My incoordination is gone; my bladder problem and constipation are gone, my lower back pain is less intense."

At subsequent follow-up visits in December 1982, February 1983 and April 1983, Ted has continued to do well. And in May 1986 he commented,

> "I'm well. No symptoms as long as I follow my diet. I took nystatin for over two years and haven't had to take it since.

Now I'd like to tell you about Dorothy, a 48-year-old office worker I've known for 20 years. Here are excerpts from a letter she sent to me:

> "In 1969 I began taking sulfa drugs and I took them continuously for the next seven years to keep from developing infection related to kidney stones.
>
> "Beginning in 1975 I noticed that I was losing strength. My head hurt most of the time and I developed problems with my vision that would come and go. In 1977 I began to have joint pains. Yet these, too, would come and go. I was able to keep on working but I seemed to get weaker each year. In 1980 an eye doctor said I had scars in both eyes and in 1981 my left eye 'went out'. The doctor said it was optic neuritis."

In the 18 months before I saw Dorothy, she developed many strange sensations, including joint pains, numbness, tingling and "electricity" feeling in her legs, jerky handwriting, mental confusion, mood changes, headaches, bladder problems and eye symptoms. In addition, Dorothy commented,

> "At times I've felt I'd scream if I couldn't 'get out of my legs.' I felt like a person with boots on who needed to take them off. I also felt drugged and weak."

Dorothy was seen by several physicians, including an ophthalmologist and a neurologist. The neurologist told Dorothy,

> "It's possible you may be developing multiple sclerosis, although my findings on examination do not warrant my making such a diagnosis at this time."

Dorothy first came to me as a patient on June 14, 1982. In reviewing her history, the long-time consumption of sulfa drugs prior to the onset of her symptoms served as a "red flag". This history made me feel her health problems could be yeast-connected. So I prescribed a comprehensive program of management including nystatin, a yeast-free, sugar-free diet and nutritional supplements, including essential fatty acids. I saw her at monthly intervals and she showed consistent improvement.

On January 26, 1983, 7 months after beginning treatment, Dorothy commented,

> "Most of my major symptoms have disappeared, including mental confusion, headaches, numbness and weakness. I'm also pleased that most of the 'electricity feeling' in my arms and legs has disappeared. I still tire easily but this, too, is getting better."

Patients like Dorothy really excite me and make me say to myself,

> "Wouldn't it be great if patients with early MS-like symptoms could be turned around and made well before an actual 'disease' developed?"

Now I'd like to tell you about Phyllis, a slender 24-year-old office worker with a different sort of health problem. I first saw Phyllis on May 3, 1982. Her main complaints included "joint and muscle aches and pains, fatigue and depression." In a letter she commented:

> "For the last 4 years I've had aches and pains in every part of my body. Yet they weren't too severe until 5 months ago. Since then, they've been almost constant. The pains seem to travel from one part of my body to another. I also don't feel as active as I used to. I can't even scream . . . it seems as though I don't have enough breath."

When I reviewed Phyllis' history I found she was bothered by many other symptoms, including fatigue, depression, "peculiar feelings" in her ears, constant runny nose, sinus trouble, canker sores, dizziness, chest pains, nausea, frequent urination, irritability, numbness and tingling.

As a teenager, Phyllis took repeated antibiotics for "bladder infections." She also took birth control pills intermittently, beginning seven years ago, and had experienced vaginal yeast infections many times. Her diet included lots of junk foods including soft drinks. She also noted that exposure to perfumes and tobacco bothered her.

Three months before I first saw Phyllis, she had been comprehensively studied by a specialist in rheumatology. This physician examined her again in March, April and May, 1982, and here are excerpts from his medical report:

> "Phyllis continues to have polyarthritis, and in one instance had an episode of tenosynovitis of one wrist. She has a strongly positive FANA. Her anti-DNA antibodies were elevated at 42% and her serum complement is abnormal at 89 . . . *I therefore feel she probably has a definite*

rheumatoid arthritis without multi-system involvement. Because of the increase in her symptoms, I've started her on Plaquenil®, 200 mgs. twice daily, and a trial of Feldene® at 20 mgs. each day."

On May 3, 1982, I put Phyllis on nystatin, 1/4 teaspoon four times a day, and a yeast-free diet with some carbohydrate restriction. A week later her anti-arthritic drugs were discontinued because of a severe skin rash involving especially her hands.

Within a few weeks, Phyllis began to improve and when I saw her again in October 1982 she said,

"I'm much better. However, certain foods disagree with me and make my joint pains worse, including yeasts, wheat, sugar, milk, potatoes and beef."

I instructed Phyllis to avoid the foods that caused trouble, to rotate her diet and to continue her nystatin, vitamins and minerals. I also prescribed calcium and magnesium complex.

When Phyllis returned on April 9, 1983 for a review visit, she said,

"I've improved 100% since starting on my anti-yeast program. What's more, I was checked by my internist and all my blood tests are now normal. I still stay away from perfumes and smokes, and I have to be careful about my diet. I find it I take 1/2 teaspoon of nystatin at each dose, I feel better."

Credit for first recognizing the relationship of *Candida albicans* to patients with severe mental and neurological manifestations goes to Dr. C. Orian Truss. And in his first paper[51a] presented in the spring of 1977, Dr. Truss told of six patients with severe health problems who improved on anti-yeast therapy, including small doses of candida extract and nystatin.

One of his patients was a 36-year-old woman who had been treated for schizophrenia for six years.

"After many courses of drug and electroshock therapy, her condition had deteriorated to the point that permanent commitment to the state mental hospital had been recommended by her psychiatrist . . . This woman was treated for one year with nothing other than the *Candida albicans* extract. Follow-up ten years later found her well."

(A second patient)

. . . "A young white woman was relatively free of health problems until 24 years of age. Then after taking tetracycline, she promptly developed yeast vaginitis which recurred intermittently during the next three years."

This patient also

> " . . . began to have episodes of marked abdominal distention, associated with anxiety and depression."

Prementrual tension also became a severe problem.

Dr. Truss treated her with oral nystatin and her symptoms, including anxiety and depression, vanished.

Another patient, a 30-year-old woman, developed a visual field defect in November 1972. A year later, she developed numbness and tingling of both lower extremities.

> "The diagnosis of multiple sclerosis was made and discussed with the patient by her neurologist . . ."

In discussing this patient, Dr. Truss commented,

> "Again, the total picture is one of lifelong allergy, chronic intestinal and vaginal symptoms, and poor hormone function. Many courses of antibiotic were administered from childhood on. The initial neurological symptom occurred during massive antibiotic therapy over a four-month period for the severe lung infection" . . . "After two years of nystatin therapy neurological examination was 'entirely normal'."

In his third paper, 'The Role of Candida Albicans in Human Illness,"[51c] presented in September 1981, Dr. Truss briefly described the successful treatment of several patients with severe and often devastating health problems. One of these was the 30-year-old woman he had reported in his first paper.

> "She is entirely well now, seven years after nystatin was begun. She went through pregnancy with no trouble and delivered a normal baby."

He also told of several other patients with multiple sclerosis who improved on anticandida therapy. One of these, like my patient, Bob, was a 31-year-old woman who started . . . "improving immediately" on nystatin and who would remain asymptomatic unless she went "on a carbohydrate binge."

Dr. Truss also told me of one case of Crohn's disease which cleared, and he commented,

> "I know of two additional different auto-immune diseases, systemic lupus erythematosus and thrombocytopenic purpura, that have responded."

At the Informal Conference on Candida Albicans in July 1982, the relationship of multiple sclerosis and other severe auto-immune diseases was discussed by the participants in attendance.

Many physicians reported successful experiences in treating patients with these disorders with an anticandida program. Yet, a number of participants pointed out that other factors played a role in causing such illnesses. They also emphasized that individuals with severe auto-immune diseases, including those with multiple sclerosis who had been confined to wheel chairs for years, could anticipate little benefit from anticandida therapy.

To obtain current information about the experiences of other physicians I sent out a questionnaire in March 1983. One question asked, "How many patients with multiple sclerosis, lupus, arthritis, Crohn's disease or other auto-immune disease have you successfully treated using an anticandida program?"

One physician listed two patients with Crohn's disease and one with multiple sclerosis. Another physician listed one patient with Crohn's disease "who did well." One physician commented,

> "These diseases are multi-factoral. The candida approach only seems to play a part."

Another physician commented,

> "I can't answer this question, as I never treat these patients with just yeast eradication. However, I often start treatment with yeast eradication and many patients show significant improvement. Yet, I've rarely seen a patient who could correct the total disease process on a yeast eradication program alone."

Other physicians have found that patients with multiple sclerosis and other severe auto-immune diseases can be helped by an anticandida program.

Dr. E. W. Rosenberg, Professor and Chairman, Division of Dermatology, University of Tennessee Center for the Health Sciences in Memphis, recently described the successful treatment of psoriasis by a program designed to get rid of gut yeast. Here are excerpts from Dr. Rosenberg's letter in a recent issue of *The New England Journal of Medicine*:

> " . . . We have become aware . . . of improvement of both psoriasis and inflammatory bowel disease in patients treated with oral nystatin, an agent that was expected to work only on yeast in the gut lumen. We have now confirmed that observation in several of our patients with psoriasis. We suspect, therefore, that gut yeast may have a role in some instances of psoriasis."

More recently, Rosenberg & associates and Sidney Baker published a report on oral nystatin in the treatment of psoriasis in the

April 1984 issue of the *Archives of Dermatology*. They described the response of four patients with long-standing psoriasis to therapy with oral nystatin. Here are excerpts from this report:

> ". . . Baker reported improvement in the condition of patients with both psoriasis and inflammatory bowel disease when treated with oral nystatin. Oral nystatin is poorly absorbed from the gut and its effect is considered to be almost solely on yeasts in the gut microflora.
>
> "We have instituted a preliminary trial of oral nystatin in patients with psoriasis and have the distinct clinical impression that it may be an important agent in the treatment of many patients with psoriasis."

Their case reports were fascinating. The first patient was a 63-year-old man, whose psoriasis began at the age of 22. After four months of treatment with 500,000 units of oral nystatin four times a day for three months and a million units four times a day for one month,. . ."he had only some pale erythema and fine scale where before large thick plaques had previously been present."

Case 2 was a 65-year-old man who had psoriasis since 1950. ". . . He had thick scaling of his hands and many small lesions on his trunk and legs." On a million units of oral nystatin four times a day, after six months . . . "he was without any lesion except for some pale redness on his legs."

A third patient, a 55-year-old man, had a 10-year history of psoriasis of his scalp, elbows, sacrum and legs. After five months of nystatin therapy, . . . "all that remained of the eruption was a slight redness of his legs."

The fourth patient, a 37-year-old man, had a 25-year history of psoriasis. ". . . After only eight weeks of the nystatin therapy and the use of a selenium disulfide shampoo, there were no longer any lesions on his scalp, trunk, arms, or legs."

Does candida cause multiple sclerosis, psoriasis, arthritis, schizophrenia and other devastating auto-immune diseases?

No, candida isn't *the* cause.

Yet, there's growing evidence, based on the clinical experiences of many physicians, that the yeast organism, *Candida albicans,* is an important strand in the "web" of causes of these and other diseases.

32

Can Candida Albicans Make A "Teetotaler" Drunk?

According to a syndicated article[†] by Don G. Campbell from the Los Angeles Times News Service, January 1983, *Candida albicans* played a role in making "poor old Charlie Swaart" drunk, even though no alcohol had touched his lips. According to the article, Charlie Swaart was picked up for drunk driving following a dinner-theater party given by a prominent Arizona politician. Yet, he hadn't been drinking. "He had a 'still' in his intestines that was capable of converting carbohydrates directly into alcohol."

In thousands of "binges" spanning 30 years, Charlie Swaart would become "a sloppy, overbearing and hostile . . . sometimes even violent . . . drunk," even though he hadn't consumed any alcohol.

"Swaart's bouts were straining his private and professional life." Then, in the mid-1960s, a clue emerged that "nature was playing a cruel trick on Charlie." On a rigid, high protein, low-carbohydrate diet prescribed to curb weight, Charlie's episodes of drunkenness decreased. Then a friend gave him an article in an old (July 20, 1959) issue of *Time* magazine. This reprint told of a 46-year-old Japanese, Kozo Ohishi, and his 25-year binge that brought him social and professional disgrace and a besmirched army record.

According to the *Time* article, Ohishi was studied at Hokkaido University Hospital in Japan where samples were taken of his digestive juices. In them, microbiologists found a flourishing

---

[†]"The Ordeal of 'Poor Old Charlie,' Drinkless Drunk" by Don G. Campbell. Copyright, 1983, Los Angeles Times. Used by permission.

growth of a yeast-like fungus, *Candida albicans*. When treated with a Japanese anticandida drug, trichomycin, Ohishi stayed sober.

Swaart's Phoenix physician ordered tests "and they showed massive colonies of the yeasts" in his intestines . . . "His subsequent research established that about 60% of the population has some yeast in the alimentary canal, and that this yeast is capable of producing some alcohol in the stomach, but never to the level of intoxication.

Swaart was then treated with mycostatin (nystatin) and improved. However, "In 1970, the mycostatin began losing its punch, and the symptoms returned—with a vengeance."

Although 30 Japanese victims, ranging in age from 3 to 74, had been identified, Swaart was the first non-Japanese to be stricken with these peculiar candida-related health problems. So Dr. Kazuo Iwata, the professor of microbiology at the University of Tokyo School of Medicine, came by to visit Swaart at his Phoenix home. Cultures and microscopic examinations of Swaart's intestinal contents showed he had a "raging case" of *meitei-sho*[†].

But Swaart ran into a problem. "The drugs recommended by Iwata and found effective in Tokyo had not been approved by the Food and Drug Administration and were not available in the United States."

Swaart's problems continued until he flew to Tokyo where studies were done which showed that a new antifungal drug developed by Hoffman-La Roche in Switzerland was effective in helping him overcome his problem.

Since the drug wasn't available in the United States, he brought a year's supply home with him. This drug discouraged the growth of candida in Charlie's intestines. After taking the drug for some months, he was able to discontinue it in September 1975.[††]

[†]*Meitei-sho* is the name given by the Japanese to the syndrome of intoxication due to candida in the gut. *Meitei* means *drunk*; *sho* means *disease*. Hence, in Japanese: "drunk disease".

[††]In a recent letter to me, Charlie Swaart pointed out that *Meitei-sho* can recur, especially if a person takes antibiotics. Charlie stated, "To save my life during a pneumonia episode, doctors gave me antibiotics . . . I got up from my pneumonia sick bed to fall flat on my face with a *Meitei-sho* return . . . This syndrome can be controlled . . . prevented . . . and attacks avoided, but the problem of freedom from candida intoxication . . . once you've been a *Meitei-sho* victim, is eternal vigilance."

Swaart pointed out that *Meitei-sho* isn't rare and that he and his wife had received hundreds of telephone calls and letters from people all over the world describing similar *Meitei-sho* attacks. "In your book, you could be a great service by alerting the medical profession of the fact that my case is NOT a 'medical curiosity' but a candida syndrome that . . . is no longer confined to Japan."

33

Overcoming Yeast-Connected Illness Isn't Always Easy

Helping people overcome yeast-connected health problems has made my life interesting, challenging, rewarding and exciting. Some 90 percent of the hundreds of my patients with yeast-connected illness have improved. Many a patient reports,

> "I'm well. No problems. And I can even cheat on my diet without triggering symptoms."

Although each patient differs from every other patient, most have been helped by the comprehensive program of management described in Sections A, B, C, and F of this book.

Because of the favorable response, I feel confident that if you're bothered by yeast-connected health problems, *you, too, will improve and you can ultimately get well.* So I urge you to take the steps needed to accomplish such a goal.

But conquering yeast-connected health problems isn't always easy. And not all of my patients improved immediately . . . or even in a few months. Moreover, some who improved initially relapsed and an occasional patient became worse. Although diet, nystatin, nutritional supplements and avoiding environmental molds and chemicals help most of my patients, some have had to struggle with their problems for months or years after starting treatment. Since most of the people I've told you about in this book are "success stories," I feel I should present the "other side of the coin."

Forty-one-year-old Sandra first came to see me in April 1980. Here are excerpts from her 4-page letter:

> "I've been married for almost 22 years, and for 15 years I've been

bothered by persistent vaginal yeast infection. For at least 10 years I've had to make myself get out of bed every morning. I couldn't hear alarm clocks, so my husband would literally have to drag me out of bed. I feel tired and dazed, like a rag doll or a wet wash rag . . . I think I could sleep 24 hours a day and still feel sleepy and tired.

Over the years I've been to all sorts of doctors because of my many complaints, including aching in my neck, joints and legs, bronchitis, nervousness, weakness, rectal itching, noises in my ears, constipation, bloating . . . I get so depressed I've thought about taking my own life.

I've been hospitalized several times, but the tests never seemed to show anything. Chemicals of all sorts bother me, including several brands of perfume and air freshener. Also, my symptoms get worse when I eat sweetened foods or drink milk."

Because of her "typical history", I put Sandra on "the program", including diet, nystatin, nutritional supplements, environmental control and immunotherapy. She has steadily improved, although there have been ups and downs. And after more than three years of treatment, she continues to experience problems.

At a visit in June 1983, Sandra said,

"I'm still taking my nystatin and I occasionally take small doses of Nizoral® which always seem to help. Yet, when I cheat on my diet, my symptoms always flare. Although I feel a lot better than I felt three years ago, many symptoms continue to bother me. Rainy weather makes my joints and legs hurt and I'm still bothered by chemicals. Just going to the grocery store 'wipes me out' and I go into a drug-like sleep when I get home."

A second patient, 31-year-old Karen, a registered nurse and mother of four, first came to see me on October 1, 1981. And because her history illustrates so many important points, I'm reproducing in full a letter she wrote me November 19, 1982, 13 months after she started on a comprehensive program of treatment:

"As I write about my problems with yeast-related illness, I've been properly diagnosed and on anticandida treatment for over a year. All of my symptoms aren't gone, but I'm confident that continuing my prescribed treatment plan will some day get me well.

"As a child, I took many unneeded *antibiotics* for colds and well-meaning neighbors provided me with too much *candy*. Knowing what I know now, I feel both of these factors set the stage for my long battle with *vaginal problems*.

"Trouble with *menstrual cramps* began when I started my period at age 12. But after my first *yeast infection* at age 17, my cramps became severe enough to spend a day in bed every month. And during the week before each period, I was irritable, bloated and generally miserable.

224

"I began on birth control pills a month before my marriage at age 19. I took them for three months, but felt so bad I had to discontinue them. I promptly became *pregnant* and was bothered by *cystitis* and *vaginal yeast infections* throughout my pregnancy.

"The next 2½ years brought two more pregnancies, one of which was spontaneously aborted. During this time I was treated with antibiotics for 10 episodes of *'cystitis.'* Recently, my doctor commented, 'Many of your symptoms were probably caused by candida irritation of your bladder outlet . . . the urethra.'

"I also experienced *joint pains and swelling*, involving especially my knees. And I was given *cortisone* and other steroids on several occasions. I began to notice, for the first time, that getting around odorous cleaning materials made me sick.

"Then early in my third pregnancy, I had my first *migraine headache* and I had no idea that it could be related to diet and my other problems.

"After the birth of my second child, I took *birth control pills* for seven months, but once again I had to stop them because I felt worse than I'd ever felt in my life. My *vaginitis* continued and my *cystitis* was so severe that my gynecologist sent me to a urologist.

"I was put on a *broad-spectrum antibiotic* for six weeks and told to take antibiotics 'for the rest of my life' . . . anytime I had urgency and frequency for several days in a row.

"At the age of 25, my *migraine headaches* became so severe that I consulted a neurosurgeon. Various drugs were prescribed to control the migraines. Yet these drugs caused so many side-effects and so much emotional upset that I soon stopped them.

"About that time, I saw another gynecologist to see if he could help me control my *vaginal infections*. Although he was kind during my first visit, he finally lost his patience and told me "not to bother him" with something as unimportant as vaginal infections! He told me I'd have to learn to live with them.

"My *fourth pregnancy* at age 26 put more pressure on what I now realize was my *weakened immune system*. I was given *progesterone* for an irritable uterus and while I was taking it my vaginal problems were aggravated. And as I've since learned, pregnancy also worsens vaginal yeast problems.

"I went into labor at around 32 weeks and was given intravenous alcohol and *steroids*. Soon afterward, I experienced severe burning in my throat, esophagus and stomach which lasted for 5 months and kept me depressed and very uncomfortable.

"I also experienced *visual disturbances*, along with *abdominal bloating* and *constipation*. My *fatigue* was full-blown by now, but I attributed it to having a new baby.

"I also noticed that turning on the *gas heat* that winter triggered my *migraine* headaches and I remember saying to myself, 'it seems crazy to think the gas heat is making me sick'. Little did I know.

"Something I haven't mentioned before is the increased *craving for sweets* which I developed over a period of many years. And during my fifth pregnancy, at age 27, I ate plenty of good foods but added a lot of junk food, too. My *visual disturbances, fatigue* and *vaginal problems* were all prominent during this pregnancy. However, after the baby was born, I began eating a high protein, low carbohydrate diet which temporarily relieved some of my symptoms.

"Then at the age of 28, all of my previous symptoms either returned or became more prominent and I experienced many new ones, including *headache* and *severe abdominal pain.* This pain was so bad that my husband took me to the doctor on two occasions because he thought I had appendicitis.

"In the meantime, my *ability to concentrate decreased,* my *memory became worse* and I got up every morning *tired.* My *vaginal symptoms* of pain, burning, itching and heavy discharge were full-blown. I was taking *antibiotics* all the time as well as using different vaginal creams and suppositories. Nothing helped me and I became increasingly miserable.

"My *depression* became a real problem and I cried so easily for seemingly no reason, and my premenstrual tension became worse. My husband was very supportive and that helped. He would assure me that I wasn't 'crazy.' (Now that I'm better, he commented recently, 'I really thought I was going to lose you.')

"My gynecologist was kind and tried everything he knew to do. I hate to admit it now, but some days the thought of death was pleasant. The only thing that helped me get through many days was memorizing the Psalms of the Bible. As I cried, I'd quote the scriptures and I'd get hope to go on.

"At the age of 29, I had a *hysterectomy.* Some of my backache and abdominal pain improved for a while, and the premenstrual symptoms were gone. However, other symptoms developed, including *numbness and tingling of my extremities,* daily *visual problems, excessive intestinal gas* and throat mucus, *joint pain* and *heart palpitations.*

"I kept a *headache* that never left. Sometimes it was mild, at other times it was severe. I felt so horrible I would pray, 'Lord, Jesus, how can I keep living this way?' My gynecologist continued to be supportive, but I never told him of my many symptoms for fear he'd send me to a psychiatrist.

"Then in October, 1981, through a sort of unique coincidence (it was definitely an answer to my prayers), I first learned about yeast-related illness. Soon afterward, I was put on a comprehensive treatment program to help me get rid of candida, improve my immune system and regain my health.

"Many different things have helped me, including nystatin, Nizoral® and the yeast-free, low carbohydrate diet. Allergy vaccines for inhalants, foods and candida have also been essential parts of my treatment program. I've also been helped by nutritional supplements, including essential fatty acids, minerals and vitamins. A blood study sent to the Medical College of New Jersey (New Jersey Medical School, 88 Ross St., East Orange, New Jersey 07018) showed I was low in vitamin A, even though I'd been taking a multiple vitamin preparation containing supposedly adequate amounts of all the vitamins. Reducing my exposure to chemicals has also helped.

"Today, November 19, 1982, my vaginal symptoms are better but they are still present and bothersome. However, all the other problems are gone all or most of the time. I feel better than I have in many years and I'm grateful for the answer to my prayers."

Karen came in for a review visit on December 21, 1982. She commented,

> "I'm slowly getting better, but I still have my 'ups and downs.' Nystatin douches help my vaginitis, but the symptoms never go away and I must take tremendous doses of nystatin to control them . . . the equivalent of 48 to 50 tablets a day. I wish I could take Nizoral® again, it really helped last year. My candida shots in the weak dilutions help most of the time and I take them two or three times a week."

I continued Karen on the same basic program with a few modifications and changes. Because her liver enzymes had returned to normal, I added a small dose of Nizoral® to her treatment program . . . ¼ tablet twice a week. Mold cultures of her home showed that the mold, *hormodendrum*, was the principle offender. Appropriate changes were then made in Karen's extracts.

Karen returned for another visit on February 9, 1983. She commented,

> "I was involved in an automobile accident in January. I received many bruises and had to have a lot of x-rays. Although I experienced no serious injuries, I've been worse since the accident. I've had more vaginal burning and my fatigue level is high again. I was also bothered by a rash on two different days last week."

After reviewing Karen's treatment program, I suggested the following additional things which I hoped would help:

1. Laxative as needed to keep her colon cleaned out and hopefully get rid of some of the candida.
2. Enemas containing ½ to 1 teaspoon of nystatin to ½ pint of water. (A report from a Florida patient plus research studies from several sources indicate that candida colonization is greatest in the colon. Accordingly, reaching and killing these organisms from below would appear especially appropriate.)
3. Because I'd also learned that the Squibb preparation, amphotericin B (see chapter 37) was available in France and Switzerland, I made arrangements to obtain some of this preparation to see if it would help. I also discontinued the Nizoral®.

On March 28, 1983, Karen again returned. Here are a few of her comments:

> "That automobile accident really set me back. My vaginitis continues to bother me and my fatigue level remains high. My prescription for

amphotericin B was filled by a French pharmacy and sent to me a couple of weeks ago. I started taking it, but so far it hasn't helped.

On May 16, 1983, Karen reported,

"I'm improving and I've finally gotten back to where I was before my accident in January. My fatigue and joint pains are better although on damp days when the mold count is high, I don't feel as good. I'm continuing the oral and vaginal amphotericin B. I dump the contents of 1 capsule in my mouth four times daily and insert the powder from 1 capsule into my vagina twice daily. This seems to work better than nystatin in doses of over a teaspoon of powder four times daily. (For a discussion of amphotericin B, see chapter 37).

"I'm also following all of the other parts of the comprehensive program of management you prescribed, including inhalant and food vaccines, linseed oil, primrose oil and other nutritional supplements. I also have restricted my diet to meats, eggs and vegetables for the past 10 days but can't tell that leaving off fruits and grains has made a significant difference.

"So to repeat, I'm really doing well with all symptoms except the vulvovaginitis which continues to cause varying degrees of discomfort and frustration."

On January 3, 1984, Karen commented,

"Everything is better. I'm even free of vaginal pain and discomfort most of the time. I feel great, lots of energy and none of the other symptoms I used to have unless I cheat on my diet. And I did cheat during the holidays and had brownies. Within twelve hours, I developed bladder urgency, frequency and pain, even though I found I don't have an infection. Also, I still can't tolerate perfumes, chemicals or mold exposure.

My next two patients came to see me early in 1983. The first of these, 31-year old Sue, first consulted me on February 8, 1983. Here are excerpts from the long letter she wrote:

"My health problems began many years ago. During my high school years I was bothered by headaches and sore throats; while in college, I developed bladder infections which have recurred many times. Nevertheless, I felt good most of the time.

"Immediately after graduation from college in May 1974, I began working with a fascinating company and I continue to work for them. In July 1974, I was married and from that time on I've been going down hill. First it was just one small illness after another and in between I felt OK. However, I began to feel tired most of the time. I was bothered by abdominal symptoms which were diagnosed as "spastic colon." During the year I was constantly plagued by one thing after another. Incidentally, I had begun taking birth control pills.

"By the spring of 1975, I was taken off the pill and I seemed to get better for a time, but then my headaches and sinus troubles returned.

Allergy testing showed sensitivity to molds and weeds. I took injections for several years but they didn't really help. Meanwhile, my general health deteriorated, with headaches, sore throats and general aches and pains. All of my friends would joke and call me 'sickly Sue'. I never felt good.

"In 1979, during my pregnancy, my headaches increased in frequency and severity. I also experienced my first vaginal yeast infection and kept it for months. Worst of all, I began having bouts of fast heart beat (the doctors called it 'paroxysmal tachycardia'). For a time after my baby was born, I felt better for a couple of months but then my fatigue returned. Most of the time I ached all over and kept a sore throat. During the years, 1980-81, I was taking antibiotics almost constantly, including Terramycin®, Vibramycin®, Panmycin®, ampicillin, Keflex® and Septra®. Finally, in March, 1982 my tonsils were removed. Infections continued.

"During the past couple of years, I've been given all sorts of tests, including cardiograms, x-rays and a glucose tolerance test. The latter test resulted in a diagnosis of 'hypoglycemia'.

"Six weeks ago, my headaches took on a new dimension. The only think I had done differently was to take a lot of a 'health-energy protein drink' which I later found contained yeast. I'm at a loss as to what's wrong with me, and I continue to have headaches, tachycardia and fatigue. I'm susceptible to every germ that comes along. I go to bed tired and wake up tired. I can sleep half the day away when the opportunity arises. Please help me get well."

Because of her typical history, I put Sue on the anticandida program, including diet, nystatin and nutritional supplements.
On March 15th, Sue said

"I'm a little better, although my headaches still come and go."

In May she reported,

"I'm still experiencing many problems and although I'm improving, all of my symptoms bother me."

Sue returned for a comprehensive checkup on July 5, 1983. And in a treatment diary she commented,

"I work every day and I'm a productive person. Yet, I'm struggling. I worry because I weigh 5 pounds less than when I started. Headaches are still my major symptoms and weakness and bouts of tachycardia continue, even though I've been taking 1/2 teaspoon of nystatin four times a day and eating mainly meats and vegetables."

Because of Sue's persistent problems, in spite of 5 months on 'the program,' I prescribe Nizoral®. In addition, because her morning temperature readings were only 96.5° to 97° (in spite of normal thyroid tests), I also prescribed a half grain of thyroid once daily. Then because Sue said,

> "Several foods, including eggs and beef bother me; yet I feel I need to eat these foods to keep from wasting away,"

I scheduled Sue for food testing and possible immunotherapy with food extracts.

Another recent patient, Matilda, a 50-year-old teacher was first seen on February 11, 1983. Here are excerpts from her 8-page letter:

> "Since September, 1980, I've been trapped in a cycle of chronic pain and intermittent depression. I've taken all sorts of medicine, including antibiotics, tranquillizers, pain pills and decongestants. My symptoms, including pain in my head and legs, anger and mood swings became so frightening, I saw a psychotherapist. I went to other physicians including a gynecologist who said my symptoms were "menopausal." In addition, I've been troubled by recurrent vaginal yeast infections, abdominal pain and extreme fatigue, and exposure to chemicals, especially fabric shop odors, causes severe symptoms."

Because of her typical history, I put Matilda on a comprehensive treatment program including nystatin, diet and nutritional supplements. At a follow-up visit two weeks later, Matilda reported,

> "I've had my ups and downs. One exciting thing . . . my ears stopped ringing. However, I continue to be bothered by strange thinking disturbances and hallucinations at night."

Nystatin and diet were continued. At a visit in March, Matilda said,

> "Although my upper respiratory symptoms are better, my cerebral symptoms are bad and my chemical sensitivity is severe. I itch all over my body. I'm wondering if my dentures and fixed bridges could contribute to my problem, since my gums have been bleeding."

At a followup visit on April 22, Matilda said,

> "I've increased my nystatin to ½ teaspoon four times a day; yet this causes a lot of 'die-off' symptoms."

At a visit on May 15, she reported,

> "My vaginitis continues to cause severe discomfort even though I'm staying on my diet, taking nystatin and using vaginal suppositories. Four or five days ago I was so confused I was running around town like a frightened rabbit. Perhaps it was related to my premenstrual hormones. I got better when I started my period."

Because of Matilda's continuing severe symptoms, including 'die-off' symptoms from nystatin, on May 15th I prescribed Nizoral®. At a visit on May 23, Matilda said,

> "I couldn't tolerate the Nizoral®, it caused severe burning in my stomach. Damp days make me feel terrible. My house also makes me sick, especially since my husband continues to smoke. I really need to be in a hospital. *I feel terribly discouraged.*"

I encouraged Matilda to "Stay the course" and to continue with her diet, nystatin, environmental control and nutritional supplements. I hope she'll soon improve. Yet, like several of my other patients with complex problems who live in homes or areas contaminated by high levels of chemicals or molds, she may have to move or make drastic changes in her home in order to improve significantly.

It should now be obvious that health problems in people with yeast-connected illness are related to a *weakened immune system.* Or, putting it in simple terms, *"lowered resistance."*

In most patients with these disorders, illness develops over a period of many months and years. Moreover, the causative factors tend to be multiple and complex.

Strengthening the immune system and regaining health may occasionally be quick and easy. *More often, it takes time, patience, persistence and careful management of the multiple factors contributing to the illness.*

Section
E

Other
helpful
information

34

Miscellaneous Measures That May Help You

Suppose you're taking antifungal medication, following your diet and are improving. Some of your symptoms have disappeared, others are less frequent and/or less severe. Yet you're wondering and asking, "How long will I need to take nystatin. . . . (or other antifungal medication)? How long will I need to stay on my diet? Are there other things I can do that may help?"

Elsewhere in this book, I've emphasized the importance of avoiding sugar and junk food. I've also pointed out that you may need to take antifungal medication for many months . . . even a year or longer. I've also talked about allergies, including especially food allergies, avoiding chemicals, taking vitamin, mineral and fatty acid supplements, and psychological support.

In this chapter, I'll review and repeat some of my comments and add suggestions I've obtained from various sources, including my patients and other physicians:

1. *Hidden Food Allergies:* Adverse or allergic reactions to any food, including such protein foods as milk, egg, beef or soy, may be contributing to your health problems. To identify such food troublemakers, try the "cave man" diet for a week and see if your symptoms get better. *In carrying out this diet you must avoid any and every food you eat more often than once a week.* Then if your symptoms improve return the foods to your diet one at a time and carefully note any adverse reactions. (You'll find complete instructions for carrying out this diet in my book, *Tracking Down Hidden Food Al-*

lergy[13]). This book is available in many health food stores. Or it can be ordered from Professional Books, Box 3494, Jackson, TN 38303.

2. *Rotated Diets:* If you're eating the same food every day, you may develop an intolerance or allergy to that food. To keep this from happening, rotate your diet (see chapter 15).

3. *Multivitamin and Mineral Supplements:* Take a yeast-free, sugar-free, color-free vitamin/mineral preparation. These supplements are available from a number of sources. I recommend a daily intake of 1000 to 1500 mgs. of vitamin C, 25 to 100 mgs. of most of the B vitamins with 30 micrograms of vitamin B-12, 15 to 30 mgs. of zinc, 50 to 100 mcg. of selenium, 5,000 to 10,000 units of vitamin A, 400 international units of vitamin E, plus other nutrients and micronutrients. READ LABELS CAREFULLY. If you're allergic to yeast, make sure the preparations you take contain no yeast.

4. *Vitamin C Powder:* In general, there are two powdered forms of vitamin C: ascorbic acid and buffered forms, including calcium ascorbate. A teaspoon of powder contains 3,500 to 4,000 milligrams of vitamin C. I've found that vitamin C in large doses (2,000 to 20,000 mgs. or more daily) helps many of my patients with immune system problems. Included among these patients are those with yeast-connected illness. The total dose can be monitored by using the "bowel tolerance" test of double Nobel Prize winner, Linus Pauling, Ph.D.[21] and Robert F. Cathcart, M.D.[54]

Vitamin C Powder

In discussing the usage of large doses of vitamin C, Dr. Pauling commented, saying in effect,

> "Persons with viral infections or under other types of stress can take gradually increasing doses of vitamin C to strengthen the immune system. If and when the vitamin C causes diarrhea or digestive upset, the dose can be decreased."

And in comments on a popular television show and in lay magazines, Dr. Cathcart told of his remarkable success in treating AIDS with huge doses of vitamin C by mouth, plus intravenous vitamin C.

Norman Cousins, in his book, *Anatomy of an Illness,*[31] describes his own personal experiences with large doses of vitamin C. Mr. Cousins took 25,000 mgs. of vitamin C each day for a number of days and his physicians felt this therapy played a significant role in his recovery from a severe illness. One of my colleagues, Susan Karlgaard, commented,

> "I take 5,000 to 20,000 mgs. of vitamin C every day. I find it especially helps when I've been exposed to chemicals or when I've eaten the wrong food."

A 13-year-old patient (I'll call him Harvey) with severe asthma came in with an attack of wheezing in March 1983. This youngster had been hospitalized many times and had received all types of therapy from pediatricians, allergists, and pulmonary specialists. Harvey's skin tests showed sharp reactions to many environmental inhalants, including especially molds. He was also sensitive to a number of foods and received many antibiotics and courses of steroids. He was taking regular, around-the-clock bronchodilators, immunotherapy, cromolyn solution inhalations, nystatin and a yeast-free diet, with intermittent injections of Adrenalin® and Susphrine®.

In spite of these measures, he was experiencing increasing difficulty during the two days prior to his visit to me. He and his mother were reluctant to go back on prednisone and enter the hospital for more intensive therapy.

I increased Harvey's nystatin from 1/8 teaspoon four times daily to 1/2 teaspoon (2 million units) each dose, and, out of desperation and more or less as a "shot in the dark," I decided to try him on large doses of vitamin C. I instructed his mother to get vitamin C powder containing 1 part ascorbic acid and 1 part calcium ascorbate . . . 4,000 mgs. per teaspoon . . . and to give Harvey 1 teaspoon in a glass of water every 1 to 2 hours if tolerated.

Harvey took 35,000 mgs. of vitamin C by mouth for each of the next three days. His wheezing began to improve in 12 hours and cleared by the end of 48 hours and no further injections of Adrenalin® were required. By the end of the third day, Harvey's stools became loose and his dose of vitamin C was decreased to 10,000 to 15,000 mgs. per day. When rechecked two weeks later, he was being continued on this same dose and his mother commented,

> "The vitamin C really made a difference."

In a follow-up conversation with Harvey's mother on May 18, 1983, she commented,

> "Even though we're right in the middle of the grass pollen season,

Harvey is doing great . . . at least great for him. He's outdoors every day running and playing. He is even planning to run in a mile race. He's still taking 12,000 mgs. of vitamin C each day plus his nystatin, cromolyn and Vaponefrin® inhalations and immunotherapy.

On July 15, 1983, I received the following report:

"Harvey continues to do exceedingly well and is going to camp for the first time in his life. The nystatin and vitamin C truly make a difference. Other therapies, including his cromolyn and Vaponefrin®, had never controlled his wheezing until he began on big doses of nystatin and vitamin C. Also, if he forgets to take either his nystatin or vitamin C, he notices chest tightness.

"Something else of interest is my other 5 children came down with a bad virus . . . high fever and vomiting. One had to be hospitalized. Yet, Harvey didn't get sick. I think the nystatin and vitamin C may have strengthened his immune system."

5. *Calcium and magnesium supplements:* Unless you take dairy products, salad greens, clams or oysters on a regular basis, chances are you aren't getting enough calcium. I recommend supplemental calcium in a dose of 1000 to 1500 milligrams a day, along with 400 to 600 milligrams of magnesium.

6. *Essential fatty acids:* Unprocessed oils, including especially evening primrose oil and linseed oil, contain vital nutrients, including GLA (gamma-linolenic acid) and CLA (cis-linoleic acid). Your body needs these substances to make a family of hormone-like compounds called *prostaglandins*. These substances play a vital role in controlling normal functions of every organ of the body.

You can obtain evening primrose oil in capsule form from many pharmacies and most health food stores. The recommended dose is 1 or 2 capsules two to three times a day. Linseed oil can also be obtained from most health food stores and I recommend 1 to 2 teaspoons a day.† It can be combined with freshly squeezed lemon juice and used for salad dressing.

You can learn more about essential fatty acids from the

---

†According to Dr. Donald Rudin, some individuals are sensitive to tablespoon-size amounts of linseed oil. Yet they respond favorably to 1/2-1 teaspoon of the oil twice daily.

pamphlet, "Evening Primrose Oil," by Richard A. Passwater, Ph.D., published by Keats Publishing Co., Inc., 35 Grove St. (Box 876), New Canaan, Connecticut 06840, and from a fascinating article by David Horrobin, Ph.D. in the June 1981 *Executive Health* (9605 Scranton Rd., Ste 710, San Diego, CA. 92121). (See chapter 43, Update for a more comprehensive discussion of the essential fatty acids).

7. *Iron supplements: If you're anemic, you're apt to feel tired and weak because you don't have enough oxygen-carrying red cells. You may also show a lessened resistance to invaders of any type, including* Candida albicans. Although I haven't found anemia to occur commonly in my candida patients, two of my consultants (in the field of veterinary medicine) found that iron supplements play an important role in helping their animal patients overcome candidiasis. (See chapter 44, Update). Whether their experiences in treating animals with iron supplements are applicable to humans with interrelated health disorders remains uncertain.

   If you'd like to learn more about the role of anemia and iron therapy in individuals with candida-related disorders, you can find additional information on these subjects on page 202 of the 1979 book[†], CANDIDA AND CANDIDOSIS[‡] by F. C. Odds, B.Sc., Ph.D., a microbiologist of the University of Leicester (England).

8. *Intravaginal nystatin:* Candida makes its home on all of the mucous membranes of the body, including the vagina. Even if you aren't bothered by vaginal symptoms, use intravaginal nystatin once or twice daily or a suppository containing anticandida medication. Here's a convenient and economical way to accomplish this: After your bath, moisten your finger and coat it with $1/8$ teaspoon of nystatin, then insert it high into your vagina. Other intravaginal, anticandida medications are also available, including Gyne-Lotrimin®,

---

[†]This book was published in the U.S.A. and Canada by University Park Press, 233 East Redwood Street, Baltimore, Maryland 21202.
[‡]*Candidosis* and *candidiasis* are used interchangeably. *Candidosis* is the term used in England and *candidiasis* in America. Moreover, *candidosis* is actually a more logical term since the names of most other fungal infections end in "..osis", while the names of parasitic infections ends in "..iasis".

Monistat-7® suppositories or cream and Mycelex G® cream.

9. *Sniffing or inhaling nystatin:* Nasal congestion occurs commonly in people with yeast-related health disorders. Moreover, candida colonization often occurs in the nose as well as in the digestive tract or vagina. Nasal candidiasis is especially prevalent in persons who've used nasal steroids.

You can often help your nasal congestion, post nasal drip and mental and nervous symptoms by inhaling nystatin. Here's how you do it: Shake your bottle of nystatin powder vigorously. Remove the cap and hold the bottle just under your nose. Sniff or inhale cautiously. Do this each time you take your oral nystatin.

If you tolerate this procedure, gradually increase the amount you inhale over the course of several days. Usually 3 or 4 inhalations of nystatin "smoke" will allow the medication to settle on your deeper nasal and sinus membranes.

A word of caution: Sometimes your symptoms worsen the first several days you try this procedure. However, stick with it and you may find your symptoms will improve within a few days.

Here's an alternate way of getting nystatin into your upper respiratory passages: Prepare a fresh solution of nystatin, adding ¼ teaspoon of powder to 4 ounces of boiled and previously cooled water containing ¼ teaspoon of table salt. Using an ordinary medicine dropper, hold your head back and fill both of your nostrils with the solution. Then swing your head forward rapidly and hold it down between your legs for 2 minutes. Then sit up and let the mixture trickle down your throat.

Here's an even more convenient way of getting nystatin into your nasal passages: Buy a bottle of Ocean Mist Nasal Spray® from your pharmacy. This is an isotonic saline nasal spray. Add ¹⁄₁₆ to ⅛ teaspoon of nystatin powder to the bottle and use one or two squirts in each nostril twice daily.

Nancy, a 36-year-old factory worker with severe yeast-connected problems including fatigue, depression and poor memory, started on a comprehensive treatment program in April 1983. Her symptoms included extreme fatigue, depression, muscle and joint pain, gastro-intestinal symptoms, vaginitis and memory problems. In a followup report on July 1, 1983, Nancy commented,

"Everything is better, I'm back at work, I've thrown away all my arthritis medicine. And sniffing the nystatin several times a day helps my nasal congestion and memory problems."

Ann, the 30-year-old daughter of Dorothy commented,

"My nose runs all the time, during every season of the year."

Ann was never without a Kleenex® and she usually carried the tissue in her hand. Because Dorothy improved so much on nystatin, she encouraged Ann to try the nystatin nose drops. After using them for a week, Ann's nose cleared. And in a recent phone call she commented,

"This is the first time I've enjoyed a dry nose in 20 years."

Your nose may run because of allergies to dozens of things ranging from cat dander to chemicals and from pollens to potatoes. However, if you're troubled by yeast-connected health problems and upper respiratory symptoms persist, a trial of intranasal nystatin may help.

10. *Nystatin enemas:* In their article on "Chronic Mucocutaneous Candidiasis," Doctors Charles H. Kirkpatrick and Peter G. Sohnle[44] described *Candida albicans* studies carried out on normal adults by Cohen and associates. The candida organisms were recovered from 30% of the cultures of the mouth and throat, 54% and 55% of various segments of the small intestine, and 65% of the fecal samples. So it would appear that more candida is found in the lower part of the bowel tract than in the upper part.

Another study by Hofstra[45] and associates showed that even after large doses of oral nystatin, many stool specimens often contain no measureable amounts of the drug. Accordingly, a nystatin enema would appear to have merit. I particularly recommend nystatin enemas for individuals with severe yeast-connected illness, especially those characterized by multiple bowel symptoms, including persistent constipation, who aren't improving using other therapeutic measures.

Here's other data which make me feel that nystatin enemas are extremely worthwhile even though I've had little experience in using them with my patients:

Nystatin acts on intact yeast cells. It binds to components of the yeast cell membranes and, in effect, chisels holes in the membrane. Contents of the yeast cell leak out and the yeast cell dies. So it's obvious that it's important to get the nystatin and the yeast germs together.

Before using a *nystatin enema*, empty your colon using a laxative or cleansing enema.† Then add ¼ to ½ teaspoon of nystatin to 8 ounces of salt water (½ teaspoon of salt to 8 ounces of water). Retain the enema solution as long as possible.

11. *"Die-off" reactions following nystatin:* When you kill out yeast germs on your intestinal, respiratory or vaginal membranes, you absorb products from these dead yeast germs which temporarily worsen your symptoms. Don't be discouraged. "Stay the course". The more yeast you get rid of, the sooner you'll get better. Many individuals who think that nystatin disagrees with them are experiencing these "die-off" reactions. And others who think garlic, onions or cabbage disagree, may be experiencing similar reactions.

Each person is different. When nystatin continues to cause symptoms, including fatigue, depression, aching, feeling "slowed down" and cold, these symptoms can often be relieved by taking a bigger dose of nystatin.

On the other hand, if you're taking ½ teaspoon of nystatin and notice that you feel feverish, flushed, stimulated, talkative and other "hyper" symptoms, try taking a smaller dose.

Some patients feel better when they start nystatin, and then weeks later nystatin disagrees. When this happens, the dose should be varied up or down until symptoms are relieved. If adjustment of the nystatin dose continues to present a problem, the efficacy of the nystatin can be enhanced by using garlic, vitamin A and other nutritional supplements, including zinc. Or the carbohydrate content of the diet may temporarily need to be lowered.

12. *Mold control in your home:* Take a look at your house or your workplace. If it's damp and moldy, take measures to reduce the mold content. (See also chapter 9.)

---

†Cleaning out the lower bowel may help even though nystatin isn't used. Why? I don't know. Yet, I've heard Dr. Denis Burkitt talk about the importance of a rapid bowel "transit time". Moreover I've read a number of reports in the medical and lay literature about toxins of various sorts that develop in intestinal contents when emptying time is delayed.

Also the recent report by Zamm (see chapter 37) suggests that a low residue diet and enemas mechanically remove candida spores and mycelia along with intestinal material these organisms thrive on. In addition I have received many other anecdotal reports from physicians, nurses and other health practitioners who have found that cleaning out the colon helps the candida patients—especially the individual who suffers from persistent constipation and bloating.

13. *Lessen your exposure to chemicals:* Make sure you're keeping your chemical exposure at a low level. Perfumes, colognes, cigarette smoke, insecticides, furniture polishes, detergents, gas cooking stoves and other chemical exposures can

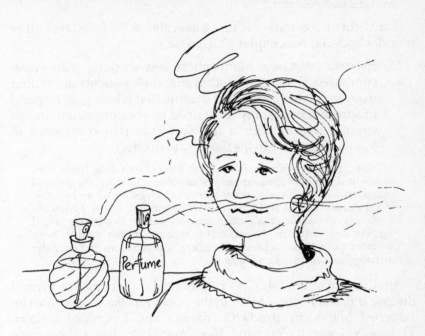

make you ill . . . especially if your immune system is already weakened by candida (see also chapter 17).

14. *Lactobacillus acidophilus* (and other friendly bacteria): The beneficial effects of these friendly germs have been recognized for a long time. They compete with and help control candida in the digestive tract. Moreover, yogurt . . . more especially home-prepared yogurt[†] . . . has been used successfully in treating vaginitis caused by *Candida albicans.*

[†]According to Professor Marvin L. Speck and associates of the Department of Food Science, North Carolina State University, Raleigh, N.C., commercial yogurt products may *not* contain appreciable numbers of *Lactobacillus acidophilus.* (As quoted by Von Hilsheimer, G. L.: "Acidophillus and the Ecology of the Human Gut," Journal of Orthomolecular Psychiatry, 11:3, 1982, pp. 204-207.)

In commenting on lactobacilli, John W. Rippon, Ph.D., had this to say,

> *"Lactobacillus acidophilus, especially if you consume it on a regular basis, restores normal flora to the intestinal tract. I feel it will help patients with yeast-connected health disorders."*

(For a further discussion of *Lactobacillus acidophilus* and other friendly bacteria, see chapter 43, Update.)

15. *Hormone imbalance:* Many physicians working with yeast-connected illness have found that their patients also suffer from endocrine (hormone) dysfunction which may respond to appropriate therapy prescribed by your physician. In discussing this subject at the San Francisco conference in March 1985, Dr. Phyllis Saifer said in effect,

> "Many patients with environmental illness, including those with yeast-connected problems, appear to have thyroiditis. Yet, the physical examination of the thyroid often shows no irregularities and routine blood studies (T-3, T-4 and TSH) may all be entirely normal. Precise diagnosis is often difficult, although measurement of T-cells may help. I suspect thyroiditis, in the difficult-to-manage, brittle patient, with symptoms of fatigue, depression, chilling, constipation, and irregular menses." (see chapter 42, Update.)

Another physician who has commented on inapparent thyroid disease is Broda Barnes, M.D. In the book *Hypothyroidism: The Unsuspected Illness,* by Broda O. Barnes and Lawrence Galton, Thomas Y. Crowell Company, New York, 1976, the authors comment,

> "The normal range of basal temperature is between 97.8° and 98.2° Fahrenheit. When symptoms of thyroid deficiency are present, the basal temperature may be 1 to even 3 degrees below normal. With thyroid therapy, the temperature will start to rise."

Dr. Barnes suggests 10-minute axillary temperatures for 7 straight days before you get out of bed in the morning. If your temperature is consistently under 97.8 to 98.2, the possibility of thyroid deficiencies should be considered and a therapeutic trial of thyroid is recommended.

If you feel you're bothered by unsuspected hypothyroidism, get a copy of the book, *Solved: The Riddle of Illness,* by Stephen E. Langer, M.D., with James F. Scheer, Keats Publishing Co., Inc., New Canaan, Connecticut, 1984.

Treatment with progesterone may be indicated in some patients with premenstrual syndrome (see chapter 27) and therapy with estrogen may be indicated in patients with menopausal symptoms.

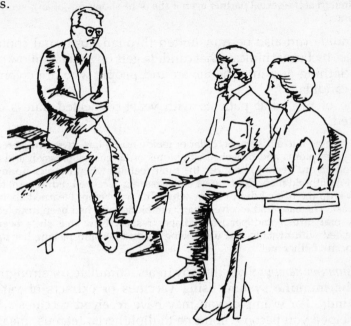

16. *Treat the marital partner and/or other family members:* Candida, like other microorganisms, can be transmitted from person to person through intimate contact of various sorts including sexual relations. Although the sexual partner with a strong immune system may not appear to be bothered by candida-related health problems, I've gradually come to feel that such a partner should be treated. So do a number of my colleagues.

In April 1986, Dr. Harold Hedges of Little Rock, Arkansas, commented:

"I always treat the sexual partner even if the partner shows no symptoms. One of my recent patients had been experiencing persistent problems which weren't responding to treatment. After she was divorced, she immediately began to improve. Although a part of her improvement may have been due to other causes, including less psychological stress, I feel that candida organisms were being passed back and forth through intimate contact."

And Dr. Richard Mabray of Victoria, Texas, commented,

> "I feel wives can infect husbands with candidiasis and vice versa. So I often treat the sexual partner even if she or he shows few, if any, symptoms."

Candida can also be transmitted through nonsexual contacts. Studies by Lucas[4] indicate that candida gets on sheets, pillow cases and clothing and into the air around people who are colonized with candida.

One of my adult patients with yeast-connected illness commented,

> "Going into a basement, cellar or moldy house has always triggered my symptoms and provoked symptoms of fatigue, depression and a 'spaced out' feeling. I noticed the same feelings when I'd pick up my 18-month-old niece. It got to be embarrassing because I didn't want to pick up the baby. I didn't know why. This was before I learned about yeast. The baby had received many antibiotics and had been troubled by oral thrush and persistent diaper rashes. Now that she's been treated with nystatin and diet, being around her and picking her up doesn't bother me!"

17. *Immunotherapy:* Such therapy treats, stimulates or strengthens the immune system using vaccines or extracts of various kinds. For example, you may have received vaccines which helped you become immune to diphtheria, tetanus, measles, polio and other diseases. *Immunotherapy* has also been successfully used since the early 1900s in treating individuals bothered by allergic rhinitis ("hay fever") and asthma caused by pollens, dusts and molds. Yet, as recently as 1961 Francis Cabot Lowell, M.D., of Boston[†] said, in effect,

> "We allergists give many of our patients shots and we keep on giving them because they seem to help. Yet, we don't understand how and why they are effective and it is possible that we're helping our patients because of other things we're doing rather than because of our shots."

Then in about 1967 two Japanese researchers, the Ishizakas, made an exciting discovery which helped put the study of allergies on a more scientific basis. They found that individuals with pollen, mold and dust allergies and severe food allergies nearly always showed elevations in a fraction of the blood which they called *immunoglobulin* E (or *Ig*E). Subsequent studies in the 1970s and '80s

---

[†]Presidential address, American Academy of Allergy.

showed that following immunotherapy these abnormal laboratory findings (in individuals with inhalant allergies) would improve. Moreover, accompanying the lower IgE levels, patients with inhalant allergies would show fewer symptoms.

Yet in spite of the "IgE breakthrough" and other breath-taking advances in allergy and immunology research, many questions have remained unanswered. In addition controversies have arisen between allergists of different persuasions.

Some allergists (I'll call them "Group A") insist that the term "allergy" should apply *only* to those disorders which can be demonstrated by presently available immunologic or laboratory studies . . . including the allergy scratch test.

Other allergists (I'll call them "Group B") agree in part with the Group A doctors and include under the term "allergy" the immunologically proven disorders which can be confirmed in the laboratory and which show a positive skin test. Yet, they feel the term "allergy" should also be used to apply to disorders caused by food and chemical sensitivities even though the mechanisms of these reactions cannot always be demonstrated.

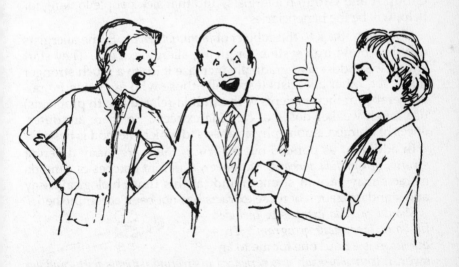

So a "tug of war" has been going on in the field of allergy. The differences of opinion have confused and frustrated many allergy sufferers; but, there seems to be a "light at the end of the tunnel." For example, in his award winning Bela Schick lecture for 1984

William T. Kniker, M.D.,[†] emphasized the importance of treating immunologically proven "classical allergies" (asthma caused by pollen and other inhalants). He also pointed out that there are other equally important mechanisms that make people sick and that such illnesses are often indistinguishable from those caused by traditional allergies. He stated:[‡]

> "In addition, there are countless millions of other individuals who have unrecognized adverse reactions to various antigens, foods, chemicals and environmental or occupational triggers . . . These agents may activate mediators of inflammation . . . by immunologic, chemical, idiosyncratic, physical, neurogenic and infectious triggering routes. The acquired disease may be limited to body surfaces or may involve a puzzling array of organ symptoms, causing the patient to visit a number of different kinds of specialists, who are unsuccessful in recognizing that an allergic or adverse reaction is going on."

Although Dr. Kniker didn't mention *Candida albicans* as one of the infectious "triggering agents" that could activate pathogenic mechanisms, I feel that the concepts that he presented will play an important role in bridging the communication gap between the Group A and Group B allergists, and that sick people looking for help, will be the beneficiaries.

Now then. Back to the subject of *immunotherapy*. Some allergists use the "build up" system for giving allergy extracts. They start with a weak dose and gradually increase it up to a much stronger dose. Yet, other allergists (especially those who are using immunotherapy for their patients with candida-related health problems) use much weaker doses of candida extracts. So there are differences of opinion among physicians as to which method is best.

In addition, as pointed out by Truss, there are many different strains of *Candida albicans*. Moreover, different batches of candida extracts may vary in strength and (at this time) biological assay and standardization of these extracts has not been accomplished.

Should candida extracts be included in your treatment program? This question is a hard one for me to answer. *If your physician is experienced in treating patients with candida-*

---

†Professor of Pediatrics and Microbiology; Head, Division of Clinical Immunology, Department of Pediatrics, University of Texas Health Science Center, San Antonio, TX.
‡Kniker, W.T. "Deciding the Future for the Practice of Allergy and Immunology". Annals of Allergy SS: 109-110, (Aug.) 1985.

related health disorders, and more especially, in using candida extracts, I'd answer "yes", they can be helpful. Yet, no precise protocols have yet been established which will suit every patient.

In my own patients with candida-related health disorders, I always recommend diet, antifungal medication, nutritional supplements, exercise, avoidance of chemicals and appropriate life style changes. I also may prescribe or administer candida extracts. However, I do not usually use them until the other measures have been carried out.

18. *Air ionizers:* The air we breathe contains molecules with positive and negative electrical charges. Research studies over a period of several decades show that those who live or work in closed spaces and in environments containing more positive ions than negative ions develop a variety of symptoms. Typical manifestations include fatigue, headache, drowsiness, irritability, nasal discharge, burning eyes and cough. These and other symptoms commonly found in individuals with yeast-connected health disorders may be helped by a negative ion generator. Such generators cost between $75 and $125 and are available from many sources. Further information on the effect of ions can be found in the medical[48a-b] and lay literature[49].

19. *Larger doses of vitamin A:* In his book *Candida and Candidosis,*[3] Dr. F. C. Odds points out that independent studies show that mice and rats are less susceptible to candida when given high doses of vitamin A. Yet, vitamin A can be toxic if used in large doses for many months.

Accordingly, when my patients aren't doing well, I usually check their blood vitamin A level. Here's why: Many patients with chronic health problems, especially those involving the gastrointestinal tracts, may not absorb nutrients they ingest.

If the vitamin A level is low or borderline low, I prescribe 25,000 International Units daily for a month and then recheck the blood level. An occasional patient will require even larger doses. (Physicians and patients interested in a comprehensive review of vitamin A may wish to consult the article by *Donald R. Davis, Ph.D.* of the University of Texas entitled, "Using Vitamin A Safely.")[†]

---

†Davis, D.R. "Using Vitamin A Safely," *Osteopathic Medicine,* 3:31-43, 1978.

20. *Wood burning stoves and fireplaces may aggravate yeast-connected symptoms:* Firewood nearly always 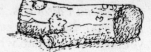 contains fungi . . . especially wood cut from dead trees. And logs that are stored often sprout fungi.

21. *Digestive enzymes:* Digestive enzymes, especially Pancreatin, seem to help many of my patients. These enzymes can be purchased without a prescription at most pharmacies and can be taken after each meal and at bedtime. Some patients experience a "die-off" reaction on enzymes the first few weeks.

22. *Clotrimazole:* This synthetic drug became available in the mid-1970s and has been found effective in treating a variety of fungous infections. In one report by Kirkpatrick & Alling[55] troches of clotrimazole were administered 5 times daily to 10 patients with persistent oral candidiasis. These individuals *had not responded to nystatin.* Yet they became *"completely or nearly asymptomatic in 5 days"* on clotrimazole therapy.

    Clotrimazole creams and suppositories have also been found to be highly effective in treating vaginal candidiasis. However, no data is presently available on the safety and effectiveness of preparations of this drug in reducing candida colonization in the gastrointestinal tract.

23. *Cleaning Foods:*† According to James A. O'Shea, M.D., of Lawrence, Massachusetts, foods can be treated in a special bath to remove fungi, insecticide sprays, bacteria and certain chemicals. Here are suggestions adapted and modified from the instructional materials prepared for his patients:

    Treat the fruits and vegetables separately. Use ½ teaspoon of Clorox® to each gallon of water.

    Step 1: Place the fresh fruits and/or vegetables into the bath. Soak frozen, leafy vegetables or thin-skin fruits for 15 minutes. Heavy-skin fruits and root vegetables require 20 minutes; a heavy-skin squash 25 minutes. Timing is important. Use a fresh Clorox® bath with each batch of food.

    Step 2: Remove foods from the Clorox® bath and soak them in a clean water bath for 15 minutes. Use fresh, clean

---

†Young S. Shin, M.D. of Atlanta comments, "I've found that chemically-sensitive patients in my practice avoid previously troublesome reactions when they soak and rinse their fruits and vegetables with baking soda and water."

water for each batch of food. Once the foods have been cleaned, they are ready for storage in freezer bags.

24. *Taheebo tea and/or other alternative therapies:* Since the first edition of THE YEAST CONNECTION was published in November 1983, I've received thousands of letters from people all over the world who've told me about various things they've found have helped them conquer candida-related health problems and regain their health. Included are the use of caprylic acid preparations, removal of mercury amalgam fillings, and the use of tea made from the bark of a South American tree (taheebo tea), plus several others (see chapter 44, Update for a discussion of alternative and complementary therapies).

25. *Mobilizing your healing resources:* Diet, nystatin, nutritional supplements, avoidance of pollutants and other treatment measures I've talked about play a role in helping you get well. But there are other important areas of healing I've scarcely touched upon. They involve resources available to every human being.

In talking and listening to my patients, I've been repeatedly impressed by those who say, "Faith, hope, and prayer, your caring and your personal interest in me and my problems played an important role in helping me get well."

In his introduction to Norman Cousin's new book, *The Healing Heart*, Bernard Lown, M.D., Professor of Cardiology, Harvard University School of Public Health, pointed out that psychological factors can affect every aspect of human illness. Moreover, Norman Cousins repeatedly documents this relationship in this book as well as in his previous book, *Anatomy of an Illness*. (See also chapter 35.)

For years I've been putting people on elimination diets for food allergy and watching them get well. In discussing my findings with my old friend, Charles May, M.D., Professor of Pediatrics, Emeritus, of the University of Colorado, Charlie replied,

> "Billy, many of your patients get better because they have faith in you and what you're doing, rather than because of the diets you put them on."

At the time (1976), I disagreed strenuously with Charlie because I knew, beyond any shadow of a doubt, that many, many patients were reacting adversely to foods, including patients who didn't like me and who hated my diets.

But now, as the years have passed, I realize that in some of these patients, at least, improvement was due in part to the interest I took in them as well as to my diets. (I haven't previously admitted this to Charlie!)

As I discussed in an earlier section of this book, countless people enjoy healthy, productive lives because medical science has provided new answers and new therapies. Yet, ever since my internship and residency days, I've been impressed and influenced by caring "people doctors," including my chief at Vanderbilt, the late Dr. Amos U. Christie, the late Dr. William C. Deamer of the University of California and many others, including physicians in my own state and my own community.

One physician I'll never forget is Dr. F. Tremaine ("Josh") Billings, a Nashville internist. In 1953, my father was hospitalized at Vanderbilt with what proved to be his last illness. Soon after my father arrived in his hospital room about 6:30 on a Sunday evening, Dr. Billings came in to check him. As he sat on the side of the bed and patted my father's arm, my mother commented, 'Dr. Jere hasn't eaten anything since lunch and the nurses tell me supper has already been served . . ." Dr. Billings asked, "What does Dr. Jere generally eat for Sunday supper?" My mother replied, "Rice Krispies and bananas with milk and cream."

I've forgotten the exact sequence of events, but Dr. Billings left the room. Then just as the nurse finished taking my father's temperature, Dr. Billings showed up again. A box of Rice Krispies was tucked under one arm, a bottle of milk and cream under the other and in each hand he held a banana. I've never forgotten Dr. Billing's compassion and concern. Certainly he knew, as did the late Francis Peabody, that *The care of the patient requires caring for the patient."*

So to get well, you'll need to:

a. Find a caring physician to supervise your overall medical care and, at the same time make sure you aren't suffering from some other organic disease.

b. Seek also the help of other health professionals who are working with patients with yeast-connected health disorders.

c. Locate a lay support group (see chapter 35). In such a group you'll usually find others who'll share their knowl-

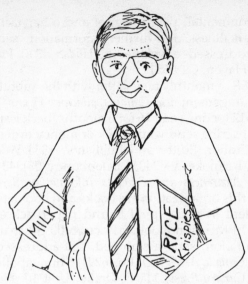

edge with you, provide you with emotional support and help you regain your health. Based on the observations of Norman Cousins, such a support group should encourage laughter, fun, creativity and playfulness. Here's why: Such emotional nutrients mobilize your pain relieving chemicals, the endorphins, and help you get well. (See *The Healing Heart*, especially chapter 34.)

Other sources of information

Other sources of information on *Candida albicans*, nutrition, and preventive medicine include:

1. *The Missing Diagnosis*, a 164-page book by C. Orian Truss, M.D. This book, published in a hardback edition in early 1983, succinctly describes correctable chronic illnesses associated with chronic candidiasis. Professionals will be especially interested in the three scientific papers of Truss which are reprinted in the Appendix of *The Missing Diagnosis*. This book is now available in paperback in many book stores. Or it can be obtained by writing: *The Missing Diagnosis*, P.O. Box 26508Y, Birmingham, AL 35226 (price . . $11.70 postpaid).

2. *Update*, a quarterly periodical published by the Gesell Institute of Human Development. Several recent issues of this periodical have discussed the role of *Candida albicans* in causing human illness. Also discussed is the role of nutritional,

environmental, psychological and other factors in causing human illness. For further information, send a stamped, self-addressed envelope to: *Update*, 310 Prospect Street, New Haven, CT 06511.

3. *CHEER*, a monthly newsletter with the subtitle, "A Shout of Encouragement for *Candida albicans* Hosts." Subscription rate $12 for one year, $6 for 6 months; back issues $1.50 each. To subscribe send your check or money order to Ms. Tamieson Cranor, Editor and Publisher, 1334 Woodbine Street, S. E., Roanoke, VA 24014, telephone (703)343-0572.

4. *PMS Awareness and Candida Information Service*. Available from this organization are books and booklets, including an excellent 81-page spiral bound paperback entitled, "Who Am I? PMS Handbook." (Price $6.00 postpaid.) For further information, send a stamped, self-addressed envelope to: *PMS/Canada AIM*, P.O. Box 6291, Minneapolis, MN 55406.

5. *Wary Canary Press*, 111 E. Drake, Unit 10, Fort Collins, CO 80525, telephone (303) 223-8816. Available from this source is a publication which deals with environmental illness, nutrition, preventive medicine and related disorders, including candidiasis. Subscription rate in U.S. is $12, in Canada $15, foreign $17.

6. *The Price-Pottenger Nutrition Foundation*, a non-profit educational foundation, incorporated in the State of California, publishes a quarterly bulletin devoted to various nutritional topics, including the relationship of *Candida albicans* to human illness. This organization has also published a 149-page book that may interest you, *The Candida Albicans Yeast-Free Cookbook*. For further information send a stamped, self-addressed envelope to: PPNF, 5871 El Cajon Blvd., San Diego, CA 92115.

7. *The Environmental Health Association of Dallas, Inc.*, P.O. Box 226811, Dallas, TX 7522. This organization provides information and support to individuals with chronic health disorders, including illness related to *Candida albicans*. They publish a newsletter, "Twentieth Century Living." For further information, send them a large self-addressed, stamped envelope.

8. *The Journal of Orthomolecular Medicine*, publication office, 2229 Broad Street, Regina, Saskatchewan, Canada S4P 1Y7. This journal provides information on a wide variety of topics

including *Candida albicans*, vitamins, trace minerals and other subjects relevant to lay persons as well as professionals.

9. *People's Medical Society*, 14 E. Minor Street, Emmaus, PA. This non-profit citizen's action group is committed to the principles of better, more responsive and less expensive medical care, and dedicated to the belief that people, as individuals or in groups, can make a difference. This society is involved in the organizing of community efforts around local health care issues and in the national debate over the future of the medical care system. Services include a bimonthly newsletter, booklets and other publications. Membership is $15 per year.

10. *The National Women's Health Network*, 224 7th Street, S.E., Washington, DC 20003. This organization is the "nation's only consumer organization devoted to women's health issues." Members have access to a large resource library and are sent information on request. They also receive a bimonthly newsletter on the latest health information. Membership fees are $25 per year for individuals and $30 per year for groups.

11. *The Center for Science in the Public Interest (CSPI)* provides a variety of excellent materials on nutrition. Their monthly 16-page publication, *Nutrition Action Healthletter*, is well-written, interesting and authoritative. They have not, however, done work on candida. For further information, send a stamped, self-addressed envelope to: CSPI, 1501 16th St. N.W., Washington, DC 20036.

12. *Allergy Information Association (A.I.A) of Canada*, Room 7, 25 Poynter Drive, Weston, Ontario M9R 1KB. This organization, founded in 1964, publishes an excellent quarterly newsletter, *Allergy Shot*, which provides information on allergies and a wide variety of related health topics.

13. *Access to Nutritional Data*, P.O. Box 52, Ashby, MA 01431, (617) 386-7002. Information about nutrition is exploding and almost impossible to keep up with. This organization publishes monthly file cards summarizing the nutritional literature. Subscription rates are $80 for six months, $150 for 12 months.

14. a. Insta-Tape, Inc., 810 South Myrtle Ave., P.O. Box 1729, Monrovia, CA 91016.

b. Creative Audio, 8751 Osborne, Highland, IN 46332.

These companies provide educational tapes for professionals and non-professionals dealing with a variety of topics relating to allergy, nutrition, environmental medicine, preventive medicine and candida-related disorders.

15. *Allergy Alert,* a monthly newsletter by Sally Rockwell which discusses food, chemical and other allergies, and yeast-connected health disorders. For further information send a stamped, self-addressed envelope to: *Allergy Alert,* P.O. Box 15181, Seattle, WA 98115. Also available from this source is *Rotation Game,* "a self-help survival kit for those with food allergies."

16. *Sara Sloan Nutra.* Available from this source is a nutrition newsletter and a variety of helpful books and pamphlets directed especially toward improving the nutritional status of children. For further information send a stamped, self-addressed envelope to: *Sara Sloan Nutra,* P.O. Box 13825, Atlanta, GA 30324.

17. *J. S. B. & Associates, Inc.* Available from this source are the following materials: A monthly audio tape service designed to alert the listener to the fast-breaking advances in nutrition by Jeffrey Bland, Ph.D. ($200 per year, $20 per copy). Also available is a magazine, *Complementary Medicine.* Six issues a year ($30). To receive further information, send your request to: *J.S.B. & Associates, Inc.,* 3215 56th St., N.W., Suite 1B, Gig Harbor, WA 98335.

18. *Brain/Mind Bulletin,* Box 42211, Los Angeles, CA 90042. This newsletter (edited by Marilyn Ferguson, author of *The Aquarian Conspiracy*) deals with medicine, psychology, learning and related subjects. $35 per year.

19. *Executive Health.* This 6 to 8 page highly authoritative publication discusses dozens of topics you need to know about if you want to take charge of your health and stay well. Published monthly by Executive Health Publications, 9605 Scranton Road, Suite 710, San Diego, CA 92121. Subscriptions are $30 per year in U.S.A., $36 foreign countries.

20. *Schizophrenia Association of Greater Washington (SAGW),* Wheaton Place Office Building North, #404, Wheaton, MD 20902. This organization was founded primarily to help individuals with schizophrenia, depression and other mental illnesses. However, it now also serves as a resource organi-

zation for both professionals and non-professionals interested in alternative approaches to health care.

21. *The International Journal of Biosocial Research*, P.O. Box 1174, Tacoma, WA 98401. This quarterly publication "is a peer-review and interdisciplinary journal devoted to research on the environmental, genetic, biochemical and nutritional factors affecting human behavior and social groupings."

22. *The People's Doctor*, an informative, stimulating and provocative newsletter by Robert Mendelsohn, M.D., an articulate advocate of preventive medicine and alternative methods of health care. For more information, write to *The People's Doctor*, P.O. Box 982, Evanston, IL 60204.

23. *The Preventive Medicine Doctor*, by M. J. Packovich, M.D. This pamphlet lists the names and addresses of 140 publications and 121 associations, including both orthodox and alternative health care approaches. Many of these offer newsletters, booklets and magazines for low cost (or without charge). It is published by Tecbook Publications, P.O. Box 5002, Topeka, KS 66605, price $1.39.

24. *Health Consciousness*. A holistic magazine for patients, public and health practitioners, by Roy Kupsinel, M.D., P.O. Box 550, Oviedo, FL 32766.

25. *Once Daily* by Jerome Mittleman, D.D.S. "A new digest of dental health for people who want sound teeth and healthy bodies." 263 West End Ave., #2-A, New York, NY 10023.

26. *Human Ecology Foundation of Canada*, John G. Maclennan, M.D., Medical Advisor, 46 No. 8 Highway, Dundas, Ontario L9H 4V9. This foundation publishes a quarterly newsletter. It was organized to provide information for those interested in obtaining safe sources of food, clothing and housing. Annual membership fee . . . $20.

27. *Yeast Tapes*. I learn something new about yeast-connected illness almost every day. Such information comes from other physicians, my patients, conferences I attend, and articles in either the medical or lay literature. To pass along some of this information, I've prepared a series of audio tapes. For further information, send a stamped, self-addressed envelope to: *Yeast Information*, P.O. Box 3493, Jackson, TN 38303.

British, Australian and New Zealand Sources of Help and Information

1. *Action Against Allergy,* 43 The Downs, London SW20 8HG, England.
2. *The McCarrison Society,* Miss Pauline Atkin, Secretary, 23 Stanley Court, Worcester Road, Sutton, Surrey SM2 65D, England.
3. *Hyperactive Children's Support Group,* 59 Meadowside, Angmering, West Sussex, England.
4. *Sanity,* 77 Moss Land, Pinner, Middlesex HA5 3A0, England.
5. *Schizophrenia Association of Great Britain,* Tyr Twr, Ooanfair Hall, Caernarvon, Wales OL55 1TT.
6. *The Journal of Alternative Medicine,* 30 Station Approach, West Byfleet, Surrey KT14 GNF, England.
7. *Clinical Ecology Society,* The Medical Center, Michael J. Radcliffe, M.D., President, Hythe, Southampton S04 52B, England.
8. *Austro-Asian Society for Environmental Medicine,* c/o Clive F. H. Pyman, M.D., 20 Collins Street, Coats Bldg., Suite 4, Melbourne, Victoria, Australia.
9. *The Allergy Self-Help Centre,* Unit 4, 42 Osborne Place, Stirling, Western Australia 6021, telephone 445-3626.
10. *Hyperactive Help,* P.O. Box 337, Subiaco, 6008, Western Australia.
11. *Allergy Association, Australia,* Adelaide Branch, 37 Second Ave., Sefton Park 5083, South Australia.
12. *Allergy Association, Australia,* New South Wales Branch, 61 Cambewaira Ave., Castle Hill (Sydney) 2154.
13. *Allergy Association, Australia,* Melbourne Branch, P.O. Box 298, Ringwood, Victoria 3134.
14. *Marlborough Allergy Association, Inc.,* 2 Surrey Street, Picton, New Zealand.

35

What You Can Do If Your Physician Is Unaware Of The Yeast Connection

If your health complaints are yeast-connected, you may experience difficulty in finding a physician to help you. Here's why: The four published articles[51a-b-c] by C. Orian Truss on *Candida albicans* and its relationship to human illness aren't available in many medical libraries. Accordingly, most physicians haven't read them. And even if a physician has heard of "the yeast connection" he may say, "There's no proof that candida plays a role in making you sick." Or "Where are the scientific studies?"

If you read medical history (or even if you take a look at medical practice today) you'll find that acceptance of new ideas has always been slow. It takes time for them to filter down through the ranks.

Moreover, Jim Johnson, a Chicago physician, recently commented that people often do not want to learn what they don't already know. Jim Willoughby, a Kansas City physician, has similarly noted that if a physician isn't "up" on a subject he tends to be "down" on it.

If your physician isn't aware of the role candida may be playing in making you sick, here are things you can do:

(1) Lend your physician your copy of THE YEAST CONNECTION. If he shows any interest, ask him to write to the International Health Foundation, Inc., P.O. Box 3494, Jackson, TN 38303. The Foundation will send him reprints from the medical literature on candidiasis, including reports published by C. Orian Truss, M.D. (Birmingham, AL), Steven S. Witkin, Ph.D. (Cornell University Medical College), Kazuo Iwata, M.D. (Tokyo, Japan), E. W. Rosenberg, M.D. (University of Tennessee, Memphis), Sid-

ney M. Baker, M.D. (Yale University), Martin W. Zwerling, M.D. & associates (South Carolina), Letters to the Editor published in the *Journal of the American Medical Association* and *Hospital Practice* discussing yeast-related illness. (Please ask him to enclose $15 to help cover costs.)

(2) Get a copy of Dr. Truss' book, *The Missing Diagnosis*, (now available in paperback) and read it. Then lend or give it to your physician. This book contains the first three Truss articles plus much additional information. You can get it from most bookstores, or you can order it from: *The Missing Diagnosis*, P.O. Box 26508, Birmingham, AL 35226 ($11.70 postpaid).

(3) Ask your physician to write to me. I'll do my best to respond.

(4) If your own physician isn't interested, send a stamped, self-addressed envelope and $5.00 to: The International Health Foundation, Inc., P.O. Box 3494, Jackson, TN 38303 and the Foundation will send you the names of physicians in your geographical area who have expressed an interest in yeast-related health disorders. However, the Foundation cannot recommend a particular physician or be certain that each physician listed will be of help to you.

(5) Send a stamped, self-addressed envelope and $5.00 to the Price-Pottenger Nutrition Foundation, 5871 El Cajon Blvd., San Diego CA 92115. This organization maintains a roster of physicians interested in nutrition and preventive medicine and in yeast-related disorders.

(6) *Take charge of your own health*. Although I hope you can find a kind, compassionate physician who is interested and knowledgeable in treating yeast-related health disorders, even without the help of such a physician there are many things you can do to strengthen your immune system and reduce the load of *Candida albicans* in your body. Here are suggestions:

A. Follow the diet instructions in this book (Section B).
B. Rotate your diet. Food intolerances or allergies are more apt to bother people who eat the same foods every day, especially if they eat them several times a day.
C. Lighten the load of pollutants in your home or work place (see chapters 21-23).
D. Exercise regularly.
E. Stop smoking. Avoid birth control pills and antibiotics (unless absolutely necessary).

F. Supplement your diet with yeast-free vitamin/ mineral preparations. Such preparations should include 15 to 30 mgs. of zinc, 750 to 1500 mgs. of calcium, 400 to 800 mgs. of magnesium (see discussion in chapter 43, Update), vitamins A, B-complex (yeast-free), vitamin C, vitamin E and selenium.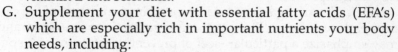

G. Supplement your diet with essential fatty acids (EFA's) which are especially rich in important nutrients your body needs, including:

1. Linseed oil, ½ to 2 tablespoons daily. This oil can be mixed with lemon juice and used as a salad dressing. Or it can be mixed with small amounts of butter and used as a spread.

2. Evening primrose oil, 1 or 2 capsules two or three times a day. This group of EFA's seem to be especially helpful during the 7 to 14 days before the start of the menstrual period.

3. Take the following non-prescription substances which help reduce the growth of candida in your digestive tract:

(1) Preparations of *Lactobacillus acidophilus, Lactobacillus bidifus* and/or *Streptococcus faecium*. Taken on a daily basis, these "friendly" bacteria compete with *Candida albicans* and help bring the flora of your digestive tract back to normal.

(2) Garlic, garlic powder, garlic oil or garlic extract. Many preparations are available. (See, also, chapter 43, Update).

(3) Preparations containing caprylic acid. (See, also, chapter 43, Update).

H. Put your "emotional house" in order. Love, touch, faith, hope and prayer are all important in helping you get well and stay well.

I. Get help from alternative or complementary health care professionals and nonprofessionals (see below).

J. Join a support group.

If you're tired, discouraged, sick and depressed, you may find it difficult to follow the above program without additional information, help and support. Fortunately, many facilities, groups and organizations . . . large and small . . . interested in nutrition, preventive medicine, allergies, environmental medicine and candida-related disorders have been established in the United States, Canada, England and Australia. Most of these organizations are staffed by volunteers and their financial resources are limited. So if you ask them for information and help, please send them a stamped, self-addressed envelope and a contribution to help defray their expenses.

Here's a list of organizations interested in one or more of the categories listed above. Each of these organizations is unique and may emphasize a particular facet of preventive medicine or a specific health problem.

For example, NOHA in Winnetka, Illinois (see below) is interested mainly in nutrition, and SAGW (see below) was founded primarily to help individuals with mental illness. However, both organizations through *"networking"* have broadened their fields of interest and could serve as a resource that would enable you to find a physician or other professional who can help you.

Another example: HEAL . . . a not-for-profit national organization (with chapters in many cities) was formed primarily to help people with environmental illnesses and allergies. Yet, most . . . and perhaps all . . . chapters are interested in individuals with yeast-connected health disorders.

Still other examples: Because PMS is usually related to *Candida albicans,* many PMS clinics and support groups may be able to help you. Also since infections with the chronic EB virus (CEBV) and candida often co-exist and may cause problems in the same person, the national or local CEBV groups may provide you with information that you may find helpful.

SUPPORT GROUPS:

1. *Candida Research and Information*. Director, Gail Frazier Nielsen, Box 2719, Castro Valley, CA 94546, (415) 582-2179.

2. *Rocky Mountain Environmental Health Association*. 420 S. Marion Parkway, Denver, CO 80209, (303) 722-3423.

3. *Human Ecology Action League* (HEAL). Ken L. Dominy, Executive Director, P.O. Box 49126, Atlanta, GA 30359-1126, (404) 248-1898.

4. *Partners in Health*. A Candida support group. Director, Margaret Corbin, M.A., 7 Portsmouth Terrace, Rochester, NY 14607, (716) 473-5400.

5. *The Well Mind Association of Greater Washington*. 2730 University Blvd., West, Suite 404, Wheaton, MD 20902, (301) 949-8282.

6. *REACTOR*. Director, Susan Malloy, San Francisco, CA (415) 331-2148.

7. *Bio-Tox Support Group*. 3888 B Calle Fortunada, San Diego, CA 92123.

8. *Environmental Health Association*. Contact person, Giovanna Medina, P.O. Box 86505, San Diego, CA 92138, (619) 571-0300.

9. *Candida Support of Bethesda*. P.O. Box 3584, Silver Spring, MD 20901.

10. *Candida Research and Information Foundation of Canada*. Contact person, Maggie Burstun, 578 St. Clair Ave., West, Toronto, Canada, (416) 656-0047.

11. *HEAL*, Sandy Anello, President, 506 E. 84th Street, Apt. 4 West, New York, NY 10028, (212) 517-5937.

OTHER CONTACTS OR SOURCES OF INFORMATION

1. *PMS Awareness and Candida Information*. Rickey Weiss, Director, P.O. Box 6291, Minneapolis, MN 55406, (612) 724-4425.

2. *Premenstrual Program, Inc.* 40 Salem Street, Lynnfield, MA 01940, (617) 245-9585.

3. *International Health Foundation, Inc.** (IHF), P.O. Box 3494, Jackson, TN 38303.

• Medical reprints, quarterly newsletter
• Telephone Hotline calls 11:30 a.m. – 12:00 noon (CST) most weekdays (901) 427-8100.
• Nationwide physician referral service

---

*For more information about IHF see pages 397–398.

4. *HEAL*. 425 E. Washington Ave., Ann Arbor, MI 48104, (313) 662-3384.

ALTERNATIVE MEDICINE AND "CONSUMERISM"

In the December 15, 1983 issue of the *New England Journal of Medicine* (309:1524-1527, 1983), John Lister, M.D., Farm End, Burkes Road, Beaconsfield, HP9 1PB England, in a commentary entitled, "Current Controversy on Alternative Medicine," had this to say:

> "For various reasons there seems to be an increasing dissatisfaction with certain aspects of conventional or orthodox medicine . . . one of the growth industries in contemporary Britain is—*alternative medicine*."

Dr. Lister told of the formation of the British Holistic Medicine Association and of the growing debate in England, especially since the *London Times* published three major articles on various aspects of alternative medicine as well as an editorial entitled, "Physician Heal Thyself."

In its editorial the *Times* supported the concept of alternative medicine and was highly critical of those who resist alternative approaches to health care, and further stated,

> "There is a growing loss of faith by the public in a purely scientific approach to medicine.
> Moreover, such an open approach seems to present the British National Health Service with an insatiable demand for all kinds of surgery and with a drug bill for billions of pounds with its inevitable component of dangerous mistakes. It is recognized that orthodox medicine has great scientific achievements to its credit but the *Times* believes that it is ungenerous in its attitude to alternative systems or treatment when scientific research has failed to provide satisfactory answers."

In his article, Dr. Lister also presented the ideas of those who defend contemporary methods of medical practice. Yet, he noted,

> "There is often an arrogant reluctance of the medical profession to accept—or even to consider—healing methods which haven't been confirmed by scientific studies."

In concluding his commentary, Dr. Lister emphasizes that the physician's "first priority" must be to make sure that he or she is not missing treatable organic diseases, especially in patients with rather vague symptoms. Having done so, he or she may then use whatever methods "are available and appropriate" and that "if such methods are unorthodox they should be considered as *complementary* rather than *alternative* to orthodox methods (see also chapter 44, Update). Nearly all emphasize better nutrition, exercise and lifestyle changes rather than relying on prescription drugs and surgery.

In his recent book, *The Healing Heart*, Norman Cousins expresses similar thoughts in a chapter entitled "Consumerism Reaches Medicine:"

> "Holistic medicine is an expression of, not a substitute for, the best in traditional medical practice . . . The new consumerism need not be regarded as a threat to medicine or as anything alien."

The rise of consumerism and the growing interest in alternative health care was also discussed recently by Marilyn Ferguson:

> "One major arena, health care, has already begun to experience wrenching change . . . For all its reputed conservatism, western medicine is undergoing an amazing revitalization. Patients and professionals alike are beginning to see beyond symptoms to the context of illness: stress, society, family, diet, season, emotions . . . Hospitals, long the bastions of barren efficiency, are scurrying to provide more humane environments for birth and death . . .
>
> "A guest editorial in *American Medical News* decried medicine's crisis of human relations . . . 'Physicians must recognize that medicine is not their private preserve but a profession in which all people have a vital stake'. . . ."
>
> "Surely, historians will marvel at the heresy we fell into, the recent decades in which we disregarded the spirit in our efforts to cure the body. Now, in finding health, we find ourselves."[†]

Ms. Ferguson also referred to the influence of Norman Cousins and pointed out that informal discussion groups on holistic approaches to medicine were meeting regularly at such medical schools as UCLA, University of Texas in Galveston, Baylor in Houston and Johns Hopkins in Baltimore.

I became personally aware of the interest of medical students in holistic and preventive medicine in May 1986. At that time, I was invited to talk at a Symposium on Preventive Medicine planned by the Humanistic Health Committee, a group of health science stu-

---

†Excerpted from *The Aquarian Conspiracy; Personal and Social Transformation in the 1980s,*©1980 by Marilyn Ferguson. Published by J.P. Tarcher, Inc., 9110 Sunset Blvd., Los Angeles, CA 90069. $15.00, $8.95 soft cover. Used by permission.

dents sponsored by C.H.I.P. (Council for Health Interdisciplinary Participation) at the University of Minnesota.

Additional sponsorship and funding for the Symposium was provided by the American Holistic Medical Association, the Public Health Student Senate at the University of Minnesota, and the American Medical Student Association. The title of the Symposium—"FIRST DO NO HARM."

On the first day of the meeting, a panel discussed perspectives on major health problems (smoking, alcohol abuse, teenage pregnancy, nutrition, and the government's role in providing preventive health care).

On the second day, I talked about the role of candida in human illness. There were sixteen different workshops. Topics included Food Allergy and Nutrition, Exercise, Homeopathy, Massage Therapy, Acupuncture, Self-Relaxation in Dentistry, and Mental Imagery.

Here's more: John Naisbitt, in his bestseller, *Megatrends—Ten New Directions Transforming Our Lives†*, noted the growing interest in health promoting diets, exercise and self care. And he commented on several major trends in health, including:

> "The triumph of the new paradigm of wellness, preventive medicine and holistic care over the old model of illness, drugs, surgery and treating symptoms rather than the whole person."

In the 1985 book, *Re-Inventing the Corporation‡* (co-authored by John Naisbitt and Patricia Aburdene), in a chapter entitled, "Health and the Corporations," the authors commented:

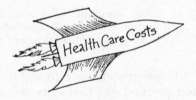

> "As health costs skyrocket, providing health care is becoming one of the highest costs of doing business . . . The most effective way to cut health care costs is to prevent hospital and doctor bills by promoting health, wellness and well being among the people in your company. Wellness programs are not just trendy anymore; they are a proven way to cut health costs."

And Margot Brown, Wellness Specialist (and recipient of the 1st

---

†*Megatrends—Ten New Directions Transforming Our Lives*, 1982 by John Naisbitt. Published by Warner Books, 666 5th Avenue, New York, NY 10103.

‡Warner Books, Inc., New York, NY, 1985.

National Wellness-in-the-Workplace Award), Nissan Motor Company, Smyrna, Tennessee, had this to say:

> "Individual health is fundamental to the well-being and productivity of any organization. At Nissan, we feel that the quality of our product is only as good as the fitness of our employees. And we're teaching them that exercise, a good diet, and other lifestyle changes will make them look good, feel good, enjoy their work and become more successful in every way."

I've heard it said, "There's nothing more powerful than an idea whose time has come." So when you take charge of your life and health, you'll be joining millions of other folks all over America.

36

Summary Of The Dallas, Birmingham and San Francisco Conferences

According to Odds[3], hundreds of articles appear each year on *Candida albicans*. Yet, until the three articles by Truss published in the *Journal of Orthomolecular Psychiatry*[51a-b-c-d] beginning in 1978 (followed by the Truss book[2] in 1983), few, if any, reports in the medical literature discussed the type of yeast-connected illnesses which are the subject of this book. And even today . . . summer, 1986 . . . only scant additional medical references are available to help physicians seeking further information.

Yet, during the years 1982-1986, interest in the relationship of *Candida albicans* to human illness has skyrocketed. This interest has also been stimulated by discussions on TV[†] and radio and in magazines and newspapers.

In spite of this tremendous demand from the public for more information, other than the articles by Truss and a number of Letters to the Editor[39-53a-b-c-d] few reports have appeared in the medical literature describing the numerous health disorders which clinical observers have found to be related to *Candida albicans.* Accordingly, I felt it appropriate to briefly summarize the discussions of three conferences on the relationship of *Candida albicans* to a variety of

---

†Dr. Truss and one of his patients, Suzi Elman, were interviewed by Sandi Freeman on *Freeman Reports* (Cable News Network) in September 1981. According to Sandi, "This program brought more mail and phone calls than any previous program."

I discussed yeast-connected health problems with Bob Braun (Braun and Company, WLW-TV, Cincinnati) in January 1983. Within 7 days, my office received 7,300 requests for more information.

human illnesses. The first of these was an informal meeting in Dallas, July 9-11, 1982. The second was a symposium in Birmingham, December 9-11, 1983. The third was a symposium in San Francisco, March 29-31, 1985.

THE DALLAS CONFERENCE,
July 9-11, 1982

Some 20 physicians who had been working with patients with candida-related illness met and presented their experiences informally. An additional 20 to 30 physicians participated in the general discussion.

Most participants agreed that *the history was the most useful tool in diagnosing candida-related illness* and emphasized the role of antibiotics in causing this illness.

Nearly all participants agreed that symptoms referrable to the nervous system, the reproductive organs (especially in adult females) and the gastrointestinal systems were especially prominent. However, involvement of every body system was reported.

All physicians used nystatin in treating patients with candida-related illness. However, experiences were varied in regard to the most effective dose. Several participants described nystatin reactions, including fatigue, depression and nausea. There was considerable discussion as to the mechanism of these reactions. The predominant feeling was that reactions were caused by yeast "die-off", caused by toxins released from killed candida organisms.

Experiences with diet were also varied. Some participants felt that an initial low carbohydrate diet (60 to 80 grams) was essential to obtain improvement. Other participants felt that the complex carbohydrates (vegetables, whole grains and fruits) could be eaten and that only sugar and other refined carbohydrates need be restricted. All participants emphasized the importance of foods with high mold content and environmental molds in triggering symptoms.[†]

---

†Many other yeasts and molds are closely related to *Candida albicans* including *Tricophyton* and *Epidermophyton*. A number of physicians treating yeast-connected health problems (including Lawrence Dickey, M.D., of Fort Collins, Colorado) have found that immunotherapy using an extract containing these two molds plus candida is often more effective than nystatin therapy or than candida extract alone. (The combined extract containing the three yeasts and molds is often termed "TCE", "TOE", or "TME").

Recently Walter Ward, M.D., an otolaryngologist and allergist of Winston-Salem, North Carolina, commented, "I'm using a great deal of antifungal therapy including nystatin, Nizoral® and immunotherapy and getting fantastic results." Dr. Ward also re-

Experiences in using immunotherapy were varied. Several physicians told of successful use of "homeopathic" dilutions of candida extract . . . one part candida to one-quintillion parts of diluting fluid†; others recommended stronger extracts, based on provocative testing and neutralization. No participants recommended the "build-up" method of immunotherapy.

All agreed that candida extracts, when used, required careful monitoring by the physician, and that no automatic protocol for use of such extracts could be provided for the physician or patient.

In discussing nystatin . . .

a. The great majority of the conference participants felt that it was an unusually safe medicine.

b. Most participants continued the nystatin and diet for 3 or more months.

c. Most physicians found they could gradually discontinue nystatin in 6 to 12 months as the patient's health improved. However, some patients required nystatin for several years.

There was considerable discussion of patients with chemical sensitivity. Several observers told of patients who recovered following anticandida treatment.

A number of physicians emphasized the importance of a comprehensive program of management. Their therapeutic approach included not only anticandida therapy, but also the avoidance and appropriate management of hidden food and chemical allergies.

Many participants noted a close relationship between the immune, endocrine and nervous systems. And hormonal imbalances in female patients often appeared to be triggered by candida-related illness. Moreover, following anticandida therapy, hormonal problems often improved, sometimes dramatically.

A few physicians reported dramatic results in treating patients with severe and often "incurable" auto-immune diseases, includ-

---

ported that extracts from the mold *Microsporum* helped some of his patients with yeast-connected illness who hadn't been completely relieved by other therapies. Among these patients were several individuals with skin problems, including psoriasis. (see also chapter 31)

---

†During 1984, 1985 and 1986, I have received additional reports describing the effectiveness of infinitesimal dilutions of candida extracts. Moreover, these extracts are being used by mouth (sublingually) and by injection. A member of the faculty of a university medical school commented, "I'm using homeopathic candida extracts. I've found them effective although I don't understand how they work. I'm now taking a look at the literature on homeopathic medicine—I hope it will give me some answers."

ing multiple sclerosis, Crohn's disease, arthritis and schizophrenia. And several physicians told of favorable results in treating severe and disabling chronic skin disorders, including psoriasis.

Many participants emphasized that candida-related illness was not a "disease" and that many factors played a role in causing people to be sick. Included among these factors were nutritional deficiencies, allergies and psychological trauma.

THE BIRMINGHAM CONFERENCE[†]
December 9-11, 1983

In his welcoming remarks, Conference Chairman Sidney M. Baker, M.D., of New Haven, Connecticut, pointed out that this was a gathering of clinicians to discuss changes in people's health "which do not follow the usual guidelines." (He pointed out that this would be a program of "show and tell" plus scientific observations, with the hope of opening up lines of communication.)

Francis J. Waickman, M.D., Akron, Ohio, showed slides demonstrating skin and other problems which were related to yeasts and molds. He also described methods for testing and treating patients with yeast and mold extracts.

John Willard Rippon, Ph.D., Chicago, Illinois (author of the comprehensive text, *Medical Mycology*[2]) reviewed the different fungi which inhabit the body and discussed the role of various foods in promoting yeast growth. (See also chapters 10, and 44 of the Update.)

Warren R. Pistey, M.D., Ph.D., Bridgeport, Connecticut, described the cultural characteristics of various yeasts and molds and described his experiences in dealing with *Candida albicans* and other molds in his role as a hospital pathologist. (He pointed out that a number of current practices lead to increased candida growth, including antibiotics, steroids, intravenous therapy, hyperalimentation and organ transplantation.)

Alan S. Levin, M.D., San Francisco, California, discussed changes in the immune system sometimes found in patients with yeast-connected health problems. He pointed out that although laboratory studies may help, the history provides the most impor-

---

†This conference, "The Yeast-Human Interaction, 1983," was sponsored by the Gesell Institute of Human Development, New Haven, Connecticut and the Critical Illness Research Foundation, Inc., Birmingham, Alabama.

tant clue in making a diagnosis of a yeast-connected health disorder. (See, also, chapters 25, and 45 of the Update.)

E. William Rosenberg, M.D., Memphis, Tennessee, discussed seborrheic dermatitis and psoriasis and presented data describing his research on the causes and therapy of these disorders. He pointed out that many factors play a role in causing psoriasis and some patients with psoriasis improve on anticandida therapy. (See, also, chapter 31.)

On the second day of the conference, Eunice Carlson, Ph.D. (Associate Professor, Microbiology, Michigan Technological University, Houghton, Michigan), described and discussed her research work on *Candida albicans*. She noted especially that when associated with or combined with infections by *Staphylococcus aureus*, candida infections became more virulent and caused greater problems. In a published article describing her observations, Dr. Carlson reported,

> "A synergistic effect on mouse mortality was demonstrated in combined infections of mice with *Candida albicans* and a *Staphylococcus aureus* strain isolated from a patient with Toxic Shock Syndrome. Mice exhibited high resistance when inoculated intraperitoneally by either pathogen alone. Dual infection with the two organisms together, however, at doses which separately caused no animal deaths, resulted in 100% mortality" . . . It must be emphasized that the study reported here was not designed as a model for human disease, but rather to determine first whether a synergistic effect on a disease process existed between these two pathogens."[†]

In a presentation entitled, *"T-Lymphocytes and Yeast Flora—Friends or Foes?"* Max D. Cooper, M.D. (Professor, Pediatrics and Microbiology, Medical School, University of Alabama in Birmingham) discussed immunological factors present in individuals with candidiasis.

Then in two one-hour presentations Kazuo Iwata, M.D. (Chairman and Professor of Microbiology, Meiji College of Pharmacy, Tokyo) described his research work on yeast toxins and the types of symptoms and diseases which he had found to be related to *Candida albicans*.

Dr. Iwata began studying *Candida albicans* in 1967. Along with his co-workers he successfully isolated a potent, lethal toxin, *Canditoxin*, (CT) from a virulent strain of C. albicans. These investiga-

---

†Carlson, E., Ph.D.; "Synergistics Effect of Candida albicans and Staphylococcus aureus in Mouse Mortality". *Infection and Immunity*. December 1982. Vol 38. No. 3, pps. 921-924.

tors isolated several high and low molecular weight toxins from *Candida albicans*.[†]

In a published report describing his studies on Canditoxin in mice Dr. Iwata commented,

> "*Canditoxin* produced unique clinical symptoms. Immediately after . . . intravenous injection (of toxin) animals exhibited ruffled fur and unsettled behavior . . . Toxicity was so acute and severe that the majority of treated animals succumbed from an anaphylactic-type reaction within 48 hours. Within 10 minutes after giving a dose of toxin, the animals became unsettled and irritable; had congestion of the conjunctivae, ears and other parts of the body and finally developed paralysis of the extremities."[‡]

In a paper published in another journal Iwata had this to say,

> "When injected into uninfected mice, *Canditoxin* exerted toxic manifestation in spleen lymphoid cells . . . This indicates the possibility that . . . *the toxin produced in the invaded tissues may act as an immunosuppressant to impair host defense mechanisms involving cellular immunity . . .*"[‡‡]

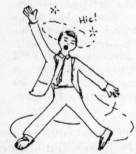

Iwata also discussed his fascinating observations on patients in Japan who were suffering from *metei-sho* or the Japanese "drunk disease" which he and other Japanese investigators had found to be related to *Candida albicans*. Here is what appeared to be happening in these unfortunate individuals: *Candida albicans* in the digestive tract—especially when massive colonies are present—is capable of fermenting sugar and other carbohydrates and producing alcohol. In some individuals the alcohol levels were sufficient to cause actual drunkenness (see also chapter 32).

Leo Galland, M.D. (Assistant Clinical Professor of Medicine, University of Connecticut) in a presentation entitled, "*Metabolic Lesions in Chronic Candidiasis*," noted deficiencies in essential fatty ac-

---

[†]Iwata, K., and Yamamoto, Y.; "Glycoprotein Toxins Produced by Candida Albicans". *Proceedings of the Fourth International Conference on the Mycoses*, June, 1977, PAHO Scientific Publication #356.

[‡]Iwata, K.,: In *Recent Advances in Medical and Veterinary Mycology*, University of Tokyo Press, 1977.

[‡‡]Iwata, K. and Uchida, K.: "Cellular Immunity in Experimental Fungus Infections in Mice", *Medical Mycology*, Flims, January 1977.

ids and magnesium. (See also Dr. Galland's comments in chapter 43, Update). He also found a need for larger amounts of other nutrients, including especially vitamin B6. Among the fascinating parts of his discussion was his observation that *in 104 patients he had studied with candidiasis, almost half showed findings on physical examination indicating mitral valve prolapse*. Moreover, this disorder was significantly associated with dry skin and other symptoms of essential fatty acid deficiency. (For a further discussion of mitral valve prolapse see chapter 42, Update).

C. Orian Truss, M.D. of Birmingham, in a presentation entitled, *"Laboratory Assessment of Chronic Candidiasis,"* told of his metabolic studies in 24 patients with yeast-related health disorders. He especially noted abnormalities of both amino acids and fatty acids in his patients as compared to a group of normals.

Truss published his findings in an article entitled, "Metabolic Abnormalities in Patients with Chronic Candidiasis," in the *Journal of Orthomolecular Psychiatry,* 1984, Vol. 13 No. 2.[†]

In studying the fatty acids Truss found a number of metabolic abnormalities in both the Omega 3 and Omega 6 series. I was especially fascinated by his descriptions of a simple test he carried out on the red blood cells of the patients. In carrying out this test using a simple suction apparatus, Truss found that red blood cells of his candida patients were less able to pass through a filter (with microscopic-size pores) than the red blood cells of healthy individuals. The explanation: The outside membranes of red cells in the candida patients had become more rigid.

Other of the Truss studies dealt with amino acid abnormalities, including glutamine, glutamic acid and asparagine. For example, in his patients with chronic candidiasis, asparagine excretion ranged from 10 to 100 micromoles per 24 hours, as compared to the expected normal range of 280 to 600.

In his presentation Dr. Truss proposed that in the metabolism of sugars by yeast organisms that a chemical substance (acetaldehyde) may be responsible for many of the biochemical abnormalities and associated health disorders seen in patients with candidiasis. (See chapter 40, Update for a further discussion of the Truss research studies.)

A panel of faculty members answered questions and made fur-

---

†A copy of this article can be obtained from *The Journal of Orthomolecular Medicine,* 222 Broad Street, Regina, Saskatchewan, Canada S4P 1Y7, Price: $2.00.

ther comments. Finally, Dr. Baker summarized the proceedings of the conference.[†]

THE SAN FRANCISCO CONFERENCE,
March 29-31, 1985

This conference, like the Birmingham Conference, was sponsored by the Critical Illness Research Foundation, Birmingham, AL and the Gesell Institute of Human Development, New Haven, CT. Participants included a number of those who presented their observations at the previous conference including Drs. Baker, Carlson, Galland, Levin, Rippon, Rosenberg and Truss.

Each of these professionals made progress reports on their continuing studies on "the yeast/human interaction" including both clinical and laboratory observations. In addition, new studies were presented by a number of other program participants.

Dr. Phyllis Saifer of Berkeley, CA in a presentation entitled, *"Endocrinopathies in Patients with Chronic Candidiasis,"* pointed out that many of her patients with yeast problems suffered from associated disturbances of hormone function including especially thyroid and ovarian abnormalities. In working with these patients she described new laboratory studies which assisted in the diagnosis. Measures she recommended in treating such patients included oral thyroid. (For a further discussion of Dr. Saifer's observations see chapter 42, Update.)

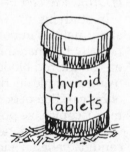

Presentations by three different groups of investigators dealt with antibody studies in patients with candidiasis. Howard Hagglund, M.D., a Norman, Oklahoma physician certified in Family Practice, and David S. Bauman, Ph.D., President of Immuno-Mycologics, Inc., Washington, Oklahoma, described their clinical and laboratory studies on candida patients. They described their findings on a new serum test, *Candida Enzyme Immunoassay (CEIA)®* which aided in the diagnosis of yeast-connected health disorders. They stated that *their patients with candida-related illness showed higher levels of antibodies than did a control group of normal individuals of the same age and sex*. They also stated that this test along

---

†Audio-cassette tapes of the Dallas, Birmingham and San Francisco conferences can be obtained from Creative Audio, 8751 Osborne, Highland, IN 46332.

with a questionnaire can greatly help the physician in making an accurate diagnosis.

F. T. Guilford, M.D. and G. DerBalian, Ph.D. described clinical and laboratory studies in patients with "low grade, chronic candidiasis." Using a test which they described as an "enzyme-linked immunosorbant assay", they determined the candida specific human antibody levels of classes IgG, IgM and IgA. *In the patients they studied, those with chronic candidiasis showed statistically significantly higher antibody levels than did a group of controls.*

In a third presentation Edward Winger, M.D., Faculty, School of Public Health, University of California, Berkeley described immune system studies in patients with candidiasis. He noted that elevations in candida specific IgA and IgM antibodies, as well as elevations in anti-endocrine antibodies, were often present in these patients. He also pointed out that *the likelihood that a patient has a candida-related health problem can be predicted using these tests.* Moreover, changes in antibody levels can help monitor the success of treatment.

Steven S. Witkin, Ph.D., associate and research professor, Department of Obstetrics and Gynecology, Cornell University Medical College, New York, in a presentation entitled, *"Lymphocyte Inhibition in Patients with Candidiasis,"* told of immune system and endocrine changes in women with recurrent vaginitis.

Witkin's observations were subsequently published in the May-June 1985 issue of *Infections in Medicine.* (See chapter 40, Update for further discussion of the Witkin observations.)

37

Potpourri

It seems that almost every day I learn things about yeast-connected illness I didn't know before. This chapter includes information I've acquired from various sources since the first and second editions of *The Yeast Connection* were published. Although some of this material is directed mainly to physicians, it should interest anyone with a health problem related to *Candida albicans*.

Observations of Practicing Physicians:[†] In October 1983 I mailed a 27-item questionnaire to a number of physicians, each of whom had treated hundreds of patients with yeast-connected health disorders. Here's a summary of their observations:

- Each patient is unique and different and no program of therapy fits every patient.
- While anticandida therapy featuring diet and nystatin is important, all patients require comprehensive management.
- Most of the clinicians emphasized the importance of the low carbohydrate diet. However, most felt that complex carbohydrates should be gradually returned to the diet as the patient improves.
- Several physicians suggested placing patients on the "Cave Man", "Stone Age" or Low Carbohydrate Diet for one week before beginning nystatin. In this way yeasts were "starved out" and die-off reactions from the nystatin were less troublesome.

[†]Doctors Jim Brodsky of Chevy Chase, Maryland; John Curlin of Jackson, Tennessee; Lawrence Dickey of Fort Collins, Colorado; Ken Gerdes of Denver, Colorado; Howard Hagglund of Norman, Oklahoma; Harold Hedges of Little Rock, Arkansas; George Kroker of La Crosse, Wisconsin; Don Lewis of Jackson, Tennessee; Allan Lieberman of North Charleston, South Carolina; Richard Mabray of Victoria, Texas; George Mitchell of Washington, D.C.; Gary Oberg of Crystal Lake, Illinois; James O'Shea of Lawrence, Massachusetts; Phyllis Saifer of Berkeley, California; and Morton Teich of New York, New York.

- Success was reported in using initial doses of nystatin of one million units ($^1/_4$ teaspoon of powder or two tablets) four times a day rather than smaller doses of 500,000 units ($^1/_8$ teaspoon of powder or 1 tablet) or "dot doses" of powder.

- Several physicians mentioned their successful use of ketoconazole (Nizoral®) in treating many of their patients, especially those who did not respond to nystatin. One physician recommended giving Nizoral® in a dose of two tablets daily for the first week of therapy to bring the patient's symptoms under control. As the patient improved, nystatin was often added to the treatment program. The dose of Nizoral® could then usually be reduced or discontinued. No serious toxic reactions were noted from Nizoral® use. (See chapters 8, and 43, Update)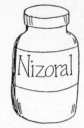

- Nearly all physicians used nutritional supplements including vitamin C in doses of 1,000 milligrams (or more) routinely. Larger doses of vitamin C were administered to patients with fever or following chemical exposure or under stress. The "bowel tolerance test" was suggested as a method of determining the proper dose (see chapter 34).

- Nearly all physicians used immunotherapy with candida extracts or candida extracts combined with 2 other molds, trichophyton and epidermophyton ("TCE" or "TOE"). Most physicians used relatively stronger dilutions of vaccine.

- Most physicians also used immunotherapy for inhalants, foods and chemicals. However, several felt that such immunotherapy was less often necessary in patients who followed a comprehensive anticandida treatment program including diet, nystatin and/or Nizoral®.

All but two of the physicians who responded to the questionnaire practice allergy and environmental medicine. Each was asked to make a statement as to how anticandida therapy had influenced or changed his/her practice. Here are representative responses:

> "Makes most other forms of treatment (except some relatively uncomplicated food avoidance) unnecessary in most cases."
> "Anticandida therapy is *only a part of my regular treatment program*. Major foods and chemicals are just as important."
> "I now regard anticandida therapy as 'the most indispensable tool.'"

Though in selected patients, chemicals and foods are equally important. I'd hate to do without either."

"Anticandida treatment is primary in 75-80 percent of my patients. Such therapy helps in a lot of patients who would have been marginally functional with food and chemical avoidance."

"I feel that anticandida therapy has revolutionized my practice in allergy and clinical ecology. I feel it is a "cornerstone" in the treatment of many chronic health problems in children."

"*I'm becoming a yeastologist.* Most patients in my practice seem to have the yeast problem. However, no one program will fit all yeast-affected patients. It is a highly individualized problem which varies from patient to patient."

"Anti-yeast therapy has dramatically helped my patients and changed my practice. Yeast control should be tried in all ecologically ill patients."

"Because of my emphasis on candida, I've attracted a large number of candida patients. Approximately 50% of the patients in my practice require anticandida therapy."

"I believe anticandida therapy is appropriate in virtually 100% of allergy and clinical ecology patients. This confirms my previous findings that seasonal gynecological problems were more often correlated with molds spore counts than with pollen counts."

"50% of my patients have some kind of yeast problem. In 10% it may be the entire problem."

"Anticandida therapy has changed my approach to patients dramatically. 75% of my practice is on anticandida therapy."

Amphotericin B: A special report to physicians. According to the *Physician's Desk Reference* (1986 edition) "This antibiotic, first isolated . . . by the Squibb Institute for Medical Research, *is substantially more active in vitro against candida strains than nystatin,* and has been widely used by the intravenous route in the treatment of many deep-seated mycotic infections. Given orally, amphotericin B *is extremely well tolerated and is virtually nontoxic in prophylactic doses.* Although poorly absorbed from the gut, amphotericin B has a high degree of activity against candida species in the intestinal tract . . ."

Yet in spite of this effectiveness and safety when given orally, such preparations of amphotericin B aren't available in the United States except in combination with tetracycline.[†] Accordingly, I hadn't thought of using oral amphotericin B in treating my patients. Then in January 1983 a physician with severe chemical sensitivity and other yeast-connected immune system problems commented,

---

†Mysteclin-F® (Squibb)

"I've been taking oral amphotericin B and it has changed my life. I suffered from severe health problems for years and had to live like a hermit. When I began sticking to my yeast-free, low-carbohydrate diet and taking nystatin, I improved significantly. Yet, chemical exposures still bothered me and I was afraid to go into public places.

"In early 1983 I became interested in oral amphotericin B and through a friend in Paris I filled a prescription for Fungizone® (the Squibb name for amphotericin B marketed in France). I've been taking 250 mg. of this drug 2 or 3 times a day for the past couple of months and have improved even more than had been possible on nystatin."

In his continuing discussion this physician commented,

"I also sniff or inhale the amphotericin powder—so it reaches the candida on my nasal and sinus membranes. This relieves my nasal symptoms and lessens my fatigue and headache. *It really is effective.*"

After receiving this anecdotal report I began to look for more information about amphotericin B. I talked to the director of the Cancer Research Program at an eastern university who commented,

"We have recently been using oral amphotericin B in special situations and are now treating 21 patients with this drug." In commenting further he said, "I wish oral amphotericin B (without tetracycline) was available in this country. Yet it seems there hasn't been enough demand for such preparations to make it economically feasible for Squibb to market them in the United States."

In investigating further the efficacy and safety of oral amphotericin B, I found a fascinating report in the medical literature by Montes, Cooper & associates of the University of Alabama ("Prolonged Oral Treatment of Chronic Mucocutaneous Candidiasis with Amphotericin B": *Arc. Derm.* 104:45-55, 1971). These investigators gave this drug orally to four patients with chronic mucocutaneous candidiasis using a total daily dose of 1,000 to 1,800 milligrams for six to fourteen months. "In all four patients oral administration of amphotericin B was free of side effects. *Likewise frequent laboratory studies failed to show abnormalities.*"

Montes, Cooper & associates also described studies of other investigators who had used amphotericin B in daily doses of 1,000 mgs. or more for many months in treating systemic fungal infections. In discussing the possible toxicity of the drug, these investigators commented,

"In the studies[†] just mentioned, as well as in our own patients, am-

---

†One study cited showed "absence of side effects when amphotericin B was given at a daily dose of 2 to 7 gms." In another study, "Patients received a total dose in excess of 1,000 gm. without ill effects. *The lack of toxic effects observed with the tablets is in contrast with the marked toxicity, particularly at the renal level, which follows intravenous administration.*"

photericin B tablets given orally showed a remarkable lack of clinical and laboratory toxicity."

In their concluding comments, these authors stated:

> "It would seem parodoxical at a time when the usefulness of antibiotic combinations has been seriously questioned that amphotericin B tablets can be prescribed in combined form designed to prevent candidiasis but cannot be obtained to be used alone to treat candidiasis."

Because of the well-known toxicity of intravenous amphotericin B, I continued to search for further information about the oral use of this drug. According to Goodman and Gilman's *Pharmacological Basis of Therapeutics* (6th Ed., 1980, pp. 1233-1236), amphotericin B, like nystatin, is a polyene antibiotic whose mechanism of action in destroying candida organisms is identical to that of nystatin. Like nystatin, amphotericin B is poorly absorbed from the intestinal tract.

Moreover, even in doses three times greater than those used by Montes, Cooper & associates, plasma levels of amphotericin B were only one-third to one-fifteenth as great as those reached on intravenous administration. These data certainly suggest that oral amphotericin B should be a safe alternative anticandida medication—especially for patients who: (1) do not tolerate nystatin, (2) fail to improve on nystatin or (3) relapse while taking nystatin after an initial period of improvement.

Between March and August of 1983, a number of patients who did not tolerate nystatin or who failed to improve while taking nystatin obtained amphotericin B from France and several showed an excellent response.

Laura, a 39-year-old teacher, had been troubled by headaches and nasal congestion for 20 years. More recently she had developed bronchitis, fatigue, nervousness, depression and peculiar eye symptoms. Study and testing by an allergist resulted in a diagnosis of "vasomotor rhinitis." Her symptoms became worse during the fall of 1982 and she received "3 rounds of antibiotics and 4 rounds of steroids."

I first saw Laura in January 1983. I put her on my usual anticandida program including diet, nystatin and nutritional supplements. She improved slightly. In March Laura developed an extensive rash. All medication was stopped including nystatin.

The rash subsided. When she resumed the nystatin the rash returned. She stopped the nystatin and the rash again subsided.

Nizoral® was then prescribed and most of Laura's symptoms improved. Yet her nasal congestion continued. She also would develop a severe headache when she cheated on her diet.

Laura ran out of Nizoral® and in May 1983, through a friend in France she obtained capsules of amphotericin B (Fungizone®). She took one-half of a 250 mg. capsule four times a day and sniffed tiny amounts of the powder.

Within two weeks she felt "much better." In a letter to me on August 3, 1983, Laura reported.

> "I'm doing great. I feel fantastically good, and my nose is clear for the first time in 20 years. I can even eat out in restaurants and cheat on my diet and not get into trouble!"

I prescribe nystatin for nearly all of my patients with yeast-connected illness. Moreover, most of them improve on a comprehensive program which features nystatin, diet, lifestyle changes, supplemental nutrients and avoidance of chemical pollutants. In addition, some of my patients require immunotherapy (allergy vaccines or extracts).

When a candida patient does not tolerate nystatin or doesn't improve while taking nystatin and following a comprehensive program of treatment, I try other antifungal agents, including Nizoral® and the nonprescription substances, especially the caprylic acid products (see chapter 43, Update). And if and when it's available, I do not hesitate to prescribe *amphotericin B*.

During 1983 and early 1984, a pharmacy in Paris, France filled *amphotericin B* prescriptions for a number of my patients. I was gratified at their response. Moreover, I received similar favorable reports from a number of other physicians, including Elmer Cranton, M.D. of Trout Dale, Virginia and Walter Ward, M.D. of Winston-Salem, North Carolina.

Then the *amphotericin B* from France became unavailable unless the prescription was signed by a French physician. So today (summer, 1986), unless you have a "French connection" (or German, Swiss or other foreign connection), *amphotericin B* remains difficult or impossible to obtain in the United States and Canada.

Yet because oral *amphotericin B* (without tetracycline) would provide an effective and safe alternative therapeutic weapon against candida, I hope Squibb[†] will soon make it available for physicians and their patients in the United States. It seems to me that if oral *amphotericin B* helps the French, Swiss and Germans, it should also be available for patients with yeast-connected health disorders in North America. If you agree, you might write Squibb a letter (E. R. Squibb & Sons, Inc., P.O. Box 4000, Princeton, NJ 08540).

Other Candida species may cause problems: At the recent Birmingham Conference, Dr. Warren Pistey pointed out that *Candida albicans* is seen commonly in the everyday practice of pathology. Yet, at times it's hard to tell whether it is normal flora, an opportunist, or a pathogen. Dr. Pistey also noted that other species of candida, including *Candida tropicalis* and *Candida krusei*, are also found in some patients.

Charles M. Swaart (the man with a "still" in his intestines . . . see chapter 32) recently wrote me and said that it seems impossible for an M.D. to say or write the word 'Candida' without also using the word 'albicans.' He emphasized that *Candida albicans* isn't the only candida species that can cause problems. He referred especially to the book by H. I. Winner and R. Hurley, *Symposium on Candida Infections* (E. & S. Livingstone, Ltd., Edinburg and London).

New Methods of Studying and Treating Patients with Mold Sensitivity: In a paper presented at the annual seminar of the *Soci-*

[†]On September 6, 1983, I received the following comments from Squibb about amphotericin B: "Until such time as there are well-controlled double-blinded multicenter studies of this use of amphotericin B, Squibb is unable to either endorse or encourage the oral use of this product. Additionally, we are very concerned to see that patients are sniffing the amphotericin B powder and must most vigorously discourage its use in this fashion and hope that you will do so also."

Physicians working to help patients with yeast-connected illness should be aware of these comments. However, as I have previously pointed out, the 1985 PHYSICIAN'S DESK REFERENCE (page 2005) states that "oral administration of amphotericin B is usually well tolerated." (No adverse or toxic reactions are mentioned.)

Also, as previously noted, the studies of Montes, Cooper and associates found no evidence of toxicity from oral amphotericin B in contrast to the marked toxicity following intravenous administrations.

Candida albicans growing on mucous membranes leads to serious health disorders. Although oral nystatin and Nizoral® have proven effective in helping many individuals with these disorders, some individuals do not tolerate either drug.

Based on available evidence it seems to me that oral amphotericin B is a safe and effective anticandida medication. Accordingly, I hope Squibb will encourage or support the "well-controlled double-blinded multicenter studies" of oral amphotericin B which they feel are needed.

ety for Clinical Ecology, in November 1983, Sherry A. Rogers, M.D., told of her yeast and mold studies. I was fascinated by her presentation and feel her observations are relevant to any person interested in yeast-connected disorders.

In studies published in the July 1982 and January 1983 *Annals of Allergy,* Dr. Rogers showed that most laboratories, hospitals and allergists use the wrong culture media to identify common fungi in the air. She found that by making minor technical changes in the media, 32% more fungi were able to be identified (malt agar was substituted for the traditional Sabouraud's media).

> "We used the results of studies to select antigens to test individually and showed before-and-after photos of diverse and severe recalcitrant conditions that were dramatically cleared with these newer fungal antigens. Discontinuing the injections was concomitant with recurrence of the conditions. An elimination diet was also required for most patients and likewise discontinuing the diet was concomitant with recurrence. The diet necessary for the majority was a *ferment-free diet.* That is, one free of products of fermentation such as yeast, bread, alcohol, cheese, vinegar, catsup, mayonnaise, mustard, salad dressing, chocolate and most factory foods."

Dr. Rogers also told of a study which was accepted for publication in *The Annals of Allergy* in the spring of 1984. This study assessed the work-leisure-sleep, or 24-hour environment of patients for 13 months. Dr. Rogers said, in effect,

> "The highlights of this study of 390 culture plates showed that the predominant class of fungi for every month was yeast. Yet, most previous studies fail to mention this because they only chart fungi which can be identified by genus and species name. Yeasts are not further differentiated by most mycologists because they require biochemical tests that take weeks to complete . . . *My studies show that we are barely scratching the surface when it comes to understanding the prevalence of yeasts in our environment."*

In summarizing Dr. Rogers' presentation, it seems to me that the following points should be emphasized:

1. Immunotherapy with yeast and mold extract often helps, but it may not help as much as we would like.

2. *When it isn't effective, it may be because the mold antigens we use do not accurately represent the fungi which are bothering a particular patient.*

3. To more accurately obtain proper yeast and mold extracts for testing and treatment often requires cultures of the patient's home or workplace.

4. Instructions for obtaining such cultures can be obtained from:

> Mold Survey Service
> 2800 West Genesee Street
> Syracuse, New York 13219

This laboratory will supply plates (Petri dishes with malt agar) and instruction for their exposure at $10 (U.S.) per plate.

Within four weeks after having mailed back the plates, your doctor will receive the results of the mycologist's findings including the type of mold that grew and the number of colonies present.

Selenium and other antioxidants: Information I've recently obtained from several sources suggests that a group of nutrients called *"antioxidants"* are important in restoring immune function and combatting what is termed "free radical pathology." Free radicals are sometimes "bad guys." Briefly, they appear to be promiscuously reactive molecules and molecular fragments which react aggressively with other molecules.

Although many free radical chemical reactions occur normally in the body and are necessary for health, other such reactions damage tissues. Substances which protect the body are called *free radical scavengers* or *antioxidants.* These include selenium, ascorbate (vitamin C), vitamin E, Beta carotene and glutathione.

The Food and Nutrition Board has recommended a dietary intake of 50 to 200 micrograms of selenium per day. However, some physicians feel a range of 100 to 300 micrograms may be optimal. Selenium-rich foods include butter, wheat germ, Brazil nuts, barley, scallops, lobster, shrimp and oats.

For further information on selenium, see the book *Trace Elements, Hair Analysis and Nutrition* by Richard A. Passwater, Ph.D., and Elmer M. Cranton, M.D., Keats Publishing Company, Inc., New Canaan, CT, 1983; or the article "Biochemical-Pathology Initiated by Free Radicals, Oxidant Chemicals And Therapeutic Drugs in the Etiology of Chemical Hypersensitivity Disease," by Steven A. Levine, Ph.D. and Jeffrey H. Reinhardt. (*Journal of Orthomolecular Psychiatry,* Vol. 12, #3, Pages 166-183, 1983)

Are selenium and other supplements important in strengthening the immune system and helping a person overcome yeast-connected illness? Although I can't answer this question with authority, a number of clinicians and researchers feel that such supplementation is appropriate and necessary, especially in patients who live in parts of the country where soil selenium is low.

Laboratory studies may help: Up to this time, the diagnosis of yeast-connected illness (as is the case with measles, arthritis and many other disorders) has been based almost entirely on the typical clinical his-
tory, followed by the favorable response of
the patient to therapy. However, immune
system studies are now becoming available which help confirm the diagnosis of
yeast-connected health disorder. In addition, blood vitamin and mineral studies,
and amino acid and fatty acid determina-
tions may help in structuring appropriate
treatment programs for patients with
yeast-connected illness, especially those who aren't improving.

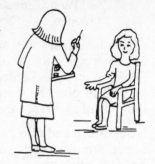

Immune system studies: Between May, 1981 and May, 1982, C. O. Truss, M.D. and Max Cooper, M.D. found changes in T cells and in the helper/suppressor ratio in patients with chronic candidiasis and associated chemical sensitivity. (Truss, C. O.: *Journal of Orthomolecular Psychiatry,* Vol. 10, #4, page 235.) At the 1983 Birmingham conference (see chapter 36), Alan Levin, M.D., San Francisco, described similar changes in his patients with yeast-related illness.

Subsequently, at a conference in San Francisco (The Yeast/Human Interaction, March 29-31, 1985) three different presentations dealt with antibody studies in patients with candidiasis. Those presenting their findings included Edward Winger, M.D., an immunopathologist, President of Immunodiagnostic Laboratory in Oakland, California and a member of the Faculty of the University of California, Berkeley; Howard E. Hagglund, M.D. a Norman, Oklahoma physician certified in Family Practice and David S. Bauman, Ph.D., President of Immuno-Mycologics, Inc., Washington, Oklahoma and F. T. Guilford, G. DerBalian and associates, San Mateo, California.

Although the studies described by these various investigators were not identical, each of them said, in effect, *"Based on our studies we can predict the likelihood that a patient has a candida-related health problem using these tests. Moreover, such tests can be carried out at the time the diagnosis is suspected and repeated after the treatment is begun. Changes in antibody levels help confirm the diagnosis in most of these patients and also help monitor the response to treatment."*

At a meeting of the American Academy of Otolaryngic Allergy in the fall of 1985 Aristo Wojdani, Ph.D., (Director of Research and Development of Advanced Allergy Research Center and faculty member of UCLA School of Medicine), Mamdouh Ghoneum, Ph.D., and Geoffrey P. Cheung, Ph.D., presented their findings on laboratory studies of a different type. According to these investigators, measurement of combinations of antibody titers along with circulating antigen and immune complexes are more helpful in the diagnosis of candidiasis than measurements of antibody titers alone.

Blood vitamin studies: Some individuals with yeast-connected illness (especially those with digestive problems) suffer from vitamin deficiencies. Such deficiencies are often related to a person's inability to absorb vitamins even though supplements are taken.

Blood studies may help in determining vitamin deficiencies or excesses. Such studies are reliably carried out in a number of laboratories including Vitamin Diagnostics, Incorporated (Dr. Herman Baker), Route 35 and Industrial Avenue, Cliffwood Beach, NJ 07735 and Monroe Medical Research Laboratory, Route 17, P.O. Box 1, Southfield, NY 10957, phone (914) 351-5134 or 1-800-831-3133.

Mineral studies: To conquer candida and get well you need proteins, carbohydrates and fats. You also need vitamins and minerals. In determining your mineral status, examinations of your hair, blood and urine are sometimes appropriate.

Physicians interested in carrying out such studies can obtain further information from Doctors Data, 30 W. 101 Roosevelt Road, West Chicago, IL, phone: 1-800-323-2784 or (312) 231-3649; MineraLab, Inc., P.O. Box 5012, Hayward, CA 94540, phone: (415) 783-5622; Omega Tech Laboratory, Medical Director: Elmer Cranton, M.D., P.O. Box 1, Trout Dale, VA 24378, phone: (703) 677-3103.

Amino acid studies: Amino acids combine in your body to form proteins. Recent clinical and laboratory studies suggest that some patients with chronic physical and mental illnesses including those who react to environmental chemicals show deficiencies or disturbances in their amino acids.

By collecting and analyzing 24-hour urine samples, data may be obtained that may serve as a guide to amino acid therapy.

Physicians interested in carrying out such studies can obtain further information from Bio Center Laboratory, 3715 East Douglas, Wichita, KS, telephone 1-800-835-3377; Bionostics, P.O.

Drawer 400, Lisle, IL 60532 (Dr. John Pangborn, Ph.D., Director); Bio Science Laboratories, 150 Community Drive, P.O. Box 825, Great Neck, NY 11022, telephone: (516) 829-8000; Monroe Medical Research Laboratory, Route 17, P.O. Box 1, Southfield, NY 10975, telephone: (914) 351-5134 or 1-800-831-3133.

Fatty acid studies: Recent research and clinical observations by Rudin, Horrobin, Baker and Galland show that you need to consume good fats and oils, if the cells of your body are to function properly. Moreover, recently published research studies by Truss show that patients with candidiasis show measurable abnormalities in their fatty acids.

Although I haven't used such studies in my own practice, I recently learned that "Essential Fatty Acid Profiles" can be determined by several laboratories including the Monroe Medical Research Laboratory, Route 17, P.O. Box 1, Southfield, NY 10975, telephone 1-800-831-3133.

Yeast-connected urticaria (hives): A famous allergist once announced at a national conference that he'd rather see a tiger come into his office than a patient with chronic urticaria. Yeasts aren't "the cause" of this devilishly difficult disorder, yet since my first candida patient in 1979 suffered from chronic urticaria and recovered completely (see page v), the subject interests me. Moreover, I successfully treated Robert (see chapter 28) and 5 other patients with chronic hives using anticandida therapy.

The yeast-urticaria connection was clearly described by G. Holti in 1966 (*Symposium on Candida Infection,* ed. Winner H. L. and Hurley R., Edinburgh: Livingstone, 1966, p. 73-81) Holti studies 255 patients with chronic urticaria, and 49 of the group reacted to candida extract. Of these 49, 27 were "clinically cured" using oral and vaginal nystatin. An additional 18 overcame their urticaria when they followed a low yeast diet for several months. In 1970 James and Warrin (*British Journal of Dermatology,* 84,: 227, 1971) confirmed Holti's observations, and so did Alfred Zamm, a Kingston, New York allergist and clinical ecologist in 1970.

More on Candida and Autism: (an anecdotal report) On January 7, 1984, I talked to Charles Swaart of Phoenix, AZ, who told me this fascinating story. (See chapter 32 for a discussion of Mr. Swaart's experience with candida)

> "Some months ago a woman called me to tell me about her 22-year-old daughter who was diagnosed as having autism when she was a young child. For almost 20 years she required total care 24 hours a day.

All the mother could do was feed her, keep her clean and shelter her. The child showed scant interest in outside surroundings and talked very little. At times she would act drunk and stagger and show other symptoms of intoxication.

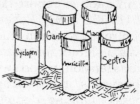

After reading the autism article by Don Campbell in the California paper (see chapter 29) she called my home and talked to my wife who told her more about candida. She went back to her doctor who ridiculed the idea. So she kept on talking and writing to my wife. Yet there was nothing my wife and I could do. Finally she called not long ago and told us her daughter was in the hospital with pneumonia and was receiving massive doses of antibiotics. She asked me if I would help her.

So I wrote her doctor and sent him all sorts of materials about the relationship of *Candida albicans* to autism and other severe mental and nervous system symptoms. This finally convinced him and he put the young woman on Nizoral® in large doses. Since then she has shown a marked improvement in her mental status.

Incidentally, Mr. Swaart tells me he has just completed a manuscript of a book (tentatively titled *Endogenous Alcohol Syndrome*) on the relationship of candida to the "drunk disease" and is looking for a publisher.

More on PMS: *Does candida cause PMS?* No. Candida isn't THE cause of the premenstrual syndrome or other problems affecting women. *Yet, there's growing evidence (based on exciting clinical experiences of many physicians) that there is a yeast connection.* And by using measures to discourage candida colonization, many women with PMS improve . . . sometimes dramatically. Yet, obviously, as with many other disorders ranging from arthritis to depression, other therapies are needed, including nutritional therapy.

Here are recent references documenting the efficacy of nutritional therapy:

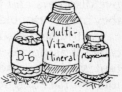

In an article in the July 1983 *Journal of Reproductive Medicine*, Guy E. Abraham, M.D. reported that all types of PMS patients may benefit from extra magnesium and B complex vitamins. In addition, tension and anxiety improve with 200 to 800 mgs. of B-6 a day. Eating less refined sugar, dairy products and arachidonic acid (in animal fats) also appeared to be helpful.

Patients with bloating and weight gain were helped by extra B-6 and by reduced sugar, caffeine and salt intake. Those with breast tenderness obtained relief with large doses of vitamin E, while those with headache, dizziness and sugar craving were helped by essential fatty acids (from vegetable oils), magnesium, zinc and vitamins B-3, B-6 and C.

In another report (*Journal of the American College of Nutrition*, 2:115-122, 1983), Robert S. London, M.D. of Baltimore described controlled research studies using vitamin E. With vitamin E there was a significant improvement in the following symptoms: nervous tension, mood swings, irritability, anxiety, headache, craving for sweets, increased appetite, heart pounding, fatigue and dizziness or fainting, depression, forgetfulness, crying, confusion and insomnia. Doses ranging from 150 to 600 I.U. of vitamin E were used; 300 I.U. per day appeared to be optimal.

In still another report in the *Journal of Reproductive Medicine* (28:465-468, July, 1983), David F. Horrobin described five studies using evening primrose oil (EPO) in women with PMS. Daily doses varied from 4 to 8 capsules, each containing 0.5 grams of Efamol® brand EPO, which contains 9% gammalinolenic acid. Significant improvement was observed in irritability, breast tenderness, ankle swelling, headache and depression. The author also suggested that addition of magnesium, zinc and vitamins B-3, B-6 and C resulted in an even greater response.

According to Leo Wollman, M.D., writing in the September, 1983 issue of *Cosmopolitan*, women need additional calcium especially during the 10 days prior to the onset of menstruation.

Marital Problems and Divorce: These unfortunate phenomena have been increasing in epidemic proportions during the past decade. Although the causes are multiple and complex, yeast-connected health disorders appear to play an important role.

Men with the "yeast problem" tend to be tired, irritable and depressed. They're often plagued by recurrent headaches and digestive disorders and their work productivity is reduced. Moreover, they may be troubled by prostatitis and a diminished sex drive.

Yeast-related disorders are especially devastating to women because yeast toxins affect hormone function. Recurrent or persistent vaginitis, menstrual irregularities, pain accompanying intercourse, fatigue, headaches, mood swings, depression and premenstrual tension occur commonly in the "yeast victim." Moreover, the problems of women are often aggravated by birth control pills, pregnancy and recurrent urinary tract infections.

Making a marriage work requires many things, including love, mutual respect and a lot of hard work. Even under ideal conditions, difficulties arise. So when one or both members of a union suffer from a yeast-connected health disorder, marital problems are an almost inevitable result.

More on Amino Acids: Amino acids are the "building blocks" found in proteins. There are 22 of them; some are essential while other are non-essential. According to John Pangborn, Ph.D.,[†] a specialist in the field, besides classical (acute) metabolism disorders, subclinical to subacute amino acid disorders are present in many diseases. Included among these are fatigue states, depression, allergic-like reactions to foods, learning disabilities, neuroses, psychoses and seizure states.

My experience in studying and treating health disorders related to amino acid metabolic defects is extremely limited. Yet because some of the symptoms associated with amino acid disturbances are found in patients with yeast-connected health disorder (especially fatigue, depression and allergic-like reactions to foods) amino acid metabolism intrigues me.

This type of metabolism involves enzymes, mineral activators, co-enzymes (from vitamin precursors) and other factors. Rapid inexpensive chromatographic procedures are now being carried out by a number of laboratories to measure urine and plasma amino acids. Moreover, corrective supplements are now available including amino acids, keto acids, vitamins, minerals and digestive enzymes.

Should your amino acid state be investigated? I don't know. Yet, if your health problems are yeastconnected and you have followed a comprehensive program of management for four months or longer and aren't improving, amino acid studies and appropriate therapy could help you.

More on Wheat and Gluten-Containing Foods: Gluten-containing foods (especially wheat, barley, oats and rye) have long been known to cause severe diarrhea and other chronic health problems in both children (celiac disease) and adults (sprue). And I've found that wheat and other gluten-containing foods also 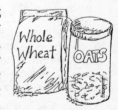 cause problems in some candida patients. So I was fascinated by a report sent to me by Lloyd Rosenvold, M.D. of Hope, Idaho describing a possible relationship of gluten intolerance and yeast

†Bionostics, Inc., P.O. Drawer 400, Lisle, IL 60532.

overgrowth to multiple sclerosis. In this report, Dr. Rosenvold commented:

"My interest in celiac sprue (CS) has been sparked (because) my wife's extended family has an inordinately large percentage of persons with multiple sclerosis and . . . individuals with symptoms compatible with a diagnosis of CS . . . We placed a number of MS patients on a gluten-free diet program. To our amazement, some of the neurological findings . . . began to lessen and disappear . . . Our MS patients (also) received some benefit from . . . nystatin and . . . gained in strength and endurance. Those that had severe diarrhea very promptly and remarkably improved. The bowel symptoms would remain under control as long as the nystatin was used . . . We know that in CS, gluten foods are improperly digested . . . (furnishing) an ideal culture medium for . . . candida yeasts. Since nystatin helps reduce yeast multiplication . . . this may be the beneficial effect of nystatin in MS."

Exercise: Many articles in the medical and lay literature tell of the beneficial effects of exercise. So this report I received from Maria shouldn't surprise you.

On March 3, 1983, Maria wrote:

"My awareness of allergy problems began in the fall of 1982 when we closed up our house for the winter. I began to develop severe headaches and depression that would come and go. I was confused and unable to sort out my thoughts. I developed paranoid feelings and thoughts of suicide kept popping into my head.

"I reflected on my life and could find no psychological or familial reason for this. I was enjoying being at home and my husband, my children and I were relating well.

"By what I consider an act of God, I found a neighbor who had experienced all sorts of allergies, including food and chemical sensitivities. She told me I was probably reacting to gas in my home. I had also noticed that my 2-year-old had become very hyper and my infant was much crabbier than he had been up to that time. We experimented with turning off the gas and, amazingly, most of our symptoms disappeared.

"Through experimentation, I've learned I feel better when I stay away from yeast-containing foods . . . less diarrhea and less fatigue. Yet, I continued to be bothered by diarrhea, stomach pains, nausea, irritability and an extreme craving for sweets and other foods as well. Please help."

Because of her chemical sensitivity, a history of vaginitis and a Candida Questionnaire score of 181, I put Maria on nystatin, a sugar-free, yeast-free diet and nutritional supplements. She improved steadily, although there were ups and downs in the ensuing months.

In January 1984, Maria wrote:

"I've gotten over the major hurdle in the treatment of my yeast problems. Since Christmas, I've felt more stable and healthier than I have in a long time. Moreover, I've been able to get off nystatin. I've also recently found I'm able to introduce offending foods into my diet, although I'm careful not to overdo it.

"I've also discovered that exercise plays a major role in keeping me well . . . maybe the largest factor at this point. I try to work out on weights, swim or exercise at least four times a week. As I begin to exercise, I can feel that tension and anger escape me and I feel more energy that day and the day after I work out."

Maria's emphasis on the benefits she derived from exercise are impressive. Her story also illustrates the importance of other factors which played a role in strengthening her immune system and helping her get well. These included prayer, avoiding chemical pollutants, diet, nystatin, nutritional supplements, and avoiding sugar and yeast-containing foods.

Here's more: In April 1986 I spent a couple of days with Harold Hedges, M.D., a Little Rock, Arkansas family practitioner who commented,

"I've successully treated hundreds of patients with candida-related disorders, and I'm gratified by their response. When people who have read your book call my office for an appointment, my office nurses tell them to begin the diet and follow the other general health measures you recommend while they're waiting to see me.

"Not infrequently, one of these prospective patients will call back and say, 'I feel like a new person. Does Dr. Hedges still want to see me?'

"Since my office appointment schedule is loaded, my nurse generally tells them, 'No, but stay on your diet, avoid chemicals, take your supplements and *exercise*'.

"Moreover, I emphasize the importance of exercise to all my patients. In my opinion, it's one of the most important ingredients of a candida control program."

More on Aspartame: Although aspartame is legal and is now being added to hundreds of foods and beverages, controversy surrounding its safety has been growing. For example in the January 13, 1984 issue of the *Wall Street Journal*, staff reporter Gary Putka said,

"The Arizona Department of Public Health is testing soft drinks containing aspartame—for possible signs that the chemical may deteriorate into toxic levels of methyl alcohol under certain storage conditions."

Storing soft drinks containing aspartame in higher than normal temperatures was of special concern to these investigators. The possible adverse effects of aspartame were also recently discussed on several national television programs.

Yet, on February 10, 1984 I talked to Laura Jane Stevens of West Lafayette, Indiana, author of the forthcoming book, *A New Way to Sugar Free Cooking* (see chapter 47, Update), who gave me a different point of view. Because sugar made her son, Jack, hyperactive for years, Laura worked to feed her family using sugar-free recipes. So when aspartame came along it helped her so much she read everything she could get her hands on (including many reports of F.D.A. research). Here are her comments:

"The breakdown ingredients of aspartame which its detractors are talking about are commonly found in fruits and vegetables in even greater quantities.

"Of course, aspartame may occasionally cause adverse effects, just as does any substance taken into the body, including commonly eaten foods. I'm aware of these food-induced reactions because I've experienced them; so have my children.

"Nevertheless, I feel comfortable about using aspartame and recommending it to others. Naturally, aspartame, like anything we consume, (whether it's milk, bananas or peanuts!) should be taken in moderation. And if it disagrees or causes adverse reactions, it can be avoided."

So what do you do? You can make up your own mind. Here are my suggestions: (1) Avoid all refined sugar products until you've conquered your candida. Also avoid or limit fruits. (2) Even after you're well, sharply limit your intake of refined sugar. Although it tastes good, it isn't good for you. To sweeten foods where sugar is called for in the recipe, use fruits as suggested by Karen Barkie. 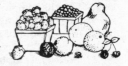 However, *wait 3 weeks before you begin trying fruits*. Then, if you tolerate them, use them in moderation. (3) You can also use Sweeta® or Fasweet® (liquid saccharin) in moderate amounts. *But don't go overboard*. (4) Avoid the powdered aspartame (Equal®) and saccharin (Sweet'N Low®) products as they contain dextrose.

What Does "Orthomolecular" Mean: About 15 years ago Linus Pauling, Ph.D., a two-time winner of the Nobel Prize, coined the term, "orthomolecular". And he published his now famous report entitled, "Orthomolecular Psychiatry" in *Science*, the journal of the American Association for the Advancement of Science. "Ortho" means to straighten. For example, the *ortho*dontist straightens teeth, and the *ortho*pedist works to provide straight bones.

Pauling used the term *ortho*molecular to convey the idea that many chronic mental disorders could be corrected by "straightening" the concentration of molecules in the brain.

Dr. Pauling's approach represents a radical change from the usual medical and psychiatric approach which deals primarily with the use of synthetic drugs which aren't normally present in the body. Orthomolecular nutrition now is applied to every part of the body and recognizes that people are biochemically different and unique (as has been frequently emphasized by Roger J. Williams, Ph.D.).

Accordingly, in evaluating and treating patients with yeast-connected illness and other chronic health disorders, I try to "straighten" my patients. One of the ways I work to accomplish this goal is by helping them obtain the nutrients they need and avoid the toxic substances which contribute to their illnesses.

More on Nutrition: About ten years ago Dr. Jean Mayer of Boston pointed out that the average physician knows about as much about nutrition as his secretary—unless his secretary belongs to *Weight Watchers*. Then the physician is apt to know half as much! About the same time I saw an editorial in the *Southern Medical Journal* which pointed out that there had been a "blackout" in nutrition education in most medical schools.

Like my peers I spent more time during my residency treating disease than preventing it. And I knew nothing about many nutritional subjects that fascinate me today. Interestingly enough, much of what I've learned about nutrition through the years has come from non-medical publications.

These include *Executive Health*, an 8-page monthly commentary which discusses topics such as magnesium, vitamin C & backache, vitamin B-6, preventing alcoholism, exercise and many other topics you need to know about if you want to enjoy good health. Moreover, the editorial board of this publication includes two Nobel Prize winners plus other scientists and academicians with impeccable credentials.

Another authoritative source of nutrition information is the *Cen-*

ter for Science in the Public Interest (CSPI). This Washington, DC based organization (headed by Michael Jacobson, Ph.D.) deserves high marks. In my opinion *it ranks at the top of the list of organizations working to improve the quality of food offered to Americans.* I support this organization and during the past 10 years I've learned a lot from their publications including, especially, their illustrated, highly readable periodical *Nutrition Action.* (see also chapter 34).

Other excellent sources of nutrition information include the health food magazines, *Prevention, Bestways, Let's Live* and *Your Good Health* which are now read by millions of subscribers. In *Prevention* I first read about the work of the late Henry Schroeder of Dartmouth College, the brilliant pioneer in the field of trace minerals. Through this same magazine I also learned of the work of Dr. Tom Brewer. This crusading obstetrician had worked untiringly to stress the importance of feeding mothers a good diet during pregnancy rather than limiting their weight and treating them with "water pills". Also, through articles in the health food magazines, I first learned that my adult patients (especially females), needed calcium and magnesium supplements to prevent their bones from disintegrating. Moreover this was 7 or 8 years before I read an editorial in the 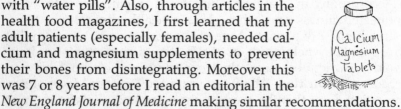 *New England Journal of Medicine* making similar recommendations.

But health food magazines aren't the only sources of nutrition information. Increasingly, informative articles are appearing in other widely read periodicals including *Reader's Digest, The Saturday Evening Post, Woman's Day, Cosmopolitan, New Woman, Family Circle, Ladies Home Journal, Redbook, American Health, The Rotarian* and many others. Such articles usually emphasize that better health doesn't always come from more doctoring, more drugs and more hospitals. Instead it is achieved from better nutrition, exercise, stopping smoking and changing your lifestyle.

If you suffer from yeast-connected health problems keep reading, studying and learning about nutrition and about yourself and your response and reactions to different foods. As I've noted previously (chapter 17) *you are unique and your dietary requirements, tolerances and sensitivities differ considerably from those of other people (including members of your own family.)*

You must change your diet to conquer your yeast-connected health problems. In fact, some people get better on dietary changes alone, even without medication. Yet, *no rules can be laid down which suit every patient*. Here's a summary of what I tell my patients today (July 1986):

1. Make sure your diet is nutritionally adequate, with fresh foods from a wide variety of sources.
2. *Diversify or rotate your foods.* (See chapter 15). Food intolerances, sensitivities or allergies develop more commonly in those who eat the same foods every day. Also, by rotating your diet you'll be better able to identify foods that disagree with you.
3. *Avoid all refined carbohydrates,* including sugar, corn syrup, dextrose and fructose. Also avoid honey, maple syrup and date sugar. Feeding sugar and simple carbohydrates to candida organisms is like pouring kerosene on a fire.
4. *Avoid refined, processed and fabricated foods.* Such foods usually contain sugar, yeasts and other hidden ingredients that may bother you. Moreover, other important nutrients including essential fatty acids, vitamins and minerals have been removed from many of these foods. In addition 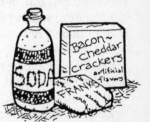 harmful (or potentially harmful) ingredients have been substituted—as for example, hardened vegetable oils and additives of various types.
5. During the early weeks of your diet *avoid fruits and milk* as the carbohydrates in these foods seem to encourage candida growth.
6. Since whole fruits are good food, as you improve try rotating them back into your diet and see if you tolerate them.
7. During the first week of your diet avoid all yeast- and mold-containing foods. Then challenge with yeast and see if it bothers you. If it does not, you can eat yeast-containing foods in moderation . . . especially if you rotate them. *But don't go overboard.*
8. Eat sugar-free *yogurt*, take nutritional supplements, including preparations of *Lactobacillus acidophilus*, vitamins, minerals, essential fatty acids and garlic.

Occasionally, if a patient isn't improving on the dietary program outlined above, I restrict the good carbohydrate grains and vegetables for a week or two. But since these carbohydrates provide so many essential nutrients, I put them back in the diet as soon as possible.

More on Die-Off Reactions: Nystatin kills the yeasts it touches. Apparently, it blasts open the capsules of the yeast spores, killing a lot of them at once. In the process, dead yeast products are released. And until your body gets rid of them, these yeast products may make you sick.

Here's how I explain these "die-off" reactions to my patients: Suppose someone throws a lighted cigarette into a waste basket full of trash. A fire results and you rush for the fire extinguisher. You put out the fire but smoke is produced which makes your eyes burn, your nose run and causes you to cough. Although the fire has been put out, it takes a while to get rid of the smoke.

Similarly, when you kill out a lot of yeast in your digestive tract, it may take a few days (or longer) to get rid of the resulting dead yeast products.

Over the past year or two, a number of people have called or written me and said, "I simply can't take nystatin. Every time I try it, it makes me sick." A number of my own patients have experienced similar reactions. However, I see fewer such reactions since I've started putting patients on the diet for 10 days before starting nystatin. In some patients, I've prescribed Nizoral® for about a week, following it with nystatin.

Recently, Alfred V. Zamm, M.D. of Kingston, New York wrote and told me of still another way of avoiding or coping with die-off reactions. In his comments, Dr. Zamm said, in effect:

> I've found I can avoid prolonged discomfort in my patients and enable them to take high doses of nystatin by removing yeasts from the digestive tract. Moreover, I've found this method to be successful in patients who had been struggling to take nystatin for a year or more. Using this plan, they were able to tolerate the nystatin within a week or two and experience less discomfort. Here's my method:
> *Day 1:* No solids. Clear broth only, made from moderately salted meat and vegetables.
> *Day 2:* Solids added, consisting of pureed meat and vegetables.
> *Day 3 to 7:* More solids added (meats, eggs, vegetables, whole grains). No sugar, corn syrup, honey, fruit, white flour products or processed foods.
> *Enemas:* On days 1 and 2, room-temperature enemas, using chlorine-free water. (By cleaning out the colon, yeasts are removed.)
> *Nystatin powder:* Begin with ⅛ teaspoon three times a day and increase to ¼ teaspoon (between the 3rd & 7th day).

"This procedure is not to be done in patients who are metabolically fragile in regard to their electrolytes, who are on diuretics or who have otherwise compromised systems incapable of dealing with a temporary stress as above outlined."

In discussing his bowel cleansing program with me in October 1984, Dr. Zamm made several additional comments. He especially pointed out that this method or procedure closely resembles that used by physicians to prepare patients for endoscopic examination of the digestive tract.

Yeasts Can Make Hormones: Yeasts have been described as being "funny little critters." Although they're like vegetables in many ways, according to Sidney Baker, "Yeasts have some very animal-like behavior when it comes to chemistry."

Nevertheless, I was surprised to read an article in the August 1984 issue of SCIENCE, telling of the observations of David Feldman, M.D., Chief of Endocrinology at Stanford University, who has spent most of his career studying steroid hormones in humans.

Recently, Feldman and his colleagues decided to look for steroid hormones in candida and they discovered what appeared to be mammalian-like receptors and steroid hormones in at least three different species of yeasts. Apparently, candida not only has receptors that have to do with cortisone and sugar metabolism, other yeasts produce the human female sex hormones, 17 B-estradiol.

The significance of these findings isn't clear to anyone at this time, but I'm pleased that more and more researchers are taking a look at *Candida albicans* and its role in making people sick.

38

What You Should Do If You Aren't Improving

Suppose your medical history (including, especially, lots of broad spectrum antibiotic drugs) suggests that your health problems are yeast-connected. And suppose you feel "sick all over" and are bothered by symptoms affecting many parts of your body (depression, headache, fatigue, digestive disturbances, skin problems, menstrual problems, etc.). Moreover, you've consulted many different specialists who have examined you and tried to help you, yet their tests have all been reported to be "normal or negative."

Then you learned about "the yeast connection" and with the help of a physician you have followed the diet and have taken one or more of the antifungal medications described in this book. Yet, after 2 or 3 (or more) months of treatment, including nystatin and/ or Nizoral®, you aren't improving . . . what then? . . . What should you do?

Although I don't have an easy answer *I feel it is essential for you to be carefully re-examined and re-evaluated.*

In my own patients who fail to improve I usually order candida immunoglobulin tests. Although these tests aren't perfect if they are elevated, I continue anticandida therapy. If I haven't used Nizoral®, I give this important antifungal medication a trial for at least a month. (Nizoral® reaches candida which may have "burrowed in" beneath the membrane surfaces of the digestive tract, vagina or respiratory tract.)

I also seek consultation from appropriate medical and laboratory specialists to help identify (or rule out) other disorders that may be responsible for my patients' continuing symptoms. Here are some of the things that may need to be evaluated or re-evaluated.

1. A careful and comprehensive review of the history[†] including any new symptoms that may have developed.
2. A careful physical examination.
3. A complete blood count and sedimentation rate to help determine the presence (or absence) of anemia, infection, and/or other abnormalities.
4. Appropriate blood and urine tests to help identify liver, kidney, thyroid and other abnormalities.
5. Other appropriate laboratory examinations including studies for the Epstein-Barr Virus (EBV) and other viruses.
6. Careful and repeated examinations of the stools may help identify infestation by microscopic parasites including *Entamoeba histolytica* and *Giardia*. (During the spring of 1986 several physicians have told me they had been able to help several of their difficult patients by identifying and treating parasitic infestations.)
7. Appropriate studies by radiology consultants (if so indicated by the patient's symptoms).
8. Nutritional deficiencies and imbalances of various kinds which may occur coincidentally or as a result of candidiasis. (See also the studies and observations of Truss, Baker and Galland.) In identifying such imbalances, a careful dietary history plus blood fatty acid and vitamin studies and blood and urine amino acid studies may help.
9. Possible sensitivities and toxicities caused by environmental chemicals may also need to be evaluated. Insecticides, formaldehyde, lead, cadmium and thousands of other chemicals are permeating our air, soil and water. The help of a specialist in environmental medicine may be indicated.

(Dr. John Laseter, Ph.D., Enviro-Health, 990 N. Bowser Road #800, Richardson, TX 75081 (214) 234-5577, conducts blood studies which measure levels of various environmental pollutants. Moreover, among the toxicities which may be causing problems are silver/amalgam/mercury fillings in the teeth. (See chapter 44, Update).

---

†See Chapter 45, Update for comments on the importance of the medical history.

Section
F

The Yeast
Connection
Update

Introduction 39

In his book, *Future Shock,*[†] Alvin Toffler talked about the rapid changes taking place in our society, including the "accelerated thrust in technology and knowledge."

In commenting on this book in his article entitled *"Deciding the Future for the Practice of Allergy and Immunology,"*[‡] William T. Kniker, M.D., Professor of Pediatrics and Microbiology, Division of Clinical Immunology, University of Texas Health Science Center, San Antonio, Texas, had this to say:

> "Before we can get used to anything, it's already obsolete; there are always more things to learn, to choose, and to decide."

In discussing the problems of today's allergists and what they should do to solve them, Dr. Kniker made many other comments which I feel are relevant.[‡‡] Here are some of them:

> "The failure of hierarchies to solve society's problems forces people to talk to one another—and that was the beginning of networks. *Networking* is a verb, not a noun, a *process of getting there . . . the communication that creates linkages between people and clusters of people. Networks exist to foster self-help, to exchange information, to change society . . . and to share resources.*
>
> They are structured to transmit information in a way that is quicker, more high tech, and more energy efficient than any process we know. One of networking's greatest attractions is that it is an easy way to get information . . . much easier than going to a library, university, or, God forbid, the government. As each person in a network takes in new information, he or she synthesizes it and comes up with other new ideas. Networks share these newly forged thoughts and ideas."

---

†Toffler, A.: *Future Shock*, New York, Random House, 1970.
‡Kniker, W. T.: "Deciding the Future for the Practice of Allergy and Immunology". *Annals of Allergy*, 55:106-113, August 1985.
‡‡This material was adapted and paraphrased by Dr. Kniker from the book, *Megatrends . . . Ten New Directions Transforming Our Lives*, © 1982, by John Naisbitt, published by Warner Books, Inc., 666 5th Avenue, New York, NY 10103.

The material in *The Yeast Connection Update* has been acquired from many, many sources. In fact, scarcely a week goes by that I do not learn something I didn't know before. Although some of this information has been acquired from the clinical observations and scientific studies of my peers in the medical profession, a lot of it has been acquired through *networking*.

The Yeast Connection Update contains much new material which should interest you and help you understand and overcome your chronic health problems, including those which are yeast connected.

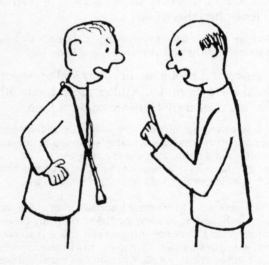

40

Is The Yeast Connection a Myth, a Fad, or Is It For Real?

The Yeast Connection Controversy

If you review medical history, you'll find countless examples of new ideas which helped sick people get well which were "stumbled on" accidentally. Some of these discoveries were made by scientists working in their laboratories and others by practitioners. Still others were made by non-physicians. But, *regardless of who makes a discovery or what the discovery is, if a full scientific explanation of the mechanism isn't forthcoming, it tends to be rejected by the "establishment"*.

As I've already mentioned, many physicians, when they hear about "the yeast connection" are apt to say, "There's no proof that candida plays a role in making you sick." Or "Where are the scientific studies?"

For example, in the March 27, 1986 issue of *The New England Journal of Medicine*, Dr. E. Richard Stiehm, a Pediatric Immunologist at the University of California-Los Angeles Medical Center and a UCLA colleague, Dr. Albert Haas, in a letter to the editor entitled, "The Yeast Connection Meets Chronic Mucocutaneous Candidiasis (CMC)", told of their experiences in treating a two-year-old with CMC, a rare candida-related disorder. The child in question had been incompletely diagnosed and inappropriately treated before coming to their medical center.

They used this single case to denigrate "The Yeast Connection" as a possible cause of fatigue, depression, headache, irritability and other symptoms in various parts of the body. Moreover, prior to the Stiehm and Haas letter, two major allergy organizations (the American Academy of Allergy and Immunology and the American College of Allergists) released an identical *Proposed Position Statement* on *Candidiasis-Hypersensitivity Syndrome* in which they stated that "the concept is speculative and unproven".

I can understand the skepticism of any physician who is faced with an idea he hasn't heard about and which he doesn't understand. Yet, in my opinion, those who reject the role of candida in making people "sick all over" aren't aware of the research studies of Iwata (see chapter 36). *These studies show that candida produces both high and low molecular-weight toxins. Moreover, Iwata found that when he injected these toxins into healthy mice, they acted as an "immunosuppressant" and caused "unsettled behavior" and other systemic symptoms.*

In addition, most skeptical physicians haven't read the four published articles by C. Orian Truss, especially his fourth article which describes his ongoing clinical and laboratory studies. These studies include laboratory findings which indicate that patients with candidiasis develop metabolic abnormalities. (See chapter 36).

And they probably haven't read the brief report of E. W. Rosenberg, M.D.[†] and his associates which was published in the *New England Journal of Medicine* (Volume 308:101, January 13, 1983). In this report these physicians described the improvement of patients with psoriasis and inflammatory bowel disease accompanying the administration of oral nystatin, "an agent that was expected to work only on yeast in the gut lumen".

Now then, I would like to digress a bit. I became interested in allergy some 30 years ago and the rejection of "the yeast connection" reminds me of the rejection of allergy (especially food allergy) by the medical establishment. In an article published in *Pediatrics*[‡] in April, 1958, I made these comments:

> Allergy—occupies a uniquely confusing and controversial position. No other field of medicine has been the subject of as much violent controversy, difference of opinion and confusion . . . It's small wonder that cynical skeptics—incorrectly consider the whole of allergy to be so much "hocus pocus" or quackery.

---

†E. W. Rosenberg, M.D., Professor and Chairman of the Department of Dermatology, University of Tennessee, Memphis, TN.
‡Crook, W. G., Harrison, W. W., and Crawford, S. E., "Allergy—The Unanswered Challenge in Pediatric Research, Education and Practice". *Pediatrics* 21:649-654, 1958.

During the past 28 years, I've written and talked about the effectiveness of elimination diets in helping people with allergy, headache, fatigue, hyperactivity, digestive problems, irritability and a host of other symptoms. Yet, my observations were usually ignored or rejected by most physicians—even though I published my observations in a peer-reviewed medical journal and included a double blind scientific study.[†]

But now after many years, "hidden" food allergies are finally being recognized and are "coming out of the closet", according to William T. Kniker, M.D. (Head of the Division of Clinical Immunology, University of Texas Health Science Center, San Antonio, TX).

In a presentation at the January, 1986 meeting of the American College of Allergists, Kniker urged the physicians in the audience to take a look at delayed food reactions and start helping their patients. Here are a few of his comments (as quoted by the February, 1986 issue of *Allergy Observer*):

> "Our patients deserve to have their food allergies diagnosed and managed in an expeditious and scientifically sound manner. We have to become experts in assessing the effects of all the things our patients drink, breathe and touch. If we don't someone else will."

In his continuing discussion, Dr. Kniker pointed out that *proving these food reactions in the laboratory was still unsatisfactory* and that diet manipulation is the best way to identify a food-related problem.

The food allergy connection resembles the yeast connection in several ways. Here they are:

1. The role of *Candida albicans* in causing fatigue, depression, PMS and other symptoms is recognized by millions of people and a handful of physicians.

2. Clinical reports clearly describe this relationship, and a few scientific studies explain it. Yet, the yeast connection is rejected by many members of the "medical establishment".

3. Although a number of investigators are now carrying out sci-

---

[†]Crook, W. G., et al.: "Systemic Manifestations Due to Allergy. Report of Fifty Patients and A Review of the Literature on the Subject." *Pediatrics*, 27:790, 1961.

entific studies, *diagnosis of the candida-human illness relationship at this time is based on a careful clinical history, followed by the response of the patient to a simple treatment program.*

I fully realize that other factors (including environmental chemicals, toxins, viruses, and allergens) can and do cause symptoms similar to those described in this book. And, as new information becomes available, I sincerely hope "the yeast connection controversy", like the food allergy controversy, will fade away.

The Tomato Effect—Rejection of Highly Efficacious Therapy

In a recent issue of *The Journal of the American Medical Association* James S. Goodwin, M.D. and Jean M. Goodwin, M.D., M.P.H.[†], Department of Medicine and Psychiatry, University of New Mexico, School of Medicine, published a fascinating article, "The Tomato Effect", which I know will interest you. Here's why: It'll help you understand why your doctor may reject what you tell him about "the yeast connection." Here are highlights from this article.

> The tomato is a New World plant, originally found in Peru and carried back to Spain from whence it quickly spread to Italy and France . . . By 1560 the tomato was becoming a staple of the continental European diet . . .
> (Yet) at the same time it was ignored or actively shunned in America . . . The reason tomatoes were not accepted . . . *everyone knew they were poisonous, at least everyone in North America* . . . Not until 1820, when Robert Gibbon Johnson ate a tomato on the steps of the courthouse in Salem, N.J. and survived, did the people of America begin, grudgingly, . . . to consume tomatoes.

According to these two medical school professors, *"The tomato effect in medicine occurs when an efficacious treatment for a certain disease is ignored or rejected because it does not 'make sense.'"*

If you review medical history you'll find many examples of the "tomato effect" in medicine. In my opinion, and that of Dr. David Edwards of Reno, Nevada, a current "tomato" is the rejection by the medical establishment of the yeast connection. They tend to reject it because they don't understand it and how it can make people "sick all over." It doesn't "make sense" to them because

---

†Goodwin, James S., M.D. and Goodwin, Jean M., M.D., M.P.H. "The Tomato Effect", JAMA Vol. 251, No. 18, pp. 2287-2290, May 11, 1984.

they haven't read the reports by Iwata, Truss, Witkin, Rosenberg and Baker which have been reviewed and discussed on many pages of this book.

In their continuing discussion Drs. Goodwin and Goodwin had this to say,

> ". . . Modern medicine is particularly vulnerable to the tomato effect. Pharmaceutical companies have . . . turned to theoretical over practical arguments for using their drugs. Therefore, we are asked to use a new arthritis drug because it stops monocytes from crawling through a filter, a new antidepressant because it blocks re-uptake of serotonin but not norepinephrine into rat synaptosomes, a new antihypertensive because it blocks angiotensin generation, or an oral diabetes drug because it increases insulin receptors on monocytes."

> "What gets lost in such discussions are the only three issues that matter in picking a therapy. *Does it help? How toxic is it? How much does it cost?* In this atmosphere we are at risk for rejecting a safe, inexpensive, effective therapy in favor of an alternative treatment, perhaps less efficacious and more toxic."

So when safe prescription and non-prescription substances (such as nystatin, caprylic acid, garlic and acidophilus) plus a special diet are rejected "in favor of a less effective treatment which is also more toxic" we see a clear example of the tomato effect.

Metabolic Studies By C. Orian Truss, M.D.

Thousands of scientific articles have been published describing infections caused by *Candida albicans*. However, most of these have dealt with membrane infections due to candida (especially vaginitis) and severe systemic infections in individuals with severe immune system disorders.

Then, beginning in 1977, clinical observations on the role of *Candida albicans* in contributing to many chronic health disorders were first presented by C. Orian Truss, M.D., at the Eighth Annual Scientific Symposium of the Academy of Orthomolecular Psychiatry held in Toronto, April 30-May 1, 1977.

Truss' observations were published in a paper in 1978 and in two subsequent papers in 1980 and 1981, as well as in a book, THE MISSING DIAGNOSIS, in 1983.

In these publications, Truss commented,

> "Because of its universal presence in the body, commonly used diagnostic techniques reveal little about it (chronic candidiasis), and the diagnosis must be suspected from the clinical picture and confirmed by the response to treatment."

Then in 1982, because of the desirability of establishing a laboratory basis for the diagnosis of patients with these problems, Truss initiated studies in 24 patients he considered "classic cases of mold sensitivity and chronic yeast susceptibility." The design of the study was to carry out a general evaluation of protein, fat and carbohydrate metabolism.

Truss' findings were presented at the conference on "Human/Yeast Interaction" in Birmingham in December, 1983 and a preliminary report was published in the summer, 1984 issue of *The Journal of Orthomolecular Psychiatry*.

A major goal of the studies consisted of testing the hypothesis that acetaldehyde produced in the intestines by the fermentation of sugars by *Candida albicans* serves as the "principal" mediator of metabolic disturbances in patients with yeast-related health disorders.

In his 27-page report, Truss reviews many biochemical interrelationships and describes the methods he used in studying both amino acids and fatty acids. Significant abnormalities were noted in both of these important components found in the human body.

How and why would these changes occur? Quite frankly, the explanation is a complex one. When sugar is metabolized in the intestine by yeast, carbon dioxide is usually released by excessive flatus, belching and bloating.

In addition, in the breakdown of sugar by yeast, other metabolic products are formed, including acetaldehyde and alcohol. Moreover, as noted by Iwata in Japan, certain strains of candida can produce alcohol in sufficient quantities to cause an elevation of a person's blood alcohol level and actual drunkenness (see chapters 29 and 32).

I don't expect you to understand all the chemistry involved. Yet, according to Dr. Truss, under the conditions existing in the gut, sugar can be converted into acetaldehyde, a toxic substance. Moreover, it would appear that the patient with chronic candidiasis cannot metabolize this substance and get rid of it. As a result, acetaldehyde (through disturbances in many biochemical and metabolic pathways) may cause the widespread systemic symptoms seen in patients with yeast-related health problems.

Dr. Truss pointed out that there are many reports in the medical literature on acetaldehyde. Moreover, some of these studies explain how acetaldehyde causes these metabolic abnormalities.

In summarizing his comprehensive study, he made these comments:

> "The results of metabolic studies in 24 patients with chronic candidiasis have been presented. An attempt has been made to consider the principal symptoms of this condition and these metabolic findings in relation to various toxic effects of acetaldehyde. Though speculative, these thoughts as to how this toxin could cause the clinical and laboratory characteristics of this illness are a vital part of this hypothesis."

The Witkin Immune System Studies

In the May-June, 1985 issue of *Infections in Medicine* Steven S. Witkin, Ph.D., published his observations on 50 women who had experienced at least three separate episodes of candida vaginal infection within a 12 month period. The title of the Witkin article, "Defective Immune Responses in Patients With Recurrent Candidiasis." Here are excerpts from this report.

> "Clinically significant infections of mucous membranes by *Candida albicans* are occurring with increased frequency . . . Recent studies suggest that the infection, itself, may cause *immunosuppression*, resulting in recurrences in certain patients. In addition to creating an increased susceptibility to *Candida* reinfection, the immunological alterations may also be related to subsequent *endocrinopathies* and *autoantibody formation*."

In his continuing discussion Dr. Witkin discusses the factors which predispose an individual to *Candida albicans* infection.

> "Antibiotic therapy can create conditions conducive to *C. albicans* proliferation by several possible mechanisms. Orally administered broad spectrum antibiotics change the microbial composition of the alimentary tract and vagina. The resulting alterations in pH and composition of available nutrients or microbial products can lead to proliferation of *Candida*."
>
> "In addition, antibiotics can also interfere with the ability of the immune system to limit fungal infections. Aureomycin, tetracycline and sulfonamides have been shown to decrease the phagocytic ("germ eating") capacity of polymorphonuclear leukocytes (white blood cells)."

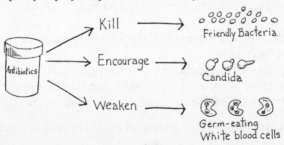

"Since an intact cellular immune system is essential for defending against fungal infections, it is not surprising that factors leading to alterations in components of this system also predispose to *Candida* infection. Hormonal imbalances due to pregnancy, corticosteroid therapy or possibly oral contraceptive use can lead to depressed cellular immunity."

As you know, many American physicians have stated that the yeast/human illness hypothesis is "speculative" and "unproven". So I was delighted to see the Witkin report as it seems to provide some of the scientific evidence that skeptics have been demanding.

More on Immune System Studies

Can laboratory studies help your physician make a diagnosis of a yeast-related disorder?

In my opinion the answer is "Yes." I often obtain blood specimens on my patients and send them to a laboratory for special candida antibody studies. Nevertheless, I continue to base my diagnosis of a candida-related health disorder on the following criteria.

1. History of repeated or prolonged courses of broad spectrum antibiotic drugs and/or corticosteroids.
2. Symptoms affecting many parts of a person's body including the nervous system, the endocrine system (especially the reproductive organs in women) and the digestive system. However, the skin, respiratory tract and musculoskeletal system are also commonly affected. (See questionnaire, chapter 6).
3. Comprehensive clinical and laboratory studies by competent medical specialists have failed to reveal the cause for the patient's symptoms. Moreover, therapies of various sorts haven't helped.
4. Heightened sensitivity to environmental chemicals (perfumes, insecticides, petrochemicals, household cleaners, tobacco, etc.).
5. Aggravation of symptoms in damp, humid weather or in moldy homes or buildings.
6. The response of the patient . . . often dramatic . . . to a therapeutic trial of a special diet (designed to decrease candida growth in the digestive tract) and antifungal medication.

Although I rely mainly on a clinical evaluation of my patients (as described above), during the years 1984-1986 I felt it was appropriate for me to support my clinical diagnosis with laboratory studies. Accordingly, I obtained blood antibody studies on over 100 of my patients; and the laboratory diagnosis in over 85% of these patients agreed with my clinical diagnosis.

Yet, at this time the results of these studies have not yet been reported in the scientific literature; moreover, there is no general agreement among physicians and researchers as to which laboratory studies are best.

In reviewing this subject recently George Kroker, M.D. of La-Crosse, Wisconsin commented,

> "Unfortunately when we attempt to apply antibody measurements to the diagnosis of (yeast-related disorders) . . . several problems arise with the antibody studies . . . Opinions on the diagnostic value of yeast antibody tests differ because of these three factors:
>
> 1. Lack of widespread standardization of testing techniques and antigen preparation.
> 2. The common occurrence of antibodies to *Candida albicans* in normal human hosts without disease.
> 3. Lack of established blood levels of candida antibodies in disorders characterized by excessive candida colonization.
>
> . . . Presently the use of candida specific antibody measurements to diagnose (chronic candidiasis) is promising but unproven."

Immune system studies on individuals with yeast-related health disorders are now being carried out by a number of laboratories including:

1. Immunodiagnostic Laboratories, 400 29th Street #508, Oakland, CA 94609 (Edward Winger, M.D.) (415) 839-6477.
2. Biological Information Systems, Inc., 101 S. San Mateo Drive #315, San Mateo, CA 94401 (415) 342-8323 (F. T. Guilford, M.D. and G. DerBalian, Ph.D.).
3. Cerodex Laboratories, Inc., 2227 West Lindsey #1401, Norman, OK 73069 (405) 288-2458 (Howard Hagglund, M.D. and David Bauman, Ph.D.) CEIA test is marketed by MEDI-TREND, Inc., Albuquerque, NM, 1-800-545-8900.
4. Advanced Allergy Research Center, 10642 Santa Monica Blvd., #211, Los Angeles, CA 90025 (G. P. Cheung, Ph.D., M. Ghoneum, Ph.D., and A. Wojdani, Ph.D.) (213) 474-6063.
5. Antibody Assay Laboratories, 805 West La Veta #201, Orange, CA 92668 (Alan Broughton, M.D.), (714) 538-3255.

Immunotherapy For Candida-Related Health Problems

Recently I reviewed articles in the medical literature (including several I hadn't seen before) which described improvement in candida-related health disorders following the use of candida extracts. Included among these was a report by an Israeli physician (*Candida albicans as an Allergenic Factor*. Liebeskind, A. *Annals of Allergy* 20:394-396, 1962). Here are excerpts from this report:

> The presence of *C. albicans* can evoke allergic reactions in a human organism . . . So far, not much has been mentioned in the literature about this allergy. The following work is based on the study of 25 cases of *C. albicans* allergy. It is divided into two groups. The first group represents seven cases of *C. albicans* allergy belonging to the classical form of respiratory allergy . . .
>
> The second group of patients presents a particular interest in that it is comprised of 18 cases of *C. albicans* allergy drawn up from various fields of medicine. *These patients were chronically ill and were treated for many years by physicians, including specialists in the various branches of medicine. They were given symptomatic treatment according to the signs and symptoms with which they presented themselves.*
>
> *The results of this kind of symptomatic treatment proved to be a complete failure.* Only by a chance subcutaneous test performed on these patients, the possibility of *C. albicans* allergy was suspected. Subsequently, these patients were treated with hyposensitization injections of *C. albicans* extracts during a period of 6 to 10 months. *Thirteen out of the above 18 patients got complete relief of their symptoms, and five showed a remarkable improvement.*
>
> Symptoms included gastrointestinal manifestations, bronchial manifestations (non-asthmatic), migraine headaches, and vulvitis . . . The relatively small number of patients studied does not permit us to draw any definite conclusions. However, the possibility of *C. albicans* allergy should be given.

I was fascinated by the Liebeskind report because it resembled the initial report of Truss (C. O. Truss, *The Missing Diagnosis*, pg. 128) in two respects. Both physicians noted a relationship between candida and a variety of systemic symptoms and both physicians appeared to ''stumble on'' this observation by what might be called a serendipitous route.

In a subsequent paper (Hosen, H. "Focal Fungal Infections Treated by Immunological Therapy with Emphasis on Vaginal Moniliasis", *Texas Medicine* 67:58, 1971) a Texas physician told of his experience in studying 35 patients with monilia (candida) vaginitis using candida extract injections. In the summary of his article he stated:

> "While local therapy eradicates the symptoms of mycotic infections,

it does not affect fungi which may have penetrated into deeper layers of tissue; therefore, recurrences are common. Immunological types of therapy produce more rapid and efficient clinical results. Local and immunological methods may be used in combination for patients with recurrent monilial infections."

In a subsequent similar report (Kudelko, N. M. "Allergy in Chronic Monilial Vaginitis", *Annals of Allergy* 29:266, 1971) an Oregon physician told of his experiences in helping patients with chronic yeast infections of the vagina using allergy extract injections. Here's a summary of his report:

"Seventy selected patients with chronic monilial vaginitis had unsatisfactory results from conventional treatments. After they were evaluated for an allergic diathesis, and *Candida albicans* allergens were included in their hyposensitization injections, 90 percent responded with good to excellent results. Gynecologists and allergists are reminded that allergy may involve the vulvo-vaginal tract and that specific anti-allergic therapy may be indicated in many resistant cases of chronic monilial vaginitis."

Two more reports on the successful use of *Candida albicans* extract in treating persistent vaginal and skin problems were reported by a Virginia physician (Palacios, H. J. "Hypersensitivity as a Cause of Dermatologic and Vaginal Moniliasis Resistant to Topical Therapy", *Annals of Allergy* 37:110-113, 1976 and Palacios, H. J. "Desensitization for Monilial Hypersensitivity", *Virginia Medical*, pp. 393-394, June 1977). In concluding remarks in his article in the *Annals of Allergy,* Dr. Palacios commented:

"Complete evaluation of respiratory and skin symptoms in patients with recurrent or chronic forms of mucosal or cutaneous moniliasis has revealed the association of a high incidence of allergies . . . *Our results indicate that desensitization with Candida albicans antigen is the mainstay in the treatment of resistant dermatologic or vaginal moniliasis and the sole form of therapy in cases of nail involvement with deep-seated lesions out of the reach of topical agents."

In an even more recent study from England (Rosedale, N. and Browne, M. B. "Hyposensitization in the Management of Recurring Vaginal Candidiasis", *Annals of Allergy* 43:250-253, 1979) investigators reported on their experiences in a study of 27 patients with recurrent vaginal yeast infections. Some of these patients received active antigens, while others received control ("blank") injections. No differences were noted in the two groups.

However, subsequently, 10 women who took part in the original trial were given a different type of immunotherapy (commercially available Allpyral®) with much greater success. Following immunotherapy, these women showed a relapse rate of once in 15.7 months, as compared to a relapse of once every 5.1 months prior to treatment. Yet, investigators pointed out that:

> "A proportion of patients . . . despite fullest investigation of predisposing factors, persistence of treatment and most sympathetic handling, remained as treatment failures. It is to this unfortunate group that hyposensitisation appears to offer a promising new therapy."

Candida-related health problems (as is the case with all chronic health disorders) never respond to a single treatment measure. So if you're bothered by recurring episodes of vaginitis and are experiencing other systemic symptoms (including fatigue, depression or PMS), immunotherapy may help. In addition, you'll be helped even more by a special diet, oral antifungal therapy, nutritional supplements and other treatment measures described in this book.

Candida Albicans—A Dr. Jekyll and Mr. Hyde

In trying to learn more about *Candida albicans*, I've read everything I could get my hands on. I've also listened to the reports and observations of both professionals and non-professionals. And many people have described the variable growth characteristics of the pesky "critter" known as *Candida albicans*.

Mycologists and other scientists have investigated these different candida forms for over a hundred years. The single cell candida is called a *blastospore*. Little buds sprout from each cell and grow. Soon two daughter cells appear. These in turn divide and continue to multiply.

Blastospore   Budding   Dividing   Daughter Cells

The second form of candida is a long, microscopic tube or *hypha*. These tubes arise from *spores* or from other *hypha*. When a *hypha* puts out branches, we call it a *mycelium*.

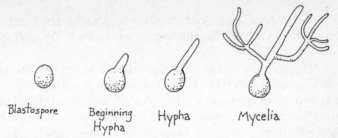

Blastospore | Beginning Hypha | Hypha | Mycelia

One reason for my interest in these different forms of candida relates to the type of treatment I prescribe for my patients.

Some investigators feel that in people with mild candidiasis, the single cell *(blastopore)* predominates (such cells are usually found on the mucous membranes). Accordingly, dietary changes, garlic, acidophilus, caprylic acid and/or nystatin help eradicate these yeasts and such patients will improve.

But suppose my patient doesn't get better on the above treatment program, what then? Maybe such treatment failures occur because single yeasts take on different forms which are more resistant to usual treatment measures.

In the fall of 1985, I obtained a 281-page book, *Candidiasis*, edited by Gerald P. Bodey, M.D. and Victor Fainstein from the Infectious Diseases Section, Department of Internal Medicine, University of Texas Cancer Center in Houston. Here are a few sentences excerpted from their preface:

> "*Candida Spp.* have emerged as important pathogens during the past few decades . . . With the advent of broad-spectrum antibiotic therapy, there has been a substantial increase in the number of patients with thrush and vaginitis. These antibiotics alter the normal flora of the body, facilitating colonization and subsequent super-infection by *Candida Spp.* . . . . Progress in the treatment of systemic candida infection has been hampered by limitations in diagnosis. . . . Unfortunately, despite intensive investigation, serological techniques as diagnostic tools remain unsatisfactory. . . .
>
> "Clearly, major additional research efforts are needed in the area of diagnosis and treatment of systemic candidiasis."

Although this book did not discuss the remote manifestations of candida overgrowth which are the subject of this book, I found many chapters of interest and professionals with a serious interest in candida-related health disorders should read this book.

I was especially interested in a chapter by Charles B. Smith, M.D., Department of Medicine, University of Utah College of Medicine, Salt Lake City, entitled "Candidiasis: Pathogenesis,

Host Resistance and Predisposing Factors."† Dr. Smith comprehensively reviewed the literature and cited 118 different references.

Dr. Smith pointed out that candida is less apt to attach to vaginal epithelial cells when the pH of the vagina is acidic (in the range of 3 to 4) and more apt to attach when it is more neutral (pH of 6). Also, the attachment of candida vaginal cells may be blocked by normal bacterial flora, such as lactobacilli. (This would explain why douches containing boric acid, vinegar, yogurt or lactobacillus often help in treating vaginitis.)

He also noted that invasion and disease due to *C. albicans* is often related to the quantity of organisms present. Accordingly, factors which increase colonization, for example, antibiotics, birth control pills and corticosteroids, promote candidiasis.

Some microorganisms (germs) stimulate the growth of candida, while others compete with candida organisms and antagonize them. Still others, such as "staph" germs as noted by Carlson (see chapter 36) may increase the disease-causing characteristics of candida. Nutritional factors may alter susceptibility to candida infection. Protein deficiency increases susceptibility, and vitamin A supplementation lessens it.

I was especially interested in what Dr. Smith had to say about the ability of *Candida albicans* to produce *hypha* (or germ tubes) which penetrate cell membranes. Once inside the cells, candida organisms continue to grow and put out new buds. And persistence of these organisms inside epithelial cells may explain why they may be resistant to nystatin, an antifungal agent which works mainly on yeasts on membrane surfaces.

In January, 1986, Saul Pilar, M.D. of Vancouver, British Columbia and Jeffrey Bland, Ph.D. of Gig Harbor, Washington, told me about new studies by investigators in the Department of Biology at the University of Iowa. Investigators there described studies showing how *Candida albicans* can "switch" from one form to another. In a presentation at the IX International Congress of the International Society for Human and Animal Mycology (as reported in the September, 1985 issue of *Mycology Observer*) the "switching"

†"Candidiasis: Pathogenesis, Host Resistance and Predisposing Factors." In *Candidiasis*, edited by Gerald P. Bodey and Victor Fainstein. Raven Press, New York, 1985, pp. 7, 53.

characteristics of candida are described. Here are excerpts from this report:

> "It may be that you can't diagnose candida as candida anymore . . . There are too many different types which emanate from a single cell . . . The ability to transform into an entirely different "being" prompted Dr. Soll to describe candida as having a Dr. Jekyll and Mr. Hyde Syndrome . . . This unusual phenomenon may play a role in the organism's capacity to invade different types of body tissues, evade the immune system or evade antibody treatment†.

What are the implications of these studies? Here are some that occur to me:

If you aren't improving on nystatin, it may be because the branching forms of candida have burrowed beneath the surface of your intestinal (or vaginal) membranes. And to get at them may require an antifungal agent which gets into your blood stream—specifically Nizoral®.

Then when you improve, you may be able to be shifted to nystatin (and other therapies) which strengthen your immune system (and your resistance). These include appropriate nutrition; use of vitamin/mineral supplements; exercise; and the avoidance of environmental chemicals. Immunotherapy with candida extracts may also help you.

---

†The experiences of Dr. David R. Soll and his colleagues were published in a recent issue of *Science* (Slutsky, B., Buffo, J. and Soll, D., *Science*, Volume 230, pp. 666-669, November 8, 1985).

41

The Yeast Connection to AIDS, Epstein-Barr (CEBV) and Other Viral Infections

AIDS and the Yeast Connection

Since the publication of THE YEAST CONNECTION, I've received thousands of letters and phone calls asking for more information. And here's a question that keeps popping up, "Is there a connection between AIDS and candida? And if there is, what is it?"

At the Dallas Candida Conference in July, 1982 (see chapter 36), C. Orian Truss, M.D. discussed the possible relationship of candida to AIDS. And in a commentary, published in the *Journal of Orthomolecular Psychiatry,* Dr. Truss had this to say:

> "*Candida albicans* seems to be at least one agent capable of at least a depressing, and perhaps a destructive effect on the immune system. Until the cause of the AIDS problem is uncovered, any approach would seem to be worth considering in a situation of such urgency." (Truss, C. O.: (Letters) J. Orthomol. Psy., 12:37, 1983.)

During the last 3 years, interest in AIDS has exploded. And almost every day I see and read reports in medical journals and newspapers discussing AIDS, including what causes it, how it should be treated, and what should be done to keep it from spreading. Similar reports are seen and heard just as frequently on TV and published in newspapers and popular magazines.

A study reported in *The New England Journal of Medicine* (Klein, R. S., et al.: 311:354-358 (Aug. 9) 1984) showed that the majority of AIDS victims develop *Candida albicans* infections in the mouth ...

just as do other patients with a weakened immune system. Included are individuals with cancer and heart transplants who have been given immunosuppressant drugs.

Accordingly, we can say there is a "yeast connection" to AIDS . . . meaning that individuals with AIDS usually develop yeast infections.

To get more information on AIDS and the yeast connection, I wrote to immunologist, Alan Levin, M.D. of San Francisco. Here are some excerpts from a letter I received in reply from Dr. Levin June 3, 1985:

> "AIDS is a disease of lifestyle and a specific virus, the HTLV III/LAV. The major connection with the *Candida albicans* organism is that this disease causes a weakening of the immune system.
>
> "Virtually all diseases which weaken the immune system are associated with the overgrowth of opportunistic organisms. The most common opportunist is *Candida albicans*.
>
> "We have found that individuals who are at risk for AIDS . . . seem to improve with lifestyle changes, the candida diet and nystatin or Nizoral®. This does not mean the candida causes AIDS. It simply means that the reduction of opportunistic overgrowth in immunocompromised patients is associated with an improvement in symptomatology. . .
>
> "We must emphasize to our patients that having the candida problem does not mean they have AIDS. Unless they are one of the 4 H's (homosexuals, heroin addicts, hemophiliacs or Haitians), they are not at risk for AIDS!."

Certainly I agree with Dr. Levin and I don't want my patients (or readers of this book) to start worrying about AIDS. Yet, because I've received so many letters and phone calls asking about a possible yeast connection to AIDS, I feel it's appropriate to discuss this subject further.

To learn more about the yeast connection to AIDS, I again sought the help and consultation of Dr. Levin in October, 1985. Here are excerpts from our conversation:

Levin: Candida occurs commonly in people with AIDS. It's more of an opportunist than anything else.

Crook: Then it comes after the AIDS, rather than predisposing a person to get AIDS?

Levin: Yes. Yet I feel that AIDS as a disease develops because of many factors. While I agree that the HTLV III virus is necessary, it takes more than this one virus to make a person get sick with AIDS. And other viruses (such as the EB virus or the hepatitis virus) may contribute to the weakening of a person's immune system. And, to repeat, when the immune system is weakened . . . regardless of the cause or causes . . . candida organisms multiply.

Crook: I understand what you're saying. But let me approach the candida/AIDS relationship from a different direction.

Suppose you're studying two groups of people and trying to decide which group would be most susceptible to AIDS.

Group A would be composed of individuals who:

1. Had taken daily broad-spectrum antibiotics (or prednisone) for a year or more.

2. Lived and worked in poorly ventilated homes and offices and were exposed to a heavy load of molds and chemical pollutants.

3. Consumed nutritionally deficient diets.

4. Consumed large amounts of sugar.

By contrast, Group B would be composed of individuals who:

1. Had taken no antibiotics or prednisone.

2. Lived and worked in well ventilated, chemically-uncontaminated homes and offices.

3. Consumed diets rich in essential nutrients.

4. Ate little sugar.

It would seem logical to conclude that *if* . . . there were other predisposing factors leading toward AIDS (as for example, hemophilia or homosexuality), a Group A individual who came in contact with AIDS virus with be more apt to develop AIDS than a B Group person following an identical contact with this virus.

Levin: I agree on that point. No question. Yet, more often, candida is an opportunist rather than a root cause. But we can all agree, once candida is present, steps should be taken to eliminate it.

So in a person with AIDS or at risk for AIDS, who contributes a history consistent with a yeast problem, appropriate anticandida therapy should be a part of the overall treatment program.

More thoughts about AIDS and other "diseases":

Identifying the HTLV III virus which plays a major role in causing AIDS is important. So is the search for a drug or vaccine that will kill or neutralize this virus.

But is this the answer . . . the only answer?

No. As emphasized by Cheraskin, Truss and Baker (see chapter

327

25), although identifying and labeling diseases is sometimes useful, other better ways of looking at people and their health problems may furnish us with better answers.

Obviously, candida isn't "the cause" of AIDS (nor is it "the cause" of PMS, depression, psoriasis, headache, fatigue or multiple sclerosis). Yet based on the research studies of Iwata in Japan and the clinical and research studies of Truss in Alabama, and the research studies of Witkin of Cornell, *Candida albicans* infections adversely affect the body in many different ways, including a weakening of the immune system. And if a person's immune system is weak, infections (and many other types of health disorders) are more apt to develop.

So if you want to lessen your risk of developing AIDS (or psoriasis, MS, depression, etc., etc., etc.), change your diet, environment and lifestyle in such a way as to strengthen your immune system. At the same time, you should avoid the factors that weaken it.

On a recent program on a major TV network, a physician from the Center for Disease Control commented and said in effect,

> "The AIDS epidemic is growing. Yet, for every person with AIDS, there are a hundred times more people with ARC (AIDS Related Complex). Such individuals have been infected by the AIDS virus. However, they show none of the major manifestations of AIDS even though they may have symptoms of various kinds. In addition, there are one and a half million people who have been infected who show no symptoms whatsoever."

I've never seen a patient with AIDS and my knowledge of it is limited to articles I've read in various scientific journals plus things I've learned from the media. Nevertheless, I feel that persons with ARC or who have the AIDS virus should be aware of the yeast connection and should follow an anticandida treatment program if his/her history suggests that candida overgrowth may be present.

Epstein-Barr and The Yeast Connection

Are you troubled by fatigue, headache, muscle and joint pains, digestive symptoms, skin rashes, and other complaints? If your answer is "yes", your problems are apt to be yeast connected—especially if you've taken many broad spectrum antibiotic drugs (or birth control pills and/or cortisone).

Yet, if you've been taking nystatin (or Nizoral®) for several months and have been sticking to your diet and aren't improving, other factors may be playing a role in making you sick. One such factor is *chronic Epstein-Barr virus* (CEBV) infection.

What is the EB virus? It's a virus in the herpes group of viruses. It is the same one that causes *infectious mononucleosis* or *"glandular fever"*. Like other herpes viruses, once it gets into your body, it stays there. Happily, this virus usually becomes inactive and your symptoms go away in several weeks.

Yet, for reasons that aren't clearly understood, some people with CEBV infections continue to be bothered by symptoms.

In an article published in the January 1985 issue of the *Annals of Internal Medicine*, Stephen Straus, M.D. and associates of the National Institute of Allergy and Infectious Diseases (NIAID), describe their research studies in twenty-three patients with a chronic illness associated with CEBV infections.

These patients were followed at the National Institutes of Health (NIH) for an average of two years. Most were over the age of 30, and thirteen of the patients gave a history of a previous mononucleosis-like disease that was characterized by a prolonged fever and swelling of the lymph glands.

Most of their patients complained of "flu-like" symptoms with muscle aching, mild sore throat, tender lymph glands, and low grade fever. However, fatigue appeared to be the major symptom.

Laboratory studies of these patients showed higher than normal antibody levels to what they termed VCA-IgG (IgG antibodies to viral CAPSID antigens and to the viral early antigens). In addition, the virus was recovered from throat washings of some of the patients.

In the discussion section of the Straus paper, the authors commented:

> It is by no means certain that Epstein-Barr virus either causes the syndrome or plays an ongoing role in its chronic manifestations.—Certainly the clinical picture is far from unique and resembles features of some other disorders—.
>
> In any case, the disorder we are considering to be chronic Epstein-Barr virus infection is not rare and warrants further investigation.

To get an additional opinion on the relationship of the Epstein-Barr viral infection, I consulted two of my colleagues. Elmer Cranton, M.D. had this to say:

"The EBV persists in the body for a lifetime once it is contracted, much like the herpes simplex virus, cytomegalovirus (CMV) and many others. Once contracted, the virus is always present but the body's immune system keeps it in check.

"In testing patients in my practice with yeast-related illness, I find that close to one-fourth have EBV disease. There is also no question that the vast majority of these patients are primarily candida related. I feel that the chronic yeast condition weakens the immunity and causes EBV to recur and to become persistent—.

"I am not certain which comes first, the chicken or the egg. That is, did the EBV lower immunity and cause a person to become more susceptible to yeast or vice versa? I am sure that it must occur in both directions."

Sidney Baker, M.D. commented:

"I think it is fairly likely that the yeast problem is more significant than the EBV problem in terms of an original etiologic factor. On the other hand, it is worth considering that there are general trends towards something interfering with immune function in people in our population and antibiotics may not be the whole answer."

In the January/February issue of *20th Century Living*, a bimonthly, environmental health newsletter published by the Environmental Health Association of Dallas, Texas, P.O. Box 226811, Dallas, TX 75222, Lawrence A. Plumlee, M.D. discussed both candida-related disorders and EBV infections. He recommended screening blood tests for both candida and for EBV to determine which factors are most important.

In an article in the February 6, 1986 issue of the *New England Journal of Medicine* entitled "Medical Consequences of a Persistent Viral Infection" (by Peter Southern, Ph.D. and Michael Oldstone, M.D.) appeared these comments:

"Numerous viruses, such as herpes simplex virus, cytomegalo virus, Epstein-Barr virus—are known to cause persistent or latent infection—. Interest is now focusing on a possible viral cause for disorders of the nervous system, the endocrine system, and the immune system."

As pointed out elsewhere in this book, "every part of your body is connected to every other part" (See chapter 26). Moreover the immune system, endocrine system, and the nervous system are closely interrelated. Viruses and candida toxins affect each of these systems. Accordingly, appropriate treatment of candidiasis should help you develop a greater resistance to the viruses which "move in" when your immune system is weak.

More on Viruses

In the May 12, 1986 issue of *Medical World News*,* reporter Richard Trubo reviewed recent research which links many chronic diseases to persistent viral infections. Here are excerpts from his article:

> "Physicians have generally been taught that most of the more than 40 viruses known to infect humans are relatively benign or become so after an acute bout. But now, investigators are discovering that many viruses don't hide away innocently after the patient's initial infection."

In his report, he talks about recent studies on EB virus, the rubella virus (which "may be an etiologic agent in chronic human joint disease"), the CMV virus, the adenovirus, the hepatitis B virus and the parvovirus. In his continuing discussion, he had this to say:

> "So far the research is turning up new questions faster than it's providing concrete evidence about chronic viral infections and where they may ultimately lead. Investigators still don't fully understand the mechanisms by which viruses are maintained or how they persist and evade the body's immune response. . . . The proliferation of research into suspected viral causes of disease can be expected to continue for the foreseeable future.
>
> "Referring to his own work with patients who may have chronic Epstein-Barr virus syndrome, Dr. Straus says, 'There's a real desperation on the part of patients. People want answers. But evaluations of these patients are very difficult, and our research tools sometimes aren't refined enough to dissect out what might be going on'."

Chronic Fatigue Syndrome (CFS)

In the March 1988 issue of *Annals of Internal Medicine*, it was suggested that the term *Chronic Epstein Barr Virus Syndrome* (CEBV) be replaced by the *Chronic Fatigue Syndrome* (CFS). In addition, some physicians have suggested still another name, *Chronic Fatigue and Immunodeficiency Syndrome* (CFIDS).

Regardless of which title is used, there's growing interest and support for the relationship of this disorder to *Candida albicans*.

At a symposium in Rhode Island on October 22, 1988, one of the conference speakers, Robert Hallowitz, M.D., discussed the relationship of *Candida albicans* to CFS**. In his presentation he noted that most of his patients improved on a comprehensive treatment program which included nystatin.

**The CFS relationship to *candida albicans* is a new illustrated book by William G. Crook, M.D.—*Chronic Fatigue Syndrome and the Yeast Connection* (April, 1992).

At a subsequent CFS conference in San Francisco on April 15, 1989, Carol Jessop, M.D., told of her experiences in treating 1100 patients with CFS. All of these patients met the Center for Disease Control diagnostic criteria for CFS.

Following their acute illness, the patients experienced many other symptoms, including dizziness, depression, difficulty in concentrating, muscle and joint pains, headache and devastating fatigue. In her comments, Dr. Jessop said, "The past medical history of CFS patients is very enlightening and may represent the key to understanding this illness."

- 80% had recurrent antibiotic treatment as a child.
- irritable bowel syndrome, vaginal yeast infections, headaches and the Premenstrual Syndrome were extremely common.

Patients were treated with a special diet (no alcohol, sugar, fruit or fruit juice). They were also given 200 mg. of ketoconazole once daily. 84% of the patients showed a greater than 70% improvement. The average length of therapy was 5 months.

In her concluding remarks, Dr. Jessop stated, "CFS may represent a multitude of symptoms which are manifested with the presence of a toxin released by *Candida albicans*.*

Here's more: At the September 1988 Candida Update Conference, John W. Crayton, Loyola Medical School, described research studies which showed that patients with fatigue, depression and other symptoms had significantly elevated IgG and IgA anticandida antibodies as compared with controls.

Candida and "ME". Individuals with a disorder which appears identical to the CFS, have been described in England, Australia and New Zealand for over a decade. The name of this syndrome, which has been popularized as: *Myalgic Encephalomyelitis*, or "ME".

And in a 1989 book, *Why Me?*, by Drs. Belinda Dawes and Damien Downing, Dr. Dawes stated,

> "I would now say that without doubt, candida infection plays a role in the ill health of all the patients I see. Although their illness may not be directly related to the candida problem, eliminating the candida from their body and its related consequences has certainly been one of the factors in their recovery."

*In her Foreword to my new book, *Chronic Fatigue Syndrome and the Yeast Connection* (publication date, July 1992) Jessop said, "This book does not claim that the yeast, *Candida albicans*, is *the* cause of CFS. However, it does explain the role of multiple entities: yeast overgrowth, intestinal parasites, unchecked viral infections, food allergies and chemical sensitivities—and how there can result in the immune dysregulation we refer to as CFS."

42

PMS, Sexual Dysfunction, Suicidal Depression and Mitral Valve Prolapse

The Premenstrual Syndrome...

According to the front cover of the book, *PMS: Premenstrual Syndrome And You* by New York gynecologist, Niels H. Lauersen, M.D. and Eileen Stukane, over 25 million women suffer violent fluctuations in mood, appetite and weight each month. And in an article in the March, 1985 issue of *The Nurse Practitioner* (Vol. 10, #3, pp. 11-22), Dr. Lauersen commented,

> "The powerful hormonal changes that occur throughout a woman's menstrual cycle have long been recognized by the medical establishment, but the acceptance of PMS as a condition meriting medical attention and treatment is a fairly recent development."

Moreover, several times each week, the average American (both male and female) reads or hears about PMS. Frequent newspaper and magazine articles, and programs and advertisements on TV have now made PMS a household word. I even ran across a cartoon showing one moppet whispering to his playmate (with an irate mother in the background), "Don't worry, mama's PMS is making her grouchy."

PMS is "for real." No doubt about it. Because I'm the father of three daughters in their 30's and because most of my patients are women, I'm especially interested in the subject. And during the years 1985 and 1986, there has been new clinical and scientific evidence which indicates PMS is yeast-connected.

In a report published in the May/June, 1985 *Infections in Medicine* ("Defective Immune Responses in Patients with Recurrent Candidiasis"), Steven S. Witkin, Ph.D., an associate research professor in the department of obstetrics and gynecology, Cornell University Medical College, New York, New York, described hormonal changes in women with recurrent vaginal yeast infections.

In my own practice during the years 1984-1986, I've seen dozens of young women who felt "sick all over." Most of these patients experienced headache, fatigue, irritability, bloating and depression . . . especially the week before their periods. Candida immunoglobulin studies were abnormal in the great majority of these patients. And their response to antifungal therapy was usually gratifying.

In a special medical report in the April, 1986 issue of *Redbook* Magazine entitled, "The Newest Mystery Illness," Pamela Morford, M.D., a Minneapolis gynecologist commented:

> "The premenstrual problems of at least ninety percent of my patients can be traced to chronic candidiasis. I have found that when I give these patients anti-candida therapy, they get better."

And in a letter to me in April, 1986, Dr. Morford had this to say:

> "I, myself, have probably had yeast problems for many years. My earliest symptom was a problem with my bladder and urinary frequency since childhood. . . . Nothing has really worked to relieve the pain in my pelvis and the urinary frequency.
> "I developed PMS in August, 1982. And in November, 1983 I developed diarrhea. That was when I decided to try nystatin. My diarrhea cleared within a week; my PMS, irritability, depression and paranoia improved quite a bit. I ran out of nystatin and my symptoms returned.

H: Headache   B = Bloating
F: Fatigue   I: Irritability
D: Depression

APRIL

1	2	3	4	5	6	7
8	9	10	11	12	13	14
15 H,F	16 H,F	17 H,I,D,F	18 H,I,D, B,F	19 H,I, D,F	20 B,I	21 B,I
22	23	24	25	26	27	28
29 START PERIOD	30	31				

After resuming the nystatin, my bladder and PMS symptoms improved. At the same time, I realized that a pain in my shoulder which had appeared at the same time the PMS began, had gone.

"I've probably treated 400 to 500 women with PMS over the past year. The majority of women I see have come in complaining of bloating, irritability and depression before their periods. Many are very concerned about being out of control and unable to handle their anger. Some have lost their self-confidence. Another major difficulty is spaciness and inability to concentrate.

"Within a month after starting anti-yeast treatment, many of these symptoms diminish considerably and occasionally disappear. Many women noticed that they cannot vary much from their strict diet without experiencing symptoms.

"Many of the sicker women improve, but have a long way to go and return periodically for reevaluation. I've frequently started some of the sicker women with Nizoral® rather than nystatin to minimize the early die-off reactions . . . fortunately with good success.

"I look forward to more work and literature to substantiate what I'm telling my patients, and also so that I may convince my colleagues that what I'm doing has some validity."

A few weeks later, I had an opportunity to visit with Dr. Morford in Minneapolis and I asked her to provide me with additional details about her program for managing her patients with PMS. Here are excerpts from her May, 1986 letter to me:

"Many of my patients who complain mainly of PMS will respond favorably to nothing more than improving their diet by cutting out refined carbohydrates, caffeine, and increasing their protein and vegetables. I also advise them to take a multiple vitamin/mineral preparation (Optivite),® usually 2 with each meal. I advise them to stay away from foods to which they're allergic and to challenge themselves with suspicious foods at a later date.

"Of course, significant stress in the patient's life contributes to making her ill. (One of my patients was married for 12 years to a man who then told her he was a homosexual. He wanted to keep their relationship unchanged. They also had 2 children. I told her I could help her as much as possible with the anticandida therapy, but that her symptoms would not likely disappear until after her divorce was finalized.)

"Other supplements I've begun to use more frequently are evening primrose oil and linseed oil. I've found that primrose oil works very well for the severe breast tenderness that some women experience.

"I first try the vitamins (especially B-6, E, magnesium) but if they don't work, primrose oil almost always does, in a dose of 2 to 6 capsules daily, beginning with ovulation and through to the onset of menses.

"The linseed oil (or other sources of Omega 3 fatty acids) has worked extremely well for skin rashes. I have used it successfully either alone or along with nystatin in patients with eczema.

"I find the sicker patients frequently have PMS as only one of their complaints. Those who score over 200 on your questionnaire, I treat more delicately. If I decide to use a drug, I will almost always use Nizoral® for 1 to 2 months prior to nystatin, hoping that the person won't get sicker before she gets better.

"Occasionally, I use only the vaccine at the outset. All of this, of course, is used in combination with diet, vitamins, exercise as tolerated, and allergy evaluation and treatment if indicated.

"*The majority of symptoms respond to the anti-yeast program.* However, some women have persistent symptoms . . . anxiety, depression, migraines . . . that do respond to Dr. Mabray's minidose progesterone regimen.† Again, we teach the women to give it to themselves so that they can use it as needed at home. I occasionally use it as a stopgap measure for people who are just beginning the anticandida therapy.

"Recently, I received a call from a Ph.D. in nutrition at the University of Minnesota who wondered why no scientific studies were done. I told him that we had designed a study that would involve 1000 patients and would follow their response to diet and/or nystatin over a year-long period. Although we don't have the computers or the funds to handle the study, I'm hoping that we can set it up soon."

A Scientific Study On The Relationship Of PMS To Candida

Several years ago, along with a practicing gynecologist interested in candidiasis, I visited a research professor in the department of obstetrics and gynecology at a leading medical school. We told him of our experiences in treating women with PMS (and other related health disorders) using nystatin and a special diet. And we persuaded him to study the problem.

Some two years later, he sent me a paper summarizing observations he and his colleagues had made in studying and treating the premenstrual syndrome with anticandida therapy. Although the paper was submitted to several scientific journals, it was not accepted. And in a conversation with me in 1985, the senior investigator said, "We feel we may need to approach the study in a different way and set up more rigid controls. Perhaps then we can come up with something which will be accepted for publication."

In spite of these negatives, I feel that the efforts and results of these investigators should be made available to others who are interested. Here is a brief summary of their study:

Several hundred women were enrolled in the premenstrual syndrome unit of this university medical school at the time of data collection. Each woman underwent an extensive history and physical examination and filled out a long questionnaire. Each woman

---

†Mabray, C. R., et al.: "Treatment of Common Gynecologic-Endocrinologic Symptoms by Allergy Management Procedures." *Obstetrics & Gynecology,* 59:560-564, May, 1982.

was interviewed for one hour by a nurse psychologist. Patients in the study were selected from the entire group because of a history of vaginal candidiasis and failure to respond to established PMS therapeutic regimens. All patients received at least a one year followup in a minimum of three visits.

In tabulating the results, several study groups were set up, including some who received vitamin B-6, some who received the elimination diet and nystatin, others who received diet alone, and others who received nystatin.

Here is a summary of their study as presented in abstract:

"33 women with severe premenstrual syndrome who failed prior therapy were evaluated for chronic moniliasis. Treatment with oral nystatin and a yeast elimination diet significantly improved physical and psychological complaints in comparison to untreated controls (p. 0.01)."

Other Hormone Problems in Women

Are you struggling to conquer your yeast-connected health problems? And are your problems continuing even though you're following your diet, and taking antifungal medicine and nutritional supplements?

If your answer is "yes", according to Phyllis Saifer, M.D. you may be "allergic to yourself".

At the conference on Yeast-Human Interaction in San Francisco in March, 1985, Dr. Saifer described a subgroup of patients with chronic candidiasis who continued to experience problems in spite of anticandida treatment, and she said in effect:

"I have found that a lot of these patients suffer from thyroid problems, while others suffer from ovarian problems. The typical patient gives a history of irregular, widely spaced periods beginning in their teens. She's also apt to be troubled by respiratory, skin or digestive tract allergies, and often gives a history of many psychiatric symptoms including depression and "nervous breakdown".

These patients often show sparse hair, a pale, pasty, puffy face, and an enlarged, bumpy or pebbly swelling just below the Adams apple.

In making a diagnosis in these patients, Dr. Saifer recommends new anti-ovarian antibody studies which are carried out by a number of laboratories, including Immunodiagnostic Laboratory, 400 29th Street, Oakland, CA 94609. She also commented,

"I feel the most important thyroid test is one that isn't usually performed . . . thyroid antibodies by radioimmunoassay. When this test is carried out, it helps in making the diagnosis."

In treating such patients, Dr. Saifer recommends small doses of synthetic or natural thyroid beginning with 0.05 milligrams (½ grain) and increasing by a half grain every two weeks until there is clinical improvement. She also recommends consultation with a "cooperating endocrinologist" because these patients may be exceedingly difficult to manage.

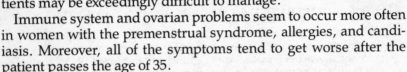

Immune system and ovarian problems seem to occur more often in women with the premenstrual syndrome, allergies, and candiiasis. Moreover, all of the symptoms tend to get worse after the patient passes the age of 35.

Symptoms that suggest ovarian problems include fluid retention, breast tenderness, recurrent yeast infections and compulsive hunger. These symptoms usually worsen the week before menstruation begins. Other symptoms suggesting hormone allergies include headache, drowsiness, spaciness, depression, chilling, nausea and stomach cramps.

If and when anti-ovarian disease and hormone imbalance are diagnosed, the patient with such problems will need comprehensive management, including a special diet, antifungal medication, avoidance of environmental chemicals, psychological support and nutritional supplements. In addition, she may also need natural progesterone as a suppository or as a sublingual powder.

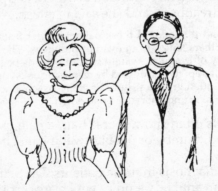

Sexual Dysfunction

During my growing-up years, I received little or no information about sex from my Victorian parents. Even during my medical training, almost no time was devoted to disturbances in sexual function. Moreover, like most men (including many of my medical contemporaries), I had been taught that women were "different." And they weren't *really* supposed to enjoy sex.

My state of ignorance continued for many years. And in spite of the sexual revolution, my adult female allergy patients rarely . . . if ever . . . discussed their sex problems with me.

Then in 1979, I learned about the yeast connection and my practice changed dramatically. By 1981, most of the patients who consulted me were women. And the majority of them were between 25 and 40. Being a pediatrician, I didn't carry out physical examinations on my adult patients. Yet I listened empathetically to their stories.

One morning in the spring of 1983, I knocked and entered the consultation room occupied by my nurse associate, Susan, and a 34-year-old mother (I'll call her Pauline). I had obviously interrupted their conversation. Then after a moment's pause, Pauline commented:

> "Dr. Crook, Susan and I were talking about something you should know about . . . sexual feelings in women. And I'd like to tell you my story. During my early years of marriage, my sexual drive and response were super. My husband and I were well matched and we had a glorious relationship.
>
> "Then came sinus infections, antibiotics, the pill, bladder infections, more antibiotics, yeast problems, fatigue, PMS, headaches . . . the whole yeast story you've heard from many of your patients.
>
> "In addition, my sex organs lost all feeling . . . all sensation. No real pain or discomfort during or after intercourse . . . just blah . . . almost numb. It was as though my bottom was made of leather! That was two years ago before I started the diet, nystatin and other parts of the treatment program. Now, most of the time, I feel like a new person and my sexual feelings have returned. My husband and I both are profoundly grateful."

As I saw more women patients, listened and showed interest, I heard similar stories (both in person and in letters). For example, a midwestern professional woman (a Ph.D.) wrote:

> "You and Dr. Truss discuss loss of libido, impaired sex drive and impotence. Yet, you weren't specific enough. And you didn't mention that candida could affect orgasm in women. Before learning about my own yeast-related problems, I lost my orgasm. Then after receiving treatment, I regained it."

Then very recently, another professional . . . 35-year-old Patty . . . wrote me a long letter. Here are a few excerpts:

"I want to tell you more about my candida 'nightmare', as I feel few are able or willing to share such experiences. My yeast problem started during my midteen years, and during my flareups I would feel 'spacey'. As time went on, I would have severe 'panic attacks.'

"About a year later, I noticed that when the infections were at their peak, I would experience bizarre homosexual feelings or intense heterosexual feelings that would persist for hours . . . or even days. By the time I was 20, this consistent state of sexual arousement became an obsession with me. I could not concentrate on anything else.

"Keep in mind that during this time some of my most severe inner conflicts were religious ones. I was raised in the Catholic Church with very strict moral standards. Moreover, I was a virgin until after I married at the age of 22. So I found the anguish of these uncontrollable urges and thoughts to be emotionally destructive.

"During times of anger or even extreme joy, my body and my emotions would respond inappropriately with intense feelings of sexual arousement. Bear in mind that this sensation was insatiable. Even 'satisfactory' regular intercourse did nothing to control or reduce this constant sexual frustration.

"I didn't know where to turn. My church didn't help. And I was condemned for having such 'horrid' and sinful thoughts. I went to dozens of doctors, including psychiatrists, all to no avail. Finally I found a doctor to help me with the yeast problem and my terrible nightmares began to improve.

"In the last four years, I'm 95% better. I no longer suffer from these horrifying sexual abnormalities and have required no more psychotherapy or mood-changing drugs. My fantastic husband and super kids have supported me through the years and my life is now gratifying and I'm working with a doctor who is helping others avoid much needless suffering."

Sexual Problems in Men

In his book, THE MISSING DIAGNOSIS, Dr. Truss pointed out that decreased libido may occur in men with chronic candidiasis, although not as often as in women. Nevertheless, a number of men who have consulted me or written me have told me of diminished sex drive and other symptoms related to their genital organs accompanying candida-related disorders.

Here are excerpts from a couple of recent letters I've received:

"My wife has yeast-related health problems with fatigue, headache, depression and recurrent vaginitis. After intercourse, even though I don't seem to develop inflammation of my genitals, I experience pain in my penis which lasts a number of days. I also tend to feel irritable and depressed."

And another man wrote,

"I've got the full yeast picture. My score on the questionnaire was 300 with symptoms of lethargy, fatigue, bloating and other digestive symptoms. Also headache, and muscle and joint pains. One of my main complaints is lack of feeling in my genitals, plus severe pain in my penis. Yet all of my lab tests are normal.

Happily, since starting on the anticandida diet and nystatin, all of my symptoms are improving. Yet I still have a way to go."

Here's more: A sexual topic which has "come out of the closet" during the last several years is homosexuality. And with the AIDS epidemic bursting on the scene, we all see and hear graphic discussions of homosexual behavior on TV and in the press almost every day.

Along with other physicians interested in candidiasis, I've begun to ask myself, "Is it possible . . . at least in some individuals . . . for homosexuality to develop because of candida-related disturbances in hormone function." Moreover, Patty's story makes me wonder if nymphomania or other symptoms of excessive sexual drive could also be related.

A lot of the questions about yeast-connected illness still can't be answered. Yet, *there's growing clinical and laboratory evidence that endocrine (hormonal) problems and sexual dysfunction occur in people with yeast-related problems and often improve when candidiasis is appropriately treated.*

Suicidal Depression

If you're like everyone else, you have your "ups and downs" . . . your good days and your bad days. Many, many factors play a role in determining your moods and how you feel. Some influences are obvious and easy to identify, including your relationship to those with whom you live or work.

Is your work, your marriage (or your relationship) truly satisfying and supportive? Is your income sufficient? Do you receive more smiles than frowns? More compliments than criticisms? And so on and on.

Then other environmental, biologic, nutritional, metabolic and hormonal influences affect you and the way you feel. Example: On cloudy, damp days with high levels of molds, chemical pollutants and/or positive ions, you're apt to feel tired or depressed. By contrast, on a clear, cool, crisp, dry, sunshiny day with lots of negative ions around and few mold spores and pollutants in the air, you're apt to feel optimistic and energetic.

Then, hormonal cycles play an important part in determining

how you feel. And you're more apt to be sluggish, bloated, irritable and/or depressed the week before your period starts (men may have hormonal cycles, too, but we don't know as much about them).

Of course, if you've been bothered by health problems of many types, you may feel discouraged. What's more, you're apt to feel frustrated and depressed, if your doctors don't seem to be able to help you. And the situation becomes even worse, if your family or friends imply you're a hypochondriac or a chronic complainer.

So, for any (or all) of the reasons listed above, you may occasionally (or even more often) feel that life isn't worth living. Yet, the will to survive, to live and to overcome your problems is deeply ingrained in you, and suicide may not be a solution you seriously consider.

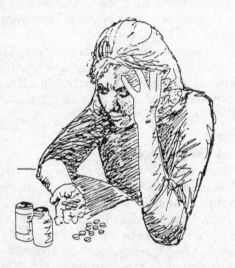

During the past three years, I've visited with hundreds of people (in person, on the phone and through the mail) who struggle with persistent or recurrent depression. Dozens of these individuals have told me of their recurrent suicidal thoughts. Here are excerpts from two typical letters:

> "I'm a 26-year-old woman who feels like 80. I'm desperate because of my severe PMS, extreme depression, *suicidal episodes,* anxiety, irritability and many more symptoms which make my life miserable. I have suffered from bladder and yeast infections for years. Please help me find a doctor who understands the yeast problem. I don't want to end up in the hospital again because of suicide attempts. Thank you!"

A woman from a midwestern state wrote:

"I'm 40 years old and have been ill for five years. Repeated respiratory infections with lots of antibiotics; vaginitis, bladder infections and more antibiotics. I suffer from dizziness, disorientation and fatigue. I would even go to sleep on a bed of nails any time during the day. *I feel so bad I think about suicide, but I haven't tried it because I'm afraid it won't work.* Please give me the name of a doctor who understands and who can help me."

On a happier note, a Tennessee woman in her late 30's wrote:

"I'm writing to thank you from the bottom of my heart for taking time to write THE YEAST CONNECTION. Before I read your book I was existing . . . not living. *I had suffered from suicidal depression for many years.* Life was just too difficult for me. I only knew I wanted out. Moreover, I had slashed my wrists on two different occasions.

"Then I got your book and was amazed at how much I fit the symptoms. I went on the diet and began to feel better. Then I was able to see a kind, compassionate doctor who knew about the yeast problem and who started me on nystatin.

"Although I still have problems, I haven't been depressed since I started the program. My attitude is so different, my energy is better. I helped two of my friends move, and I cleaned the carpets in my house and two of my friends' houses. My mind is clear, I can read more easily and my concentration has improved.

"I have a new life now . . . I never knew it could be possible for me to feel this way."

Candida toxins affect the nervous system and play a part in causing symptoms of many sorts. Headache, irritability, memory loss and a feeling of being "spaced out" and confused occur commonly. Yet, depression ranks near the top of the list of nervous system symptoms in my patients with candidiasis.

Several times, during the years 1984 and 1985, I've heard reports in the media about "epidemics" of suicide among teenagers in Texas, Iowa and elsewhere. Could these suicides be yeast-connected? I think so. Here's why:

About a year ago, a couple in a western state sent me a copy of the church service at their daughter's funeral, along with this note:

"Our daughter, Mary (not her real name) committed suicide. We now know that candida and PMS were contributing factors in her death. Thank you, Dr. Crook, for writing THE YEAST CONNECTION. We feel it will help others avoid such a fate."

Then in mid-May, 1986, just as my manuscript was going to the typesetter, I received a letter which told me of the May 1985 suicide of a 19-year-old college girl. This young woman (I'll call her Joan) had been troubled with many complaints. Here are excerpts from Joan's 10-page letter (written in the summer of 1984) that her mother sent me:

"Between the ages of 1 and 5, I had *countless ear infections,* colds and allergies. At the age of 6, I missed two months of my first grade due to these illnesses. During my grammer school years, I had recurrent abdominal pain and *severe athlete's foot* which continued on until highschool. During these early years I also continued to have frequent sore throat and ear infections for which *antibiotics* were prescribed.

In 1979, my freshman year of high school, I missed five weeks of school because of recurrent infections. Again, I was on heavy doses of *antibiotics.* I was always tired, had *constipation, gas* and *diarrhea;* also *sugar cravings.* Controlling my weight was a major problem.

"I'm only 18 and I'm passing through life in a fatigued, unrealistic way, with waves of *depression.* Doctors have always dismissed my symptoms and, after running the usual tests, find nothing. Some say that my problems are all mental, others say it's because I'm overweight.

"I've grown tired of being dismissed with diet in hand and hopes of not seeing my case again. All these symptoms from childhood to present have left me feeling like a hypochondriac. Sugary foods and breads leave me drowsy after consumption.

"Also *chemical* and *industrial odors,* gasses, fabric softeners and detergents really bother me, and my headaches never go away; the *nausea, tiredness, burning* and tearing of eyes just hit me.

"I don't know what it's like to feel well. . . . I find myself on the edge of a steep precipice, waiting to see if I can gain complete control. I can do it . . . I just need help."

In the summer of 1984, Joan got a copy of THE YEAST CONNECTION and filled out the long questionnaire. Her score was 348. A physician then started her on anticandida treatment including a special diet and nystatin. She improved significantly for a couple of months. But, then, other stresses and problems arose. Her antifungal therapy was discontinued and she was hospitalized in a mental hospital for several months in the spring of 1985. The day she was released, she took her life.

Obviously, psychological stresses at home, at school, on the job and in the world in which we live may play a part. And other factors, too, including genetic, nutritional, allergic, toxic, metabolic and environmental may cause changes in neurotransmitters (brain chemicals), resulting in depression . . . and possibly suicide. On top of all these is the "copy cat" factor.

Yet, based on my experiences with dreams of depressed patients, I feel a yeast connection should be considered in every depressed person . . . especially those with suicidal depression. *Such a connection should be suspected, especially in the individual who has received multiple courses of broad-spectrum antibiotic drugs and who complains of being "sick all over," even though the cause hasn't been found.* (I commented on my feelings about the role of candida in causing depression in Letters to the Editor in *The Journal of the American Medical Association* and in *Hospital Practice*. Dr. David A. Edwards of Nevada also supported my view. Yet, other physicians expressed skepticism.[†])

Mitral Valve Prolapse (MVP)

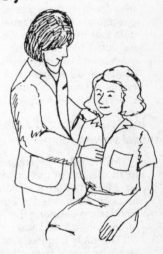

When a doctor listens to your heart, she hears sounds that have been described as "lub-dup, lub-dup, lub-dup." These sounds are made by opening and closing of the heart valves. However, if a person has a congenital valvular defect of the heart, or has had rheumatic fever or some other disease of the heart which damage these valves, the physician may hear different sounds that we call "murmurs." Yet, murmurs can be heard in many healthy people, especially children. And the term "innocent" is applied to such murmurs in normal hearts.

During recent years, heart specialists have been able to hear a little "click" when they listen to the hearts of 6% of "normal" men and some 10% to 20% of "healthy" women. Moreover, in some individuals, they hear an accompanying small murmur. Such clicks and murmurs are usually thought to be caused by abnormal closing of one of the heart valves . . . the mitral valve.

According to Isadore Rosenfeld, M.D.,[‡]

"We're still not sure what causes this condition. It is sometimes

†Crook, W. G.: *Depression Associated with Candida Albicans Infections*. JAMA (Letters) 251:2928, 1984.

Edwards, D. A.: *Depression and Candida*. JAMA (Letters) 253:3400, 1985.

Coleman, W. P., III: *Depression and Candida*. JAMA (Letters) 253:3400, 1985.

Crook, W. G.: *Candidiasis and Depression*. Hospital Practice, January 30, 1985.

Crook, W. G.: *Is Remote Disease Associated With* Candida *Infection a Tomato?* JAMA (Letters) 254:2891-2, 1985.

‡SECOND OPINION, by Isadore Rosenfeld, Bantam Books, New York, pp. 120-122.

present at birth or it may first be heard later on. It goes by a variety of names. . . . Barlow's syndrome, *Mitral Valve Prolapse (MVP)*. . . . but the most popular designation is 'Floppy Valve'. *In the vast majority of cases, such a valve neither interferes with normal heart function nor reduces life expectancy."*

What causes mitral valve prolapse? I don't know, but I've been impressed by the observations of Leo Galland, M.D. of New York. In a recent paper, "Nutrition and Candidiasis,"[†] Dr. Galland commented:

"While treating several hundred patients with candida-related illness over the past three years, I have seen that invasive, allergic and toxic effects may exist separately or together in an individual patient. Candida toxicity often appears after evidence of invasive candidiasis (e.g., vaginitis) has subsided. I've also been impressed with the high frequency with which a specific constellation of nutritional deficiencies accompany all forms of chronic candidiasis. A triad of magnesium, essential fatty acid and vitamin B-6 deficiencies appears to be the rule, especially when toxic or allergic manifestations are present."

In a continuing discussion, Dr. Galland had this to say about mitral valve prolapse:

"Mitral valve prolapse (MVP) is the commonest form of valvular heart disease in the United States, with a prevalence of 7-15%. . . . I have found a high prevalence of MVP among patients with candidiasis, an association noted by other clinicians as well (Truss . . . personal communication). Among the 104 patients in the present study, physical examination revealed auscultatory findings of MVP in 46. . . .

"The high frequency of prolapse among patients with candidiasis suggests that there are individuals whose genetic endowment predisposes them to chronic candida infection, possibly because of disturbances in Mg. or EFA metabolism. . . .

"A number of symptoms have been attributed to MVP both by patients and clinicians. These include chest pain, palpitation, fatigue, dizziness, poor exercise tolerance, anxiety and hyperventilation. *My experience with treatment suggests that these symptoms are usually due to candida allergy or toxicity, and occasionally to Mg. or EFA deficiency;[‡] they rarely have any direct relationship to the valvular lesion."*

If you have MVP and require dental work, most physicians and

[†]"Nutrition and Candidiasis", by L. Galland, *Journal of Orthomolecular Psychiatry,* First Quarter, 1985, Vol. 14, .1, pp. 50-59.

[‡]Galland, L.: Magnesium Deficiency in Mitral Valve Prolapse. (Accepted for publication in 1986 in the journal, *Magnesium*.)

Halpern, Durlach (EDS.): Magnesium Deficiency. First Eur. Congr. in Magnesium. Lisbon, 1983, pp. 117-119 (Karger, Basel, 1985).

"Magnesium Deficiency in the Pathogenesis of Mitral Valve Prolapse," by Leo D. Galland, Sidney M. Baker, and Robert K. McLellan.

dentists recommend a short course of antibiotics. Here's why: bacteria from the mouth may be "stirred up", enter the blood stream and set up an infection on a damaged heart valve (the condition is called bacterial endocarditis).

If penicillin V or penicillin G is prescribed for a short time (such as two or three days) candida overgrowth is less apt to occur. However if a broad-spectrum drug (such as Keflex®, amoxicillin or Ceclor®) is prescribed, I'd recommend nystatin and/or Nizoral® to control the candida.

I received many letters and phone calls from people with MVP who ask,

"Do I always need to take an antibiotic when I go to the dentist to have my teeth cleaned or worked on?"

I wasn't sure how to answer this question so I passed it along to Dr. Leo Galland who said, "If a person has *mitral regurgitation* or other definite valvular heart damage, I recommend penicillin prophylaxis before and after a trip to the dentist. But in the usual person with MVP, I do not feel that antibiotics are needed."

43

Prescription and Non-Prescription Therapies

The Fascinating Story of Nystatin

If your health problems are yeast-connected, especially if you've been helped by *nystatin*, you'll be interested in knowing how it was discovered and where it got its name.

You'll be especially interested if you're a woman. Here's why: Two brilliant pioneer female scientists collaborated in discovering this remarkable anti-fungal substance. The story of nystatin is told in a 1981 book, *The Fungus Fighters*, by Richard S. Baldwin.[†]

In the foreword of this book, Gilbert Dalldorf recalls the story of the "wonder drug", *penicillin*. He said,

> "Medical history was changed by what appeared to be at first a chance discovery: a mold growing on a culture plate kept common bacteria from growing."

Soon afterward (in 1943) bacteriologist Selman Waksman, after years of searching, found a second antibiotic in the soil. Its name . . . streptomycin. In his continuing comments, Dalldorf had this to say,

> "Sparks from the Fleming and Waksman discoveries started a blaze in the Albany laboratory of the New York State Department of Health. There mold researcher Elizabeth Lee Hazen began to look for an agent that might be useful in controlling fungus diseases."

Working with organic chemist Rachel Brown during the years 1948-50, Hazen found many antifungal substances in the soil; however, most of them proved toxic not only to yeasts but to laboratory animals.

[†]Cornell University Press, 124 Roberts Place, Ithaca, New York 14850.

Then while vacationing with friends on a farm in Warrenton, Virginia, Elizabeth Hazen dug a soil sample and took it back to her laboratory. In this soil she found a mold which "knocked out" other yeasts and molds (including *Candida albicans*). Moreover, tests showed that this substance did not harm the animals.

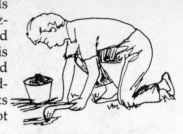

Soon afterward, E. R. Squibb & Sons met with Hazen and Brown and arranged to take this new fungus fighting substance, study it, patent it, and produce it.

Early in 1951 Hazen and Brown signed an agreement with Squibb to develop the new drug. They named it *nystatin* (pronounced *ny-state-in*) in honor of the New York State Department of Health. In their agreement with Squibb their royalties were put in a special Brown-Hazen scientific and educational fund. Neither of these women asked for or received any personal financial gain from their discovery.

During the next decade nystatin was produced in 18,000 gallon vats and marketed in many forms, including vaginal suppositories, foot powders, oral tablets and ointments. It was made available to physicians and patients (on prescription) all over the world. A patent, obtained in 1957, continued in force until 1974.

During these years royalties totaling 6.7 million dollars were paid to the Brown-Hazen fund and used to fund research on fungous diseases throughout the world.

Elizabeth Hazen died at the age of 89 in 1975; Rachel Brown died in 1980 at the age of 81. They were gratified by the help nystatin afforded women with vaginitis, and people of both sexes with yeast-related digestive disturbances. Yet neither lived long enough to learn that their discovery would help millions of people with candida-related health disorders.

A special word to physicians about nystatin powder:

If you're prescribing nystatin powder for many of your patients, ask your pharmacists to order it in bulk. They can obtain it by calling 1-800-LEDERLE. It comes in one billion and five billion unit containers.

If you're prescribing nystatin for your patients only occasionally and your pharmacist does not wish to stock it, your patients can fill their prescriptions from the following pharmacies:

Wellness, Health and Pharmaceuticals
(formerly Bob's Discount Drugs)
2800 South 18th Street
Birmingham, AL 35209
(800) 227-2627

Freeda Pharmaceuticals
36 East 41st Street
New York, NY 10017
(212) 685-4980
(800) 777-3737

Bio-Tech Pharmical
P.O. Box 1992
Fayetteville, AR 72702
(501) 443-9148 (ask for Dale Benedict)
(800) 345-1199

Medical Tower Pharmacy
1717 11th Avenue South
Birmingham, AL 35205
(205) 933-7381

N.E.E.D.S.
527 Charles Ave.
Syracuse, NY 13209
(800) 634-1380

Willner Chemists
330 Lexington Avenue
New York, NY 10016
(212) 685-0441

$1/8$ tsp. of powder = 500,000 units = 1 tablet. The approximate cost for 500,000 units of nystatin in powder form ranges from 15¢ to 20¢ per dose.

If your patients have trouble in obtaining insurance coverage for their nystatin, refer your health insurors to the reports by Rosenberg, etc. (see chapter 31).

More on Nizoral®

Nizoral® is a potent anticandida medication obtainable only on prescription. Using it in my practice I've been able to help over 150 of my patients; moreover, many of these patients had not improved on other treatment measures.

As you've read elsewhere in this book, Nizoral® (like any medication) may rarely cause severe adverse side effects. However, as I pointed out previously, "Everything you do carries a risk."

Because Nizoral® is such an effective anticandida medication, during the years 1984-1986 I have used it as the initial drug in treating many patients. Moreover, many other physicians are doing the same. One such physician, Allan Lieberman, M.D. of North Charleston, South Carolina, commented:

> "I use Nizoral® as my drug of choice in treating every patient in whom I suspect a candida-related health disorder. I have treated hundreds of patients in this manner and have never experienced a severe reaction. Nizoral® acts promptly . . . and sometimes a patient feels better after the first dose and often the response is dramatic."
>
> "I treat the average patient with Nizoral® for seven days; occasionally in a patient with severe problems I continue the medicaton for ten days. On the fifth day I add nystatin while continuing Nizoral®."

"A significant advantage of Nizoral® is that it provides a prompt therapeutic trial which helps me determine if my patients' health problems are related to *Candida albicans*. In addition, it causes fewer "die-off" type reactions. *It is an extremely useful drug.*"

"I give adults one 200 mg. tablet once a day; children who weigh from 44 to 88 pounds I prescribe ½ tablet once a day; and those who weigh under 44 pounds I prescribe ¼ tablet daily."

In May, 1986 I talked to Francis Waickman, M.D. of Cuyahoga Falls, Ohio, a physician who has treated hundreds of patients with Nizoral®. Here is what Dr. Waickman had to say:

I put all of my patients with polysystem chronic candidiasis immediately on Nizoral®. I give them 200 mg. once a day for two weeks and 90% of them show significant improvement. It is remarkable! I then switch them over to nystatin.

In my opinion the much greater improvement on Nizoral® takes place because hyphal forms of candida burrow into the deeper tissues of a person's body and nystatin simply doesn't get to them.

Treatment with Nizoral® is also cost effective since I do not feel it is necessary to put my patients through the expense of the blood tests unless I plan to keep them on this medication for many weeks.

Because during my years of practice I have seen many patients who experienced severe drug reactions to medications, I hesitate to give any drug that can cause side effects, especially severe ones. Moreover, I have personally experienced several adverse drug reactions; so have other members of my family.

But, if you're troubled by significant candida-related health problems, the slight risk of an adverse reaction to Nizoral® may be much less than the risk of doing without this medication.

Obviously, Nizoral® isn't a "magic bullet" which will solve every health problem. Yet, if your health problems are candida-related and are continuing, your physican may wish to prescribe a therapeutic trial of Nizoral®.

Another Antifungal Medication . . . Caprylic Acid

In the summer of 1984, I began receiving information about a new, yet old, antifungal medication. Its name: *Caprylic Acid*. This substance, a short-chain, saturated fatty acid had been studied some 30 years ago by Dr. Irene

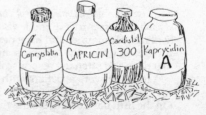

Neuhauser of the University of Illinois and found to have anti-fungal activity (*Arch. Int. Med.*, 93, 1954).

Because caprylic acid is a food substance, it is available without a prescription. Moreover, it is now being marketed by a number of different companies under various brand names.

In the preparations, Caprystatin,® Capricin®, Candistat-300®, Kaprycidin-A, and Mycopryl† 400 or 680, the manufacturers described clinical studies (unpublished) which show complete disappearance of candida from the stool specimens during treatment. Moreover, they reported that patients included in these studies experienced a remission of symptoms of their candida-related health problems. In addition, caprylic acid products are also being marketed in combination with other substances, including taheebo tea and *Lactobacillus acidophilus*.

Then in 1985, along with other physicians interested in candidiasis, I received information about new formulations of caprylic acid which are said to provide more "bioavailability" of caprylic acid in the intestinal tract. Brand names include Capricin® and Candistat-300®. Are these caprylic acid preparations effective? Are they as good as nystatin . . . or as nystatin and Nizoral® in controlling candida? What are their side effects? Are they safe? Which preparation is best?

These preparations appear to be safe and effective and I know of no serious side effects. However, as in the case with nystatin and other antifungal medications, temporary "die-off" symptoms may occur (see chapter 34 and 37). In addition, some patients experience digestive complaints while taking them.

How effective? Since I haven't used caprylic acid in treating many of my own patients, I sought help and consultation from other physicians whose opinions I respect. Here's what they told me:

Leo Galland, M.D.: "Capricin® in doses of 3-12 a day has worked very well for some patients and I believe it is a useful antifungal. Its efficacy approaches that of nystatin. The other products have been less consistent. Side effects may occur with all of them, especially gastric irritation, which is most common, incidentally, with Capricin."®

James O'Shea, M.D.: "For those who are sensitive to nystatin,

---

†Mycopryl is manufactured by T. E. Neesby Co., 2227 N. Pleasant Ave., Fresno, CA 93705 1-800-633-7294.

we use Caprystatin® and have used it very successfully. It is reasonably well tolerated."

Morton Teich, M.D.: "We've used Caprystatin® intermittently and it seemed to help a number of our patients."

Richard Mabray, M.D.: "We've found that Caprystatin® helps some of our patients. We haven't yet used Capricin®."

Don Mannerberg, M.D.: "We've had good luck with Capricin®, using it alone. No problems so far."

Pam Morford, M.D.: "We've found that Caprystatin® helps some of our patients."

Dave Buscher, M.D.: "Capricin® has helped a number of my patients. In fact, in several there has been a dramatic improvement. One patient felt the effect of Capricin® was better than that of Nizoral®. However, I've seen some die-off reactions and some intestinal intolerance. I certainly think that Capricin® is more effective than Caprystatin®, at least so far."

Gary Oberg, M.D.: "I have used Capricin® in several dozen patients, and it generally has given me as good results as nystatin (my previous favorite) or Nizoral®. There have been almost no side effects. Side effects seem to include 'heartburn,' bloating and a soapy aftertaste. These are usually avoidable by taking it after meals.

"I now start all new candida patients on Capricin® with generally gratifying results, followed by nystatin, then Nizoral® if needed, which is seldom. Yet I feel this substance is no 'cure-all' for the chronically sick patients with complex ecologic illness. *Self-treatment of such patients with over-the-counter caprylic acid products, without the supervision of an interested, knowledgeable physician, could lead to a self-made misdiagnosis of a non-candida-related problem.*

"It could also result in omission of other parts of a comprehensive ecologic illness treatment program. And in such a program, attention should be paid to endocrine problems and/or food, chemical and inhalant sensitivities. So attention to these other areas is also needed for overall good longterm results."

Elmer Cranton, M.D.: "Some patients do respond quite well to caprylic acid supplements. I believe that if caprylic acid is properly formulated for release in the colon, where most yeasts reside, that many patients do benefit. The formulation must prevent the digestive process from absorbing the caprylic acid in the small intestine, before it reaches the colon. I personally prefer to use Candistat-300®, which has been proven to have good clinical effectiveness in the treatment of my symptomatic patients, but as an adjunct to nystatin, not a replacement. It is also useful alone as a preventive, after treatment. Candistat-300® and Capricin® have very similar formulas.

George Borrel, M.D.: "Personally, I think Capricin® is a broad-spectrum and non-toxic fungicide that can be used by physicians who want to avoid the side effects of Nizoral® or use it in conjunction with nystatin to treat their patients with candidiasis."

Ken Gerdes, M.D.: "The caprylic acid products are my last drugs of choice. Two out of three of the patients on whom I've used this substance do not seem to be helped."

From these reports, I feel we now have another safe substance which helps control candida in the digestive tract. Perhaps in the year to come, clinical and laboratory studies will provide us with further information.

Garlic May Help Control Yeasts

Garlic has been widely used for medicinal purposes for centuries; for example, Virgil and Hippocrates mentioned it as a remedy for pneumonia and snake bite. In looking through the *Index Medicus*, I found numerous articles from the American and foreign literature describing the inhibitory action of garlic (Allium sativum) on candida organisms. Included among these was an article telling of the effect of garlic juice on two types of bacteria (*Staphylococcus aureus and E.coli*) as well as on *Candida albicans*. *Candida albicans* was found to be 'the most sensitive' of these three organisms to garlic juice.

Another paper commented,

> "Garlic possesses a broad antifungal activity, both on agar plates and in broth. Neither nystatin, nor amphotericin B . . . displayed such a high activity as garlic juice."

Still another article noted that all but 2 out of 26 strains of *Candida albicans* were sensitive to aqueous dilutions of garlic extract.

In spite of these studies . . . and there are many of them . . . Sanford Bolton and Gary Null and associates, writing in the *Amer-*

Capricin® is available from: Professional Specialties, 1800 132nd Ave., N.E., Bellevue, WA 98005, 1-800-426-1047;

Caprystatin® and Kaprystatin-A® are available from Cardiovascular Research, Ltd., 1061-B Shary Circle, Concord, CA 94518, 1-800-351-9429;

Candistat-300® is available from AMNI, 2247 National Ave., P.O. Box 5012, Hayward, CA 94540, 1-800-437-8888 (wholesale to doctors and distributors, and retail by mail to consumers) and Professional Nutrition Products, P.O. Box 31, Trout Dale, VA 24378, (703) 677-3102.

ican Pharmacy ("The Medical Uses of Garlic . . . Fact and Fiction", August 1982) pointed out that large scale controlled clinical trials of garlic still had never been conducted by the Food and Drug Administration. Moreover, such trials are time-consuming and extremely expensive.

During the past several years I have received many favorable reports on the beneficial effects of garlic and garlic extracts from individuals with candidiasis. Several people who have written me have reported that garlic helped even more than nystatin.

I have also received literature from several companies who produce and distribute garlic preparations. These include: Arizona Natural Products, 7750 East Evans Road, Suite 3, Scottsdale, AZ 85260, (612) 991-4414; Pure-Gar, Inc., P.O. Box 98813, Tacoma, WA 98499, (206) 582-6241; Wakanuga of America Company, Ltd., 23510 Telo Avenue, Suite 5, Torrance, CA 90505, (213) 539-3381; Professional Nutrition Products, Inc., P.O. Box 31, Trout Dale, VA 24378, (703) 677-3631; Miller Pharmacal Group, Inc., 245 W. Roosevelt, P.O. Box 279, West Chicago, IL 60185, 1-800-323-2935. Products marketed by these and other companies can be found in most health food stores and in some pharmacies.

To learn more about the effect of garlic on *Candida albicans* in February 1986 I consulted Moses Adetumbi, Ph.D. of the Department of Biology, Loma Linda University, Loma Linda, California. Dr. Adetumbi also sent me two reprints and several abstracts on the effectiveness of garlic as an antifungal, antimicrobial and pharmacological agent. The abstracts were presented at the American Society for Microbiology in 1983, 1984, and 1985.[†]

In a telephone conversation with me, Dr. Adetumbi commented,

> "Garlic is a highly effective antifungal agent. Even small amounts will have beneficial effects. By taking small amounts you won't have so much on your breath that it will create a social problem.
>
> "The major chemical constituent of whole garlic which is responsible for its therapeutic qualities is *allicin*. *Allicin* is also responsible for most of the strong odor it gives to the breath. So if you remove the *allicin*, you lose a lot of your antifungal effect although there are other components in garlic that affect cholesterol and lipid metabolism."

[†]Adetumbi, M.A., Javor and Lau, B.H.S., Loma Linda University Medical School, Loma Linda, California 92350. "Anti-Candidal Activity of Garlic—Effect on Macromolecular Syntheses." Presented at the American Society for Microbiology, 1985.

Almost all the promotional literature I receive from companies marketing garlic preparations describe "odorless" garlic. Moreover, data they sent me indicate that new techniques reduce or eliminate the odor without destroying the therapeutic value of the garlic. As you might guess, each company says, "Our product is best."

Can garlic help control your candida? Yes, no question about it; . . . especially whole garlic cloves or garlic powder. Moreover, based on reports I've received from patients, the odorless preparations seem to help, too. At least they're worth trying.

Lactobacillus Acidophilus and Other Friendly Bacteria Help Control Candida

The first bacteria of the lactobacillus group were identified over a hundred years ago. Then in 1908 Metchnikoff, a Bulgarian, recommended lactobacillus-containing yogurt in gastrointestinal and other disorders. He also felt this friendly germ played an important role in prolonging life.

During the years since that time, lactobacillus preparations have been used by both physicians and non-physicians to treat complaints ranging from constipation and diarrhea to skin problems. Moreover, when I was an intern and resident at Vanderbilt almost 40 years ago, we treated some of our babies with resistant diarrhea with human breast milk (which contained lots of lactobacilli).

In the '60s and '70s along with my pediatric peers, I often prescribed a powdered lactobacillus preparation to control diarrhea that developed following broad spectrum antibiotic drugs. Then, in the '70s I read a medical article which stated that yogurt douches can serve as an effective way of treating resistant vaginitis.

At the Dallas candida conference in 1982 the role of lactobacilli in competing with candida was discussed and a knowledgeable participant, during an informal luncheon address, commented,

"Giving preparations with lactobacilli may help your patients with overgrowth of candida in the digestive tract, especially if you give them every day."

Not long after that, I read an article by George Von Hilsheimer, Ph.D., entitled, "L-Acidophilus and the Ecology of the Human Gut." In this article, the author noted that "a long series of psychiatric patients (showed) a deficiency of *Lactobacillus acidophilus* (LA) in their stools . . . Supplementation with high levels of LA resulted in . . . observable changes in stools . . . and reduction of symptoms associated with food." Von Hilsheimer also noted that LA helped antagonize *Candida albicans* in the vagina of depressed women and other psychiatric patients.

So I began recommending yogurt and *Lactobacillus acidophilus* powders for my patients with yeast-related health disorders. Moreover, I read and heard reports from others who found that lactobacillus preparations (by mouth or in the vagina) helped their patients with candidiasis.

Then in the fall of 1984 James P. Carter, M.D., Chairman and Professor, Department of Nutrition, School of Public Health and Tropical Medicine, Tulane University, New Orleans, LA, sent me material about acidophilus and another friendly bacterium, *Streptococcus faecium* (C68).[†]

In research studies these bacteria had been fed to pigs who were then challenged with diarrhea-causing germs *(E. coli)* while a control group, given the same diarrhea germs, were not given *S. faecium* (C68). The pigs who received the friendly *S. faecium* "exhibited less severe diarrhea, recovered earlier and showed better weight gain than did pigs given *E. coli* only." *S. faecium* has also been shown to inhibit the growth of another diarrhea-causing germ, *C. difficile*.

In still another article by Italian researchers from Milan University, the colonizing ability of *Streptococcus faecium* SF68 was assessed in ten patients. And in all patients, *this friendly germ appeared to have some beneficial effects*.

Dr. Carter also referred me to the research work of Dr. Khem Shahani of the University of Nebraska, who is considered to be an authority in the area of the nutritional and therapeutic aspects of lactic acid bacteria, particularly *L. acidophilus, bifidobacterium bifidium* (also known as *Lactobacillus bifidus*) and *Streptococcus faecium*. I

[†]Underdhal, N. R., Torres-Medina, A., and Doster, A. R.: "Effective Streptococcus Faecium (C68) in Control of Escherichia Coli-Induced Diarrhea in Gnotobiotic Pigs." *American Journal of Veterinary Research*. 43:2227-22232, 1982.

Malamou-Ladas, H., and Tabaqchali, S.: "Inhibition of Clostridium Difficile by Fecal Streptococci." *Journal of Medical Microbiology,* Vol. 15 (1982), pp. 569-574, The Pathological Society of Great Britain and Ireland.

Lewenstein, A., Frigerio, G., and Moroni, M.: "Biological Properties of SF68, A New Approach for the Treatment of Diarrheal Diseases." *Current Therapeutic Research,* December, 1979, p. 967.

took this opportunity to visit with Dr. Shahani whom I had known before and got reacquainted with his research findings and their applications in the medical field.

Although Dr. Shahani and his associates have published some thirty or forty scientific papers in this area, several references[†] summarize some of their important observations.

Although I haven't done stool studies on my patients with candida (and I don't know of anyone who has), excessive numbers of *Candida albicans* in the intestinal tract seem to play a role in making people sick. So it seems appropriate to "crowd out" candida with friendly bacteria.

Moreover, Witkin in summarizing his research report said,

> "Candida albicans infection, often associated with antibiotic-induced alterations in microbial flora, may cause defects in cellular immunity."

Witkin noted that the immunological alterations may also be related to endocrine dysfunction and auto-antibody formation. So Witkin seems to be saying, in effect,

> "Antibiotics knock out the friendly "good guys" while they're killing off the bad guys. As a result, *Candida albicans* comes in and "takes over" causing a person to develop immune system and hormone problems."

Information I've received recently from several sources suggests that when you take preparations of these friendly bacteria they become "implanted". This means they will start multiplying. And in so doing they help bring about a more normal balance of germs in your digestive tract.

Many excellent preparations of these friendly bacteria can be found at your health food store (and in pharmacies and other stores too). Yet all preparations aren't identical. Moreover, (as in the case with garlic products) each company says, "Our product is best."

Can friendly bacteria help control your candida? Based on many

---

†Shahani, K. M., Vakil, J. R., and Kilara, A.: "Natural Antibiotic Activity of *Lactobacillus Acidophilus* and *Bulgaricus*. II. Isolation of Acidophilin from *L. Acidophilus*." *Cultured Dairy Prod. J.*, 12(2), 1977, pp. 8-11.

Reddy, G. V., Shahani, K. M., Friend, B. A., and Chandan, R. C.: "Natural Antibiotic Activity of *Lactobacillus Acidophilus* and *Bulgaricus*. III. Production and Partial Purification of bulgarican from *Lactobacillus Bulgaricus*." *Cultured Dairy Prod. J.*, 18(2), 1983, pp. 15-19.

Friend, B. A. and Shahani, K. M.: "Nutritional and Therapeutic Aspects of Lactobacilli." *J. Applied Nutrition*, 36, 1984, pp. 125-153.

studies in the medical literature plus reports from countless patients, my answer is "Yes".

Which acidophilus or other friendly bacteria products are best? I don't really know from my own personal experience. Perhaps further clinical and research trials in months and years to come will give us the answer.

The Essential Fatty Acids (EFA's), Minerals and Vitamins

Although I had learned a smattering of information about fatty acids when I was in medical school, the subject had long since been buried somewhere in the dusty cobwebs of my brain. Then, about five years ago, I began to read and hear more about these substances from various sources, including an article in *Executive Health* by David Horrobin, Ph.D.*

A year or two later, while attending a conference in Montreal, I met and had dinner with Dr. Horrobin who told me about his fascinating work with oil of evening primrose . . . a rich source of Omega 6 fatty acids. So my interest in these nutritional substances began to increase.

Then at the Dallas Conference in July 1982 (see chapters 17 and 34), I heard Dr. Sidney Baker describe deficiencies in essential fatty acids in his patients with yeast-connected health disorders. The following year at the Birmingham Conference (see chapter 36), Dr. C. Orian Truss presented research studies on his candida patients showing abnormalities in essential fatty acids. Moreover, following appropriate treatment, these abnormalities showed significant improvement.

I also listened to audio tapes of a conference on fatty acids which featured presentations by a number of fatty acid investigators, including Dr. Baker, Dr. Leo Galland, and Dr. Donald O. Rudin (author of a new book, *The Omega Factor: Our Nutritional Missing Link*). Yet, I still found the whole subject of fatty acids and their chemistry hard to understand.

Then in the Winter/1984 (Vol. 3, #2) and Spring, 1984 (Vol. 3, #3) issues of *Update*, published by the Gesell Institute of Human De-

---

*Horrobin, D. F.: "Alcohol—Blessing and Curse of Mankind!" *Executive Health*, Vol. XVII, 9, June, 1981. (Dr. Horrobin's two books on the subject are *Prostaglandins* and *Clinical Use of Essential Fatty Acids*, Eden Press; Montreal, London.)

velopment, Dr. Sidney Baker** and Dr. Leo Galland published essays on essential fatty acids which made this important and complex subject a lot easier to understand.

In his essay entitled, "Fat Is Not Just to Hold Your Pants Up," Baker pointed out that . . .

> "Fifteen percent of your body weight is fat even if you don't have 'an ounce of fat on you'." . . . "Too much of the wrong kind (of fat) is bad. . . . But too little of the right kind is just as bad. In no other area of nutrition is the adage 'You are what you eat' more true. . . . The key to the whole issue is that oils are not just the 'padding' of your body, but are the structural core of the wall of each of the body cells and the raw material for crucial hormones". . . .

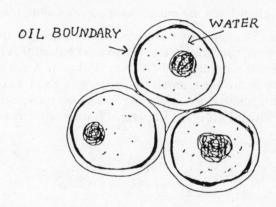

Baker then pointed out that our bodies are composed of billions of cells of various sizes, shapes and functions. Moreover, each cell contains water (and many other substances) and a water-proof boundary. This boundary is made of oils. And Baker continued:

> "Whether we're talking about a single cell or a whole human being, a kind of water-proofing is provided for each cell by oil. It gives boundary between two kinds of water: That inside the cells, where life activity takes place, and that outside or between cells."

In his continuing discussion, Baker pointed out that fat and oil molecules also play an important role in storing food energy. Then he discussed another important role of the essential fatty acids, i.e., they furnish the raw materials for making hormones—not the

---

**Dr. Baker gives credit to both Rudin and Horrobin, and also to Neil Orenstein, Ph.D. and Leo Galland, M.D. for providing him with "information and insights" on the essential fatty acids.

long distance messengers that travel between the various endocrine glands, including the thyroid, pituitary, adrenals, ovaries and testicles.

> ". . . only in the last 20 years have another group of hormones been recognized. These are the *prostaglandins*. They are short-distance message carriers that are made by all of the cells of the body. They are made from the oil molecules in the . . . cell membranes."

To learn more about these fascinating, but hard to understand essential fatty acids, I interviewed Dr. Leo Galland of New York City, an authority on the subject. Here's a summary of my interview:

Crook: Dr. Galland, tell me more about these essential fatty acids.

Galland: The diets eaten by our ancestors hundreds of thousands of years ago were very low in fat. Yet, almost half of this fat was in the form of essential fatty acids (EFA's). Today in America we eat high fat diets and only a small percentage of the fat consists of EFA's. And this relative deficiency of EFA's keeps us from forming a recently recognized group of important hormones, the *prostaglandins*.

When we look at the chemistry of these EFA's, we find they are what we call "long-chain" polyunsaturated fatty acids. And they're composed of a string of 18 to 20 carbon atoms . . . sort of like a string of pearls. Most of these "pearls" are linked by a single link, but 2 to 6 of them are hooked together by what we call "double bonds."

Crook: Are there many types of EFA's, and which ones are important for the person with a yeast problem?

Galland: There are two general classes of EFA's. One group we call *"Omega 6"* fatty acids, and the other group are the *"Omega 3"* fatty acids.

Crook: What does this mean, and how do we know which is which?

Galland: Let me explain. Each long chain of fatty acids begins with a carbon atom which has 3 hydrogens hitched onto it . . . we call it the CH 3 end of the molecule. The Omega 3 fatty acids have the first double bond on the third carbon atom from the CH 3 end of the molecule, and the Omega 6 fatty acids have the first double bond on the 6th carbon.

Crook: Sounds complicated, but I'm glad to know about this difference, even though I'm not sure I completely understand it. Now tell me about some of the physical findings you see in patients with EFA deficiencies.

Galland: Well, they include dry skin, flaky, painful skin rashes, hard, dry, bumpy spots on the skin, brittle nails and dry, straw-like hair. What's more, I found 2 or more of these findings in 65% of 104 candidiasis patients that I studied.

Crook: Are there laboratory tests to determine EFA deficiencies?

Galland: Yes. We studied levels of circulating EFA's in 37 of our patients. Some of these studies were carried out by the Monroe Medical Research Laboratory, Southfield, New York, and others were studied by the Efamol Research Laboratory, Kentville, Nova Scotia.

Crook: What were your usual findings?

Galland: The commonest finding was a general depression in all components of the Omega 3 family. What's more, the clinical importance of this type of deficiency has been well documented by Donald Rudin. However, there were also abnormalities in the metabolism of Omega 6 fatty acids in two-thirds of the patients we studied.

Crook: How do you help your patients bring these fatty acids up to a more normal level?

Galland: By making changes in their diet and by prescribing vegetable and fish oil supplements. I tell my patients to start by pruning out sugar, alcohol and fat. I ask them to especially shun the partially hydrogenated vegetable oils and saturated fats, including coconut oil and the margarines.

I also ask them to avoid the deep fried

foods, potato chips, corn chips, bacon and other fatty cuts of meat, luncheon meats, fatty cheeses, creams and cream sauces. They also need to avoid the hundreds of processed and packaged foods containing hydrogenated or partially hydrogenated vegetable oils. These fats are the "bad guys."

Then I recommend cold-pressed linseed oil . . . 1 to 2 tablespoons daily. In the underweight person, I may increase the linseed oil up to 3 tablespoons a day. Salmon, mackerel, sardine, tuna, herring and other cold-water fish also serve as an important source of the Omega 3 fatty acids. In addition, I sometimes prescribe 2 to 4 fish oil capsules each day. These contain eicosopentanoic acid (EPA), another of the Omega 3 fatty acids.

Crook: And for your patients who are deficient in Omega 6 fatty acids?

Galland: The main Omega 6 fatty acid, linoleic acid (LA) is found in the seeds of plants, especially in corn, sunflower and safflower oils. So making the dietary changes we just talked about helps. I also prescribe capsules which contain oil of evening primrose. The usual dose is 1 to 2 capsules three times a day. These primrose oil supplements seem to especially help women . . . especially those with the premenstrual syndrome.

Crook: That has certainly been my experience, too, and many of my PMS patients have told me, "I can't get along without primrose oil."

What other nutrient deficiencies have your uncovered in studying your candida patients?

Galland: We found a lot of them . . . especially deficiencies of vitamin B-6 and magnesium. Also, of zinc, vitamin A and vitamin B-3.

Crook: What symptoms do you see in your magnesium deficient patients?

Galland: Nervousness, irritability and jitteriness.

Crook: Is magnesium deficiency common?

Galland: Yes. Very common . . . and it occurs a lot more often than generally recognized. Human beings the world over used to eat a lot of magnesium. Not any more. Grains are stripped of their minerals in milling; three-fourths of the U.S. population consume less than 2/3 of the recommended daily allowance of magnesium. Over-consumption of phosphorus and phosphate-containing foods also contributes to magnesium deficiency. So does consumption of the wrong kind of fats . . . the ones we call hardened or hydrogenated fats.

Crook: Are there other reasons why people become magnesium deficient?

Galland: Yes. Yeast infections which appear to wreak havoc with the way a person handles magnesium. Some of my yeast patients seem to be "sieves" for magnesium. And they require huge doses to maintain a normal body level.
Moreover, one reason why a chronic yeast infection causes magnesium problems is that such an infection creates a deficiency of vitamin B-6. And vitamin B-6 appears to play an important role in magnesium utilization. So to get your magnesium and B-6 requirements back toward normal, you've got to treat your yeast problem.

Crook: How do you decide whether or not a person is magnesium deficient? Do laboratory tests help?

Galland: Common laboratory tests don't help very much. A magnesium loading test can clinch the diagnosis, but it is time-consuming and cumbersome. So we base our diagnosis on a history of a deficient diet plus symptoms such as fatigability, muscle cramps, irritability, poor concentration and depression which improve with magnesium supplementation.

Crook: Is there some other sort of test that could be done . . . other than a laboratory test?

Galland: Yes. A good functional test of calcium and magnesium status is a Chvostek's test.

Crook: Chvostek's test? How do you do this? What does it mean?

Galland: You can do a Chvostek's test on yourself rather simply. All you have to do is to tap lightly in the hollow of your cheek, halfway between the bottom of your ear and the corner of your mouth. If the top of your lip beneath your nose twitches or if you grimace or jump, the test is considered positive and usually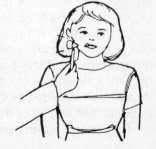

shows that you have a magnesium deficiency. A Chvostek's test can be confirmed by a test of muscular irritability called an *electromyogram*.

Crook: What are some of the food sources of magnesium?

Galland: The richest dietary sources of magnesium are also the richest dietary sources of essential fatty acids. . . . seed foods (including the whole grains, nuts and beans) and seafoods. What's more, you can protect your magnesium stores by avoiding the magnesium wasters; saturated fats and soft drinks, especially those containing caffeine.

Crook: How do yeast patients get their magnesium back up to normal?

Galland: First, they eat a good diet of the sort we've just been talking about. Then I prescribe magnesium supplements containing 300 to 600 or more milligrams of magnesium. I also prescribe calcium.

Crook: Can a person get too much magnesium? What are the symptoms of magnesium overdose?

Galland: Too much magnesium produces diarrhea of the sort you get by taking a big dose of Milk of Magnesia. This limits absorption. And when this happens, you can cut the dose down. Also, if you develop muscle cramps while you're taking magnesium and they haven't been present before, you may need less magnesium and more calcium.

Crook: Tell me more about calcium.

Galland: Calcium deficiencies are common in people who eat fabricated, processed and refined foods. Diets which feature such foods usually leave little room for an adequate intake of green leafy vegetables, whole grains, nuts, seeds and fresh fruits. Although cow's milk, yogurt, cheeses and other dairy products furnish sig- 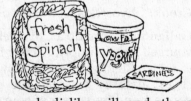 nificant amounts of calcium, many people dislike milk and others develop adverse reactions when they drink milk. So unless your patients take in a lot of dairy products, greens or sardines, chances are they aren't getting enough calcium.

Crook: How much calcium does a person need a day?

Galland: The needs of an adult for calcium vary considerably. Usually, it's somewhere between 600 and 1500 milligrams a day. A larger calcium intake is especially appropriate in people with deficiencies of magnesium, essential fatty acids and vitamin A. Adequate calcium intake is also important in women who commonly develop thinning of the bones as they grow older and more especially after the menopause.

Crook: What forms of calcium do you recommend?

Galland: There are many forms on the market. I use calcium lactate more than any other form. Other acceptable forms include calcium gluconate and calcium carbonate, although absorption of the calcium carbonate is sometimes poor. I do not recommend dolomite and bone meal supplements because they may be contaiminated with lead and other toxic minerals.

Crook: Dr. Galland, let's talk a little bit about the B vitamins.

Galland: As you know, there are many members of the B vitamin family, including B-1, B-2, B-3, B-6, B-12, B-15 and pantothenic acid. These vitamins play an important role in many biochemical and metabolic reactions in the body. Moreover, they act as a team. And although vitamin B-6 is important in yeast patients, I recommend that my patients with yeast-related health disorders take supplements containing all the B vitamins.

Crook: What doses of B vitamins do you generally recommend?

Galland: Usually from 10 to 50 milligrams of the B vitamins in a balanced formula. However, some individuals appear to need larger doses.

Crook: Can you test for vitamin deficiencies?

Galland: Yes. In evaluating a person's vitamin status, I often order blood tests to determine vitamin levels. Moreover, such a test is cost effective and reliable. For about $125 to $150, Vitamin Diagnostics, Inc.* will analyze a blood sample for 12 vitamins (B-12, folic acid, B-6, thiamin, niacin, biotin, riboflavin, pantothenic acid, Beta carotene and vitamins A, C & E). In evaluating vitamin B-6 status, I find it useful to measure levels of the active form of

---

*Herman Baker, Rt. 33 and Industrial Avenue, Cliffwood Beach, New Jersey 07735.

vitamin B-6. This form of B-6 is called pyridoxal-5-phosphate and its level can be determined by several laboratories, including the Monroe Medical Research Laboratory.*

So if you're bothered by patchy, dull, dry skin, dandruff, fingernails that are soft and break off easily, lusterless, straw-like or touseled hair, PMS depression and/or many other chronic health disorders (many or most of which are yeast-connected), Drs. Baker and Galland suggest that it's time for "an oil change." And if you'd like to learn more about this fascinating and important subject, read the Baker and Galland essays. You can obtain both by sending $3.50, and a long, stamped (39¢), self-addressed envelope to UPDATE, The Gesell Institute of Human Development, 310 Prospect St., New Haven, CT 06511.

Nutritional Supplements Help—And Are Gaining Credibility

Until the early '70s, like most physicians, when asked about vitamin, mineral and other nutritional supplements, I usually said:

"If you eat a good diet, (including foods from the basic four groups) you don't need supplemental vitamins. They're a waste of money."

But gradually, I began to change my mind based on things I read in the lay literature. Included were articles in *Prevention, Bestways, Let's Live,* and other magazines. (My mother, an organic gardener, faithfully read these magazines and passed relevant articles on to me.) I also began to receive favorable reports from my patients who were taking vitamins, minerals, and other nutritional supplements. Included were many of my patients with food and chemical sensitivities.

Then in the mid '70s, one of my patients brought me a copy of *Executive Health,* a monthly periodical which I had seen advertised in the *New York Times* and the *Wall Street Journal.* Consultants listed on the front page of this newsletter included two Nobel prize winners (Linus Pauling, Ph.D. and Albert Szent-Györgi, Ph.D.) along with the late Alton Ochsner, M.D., (founder of the world famous Ochsner Clinic in New Orleans) and other scientists with impressive credentials.

Among the subjects covered were the importance of vitamins and minerals including doses much larger than the AMA and

_____
*Route 17, P.O. Box 1, Southfield, New York 10057.

other medical organizations had been recommending. I also began to read articles in scientific journals indicating that many Americans were deficient in zinc, magnesium and other nutrients. And by the early '80s, our most conservative medical journals began to talk about *osteoporosis* and the need for calcium supplements.

Then in 1981, Mary Ware, President of Southwestern Health Organization (SWHO) invited me to talk at a conference in San Antonio, Texas. My subject—food allergies. I was impressed by the integrity, dedication, sincerity, knowledge, and expertise possessed by many of the people I met there. Included were health food store owners and distributors of many types of products including vitamins, minerals, acidophilus, whole grains, unrefined vegetable oils, and garlic.

About the same time, I became reacquainted with Elmer Cranton, M.D., of Trout Dale, Virginia, a graduate of Harvard Medical School and a pioneer in preventive and holistic medicine. Dr. Cranton and I had served together on the Advisory Board of the Pritikin Research Foundation in California. Yet, I hadn't seen or talked to him in several years. Dr. Cranton had co-authored with Richard Passwater, Ph.D., a book on minerals, TRACE ELEMENTS, HAIR ANALYSIS AND NUTRITION. He had also written a number of papers about the importance of antioxidants and other nutrients in combating *free radical pathology*.

During the years 1982-1986, I began to prescribe nutritional supplements for my patients and my family. Moreover, I began to take them myself. These included products which contained 20-100 mg. of the different B vitamins, 1,000-1,500 mg. of vitamin C[†], 50-200 mcg. of selenium, 1,000-1,500 mg. of calcium and 500-800 mg. of magnesium, 15-30 mg. of zinc plus a number of other nutrients and micro-nutrients. Then, after learning about the importance of the essential fatty acids from David Horrobin, Donald Rudin, Ph.D., Sidney Baker, M.D., Leo Galland, M.D., and Orian Truss, M.D., I began to prescribe and take supplemental *"Omega 3"* and *"Omega 6"* fatty acids including linseed oil, fish oils and evening primrose oil.

[†]In a report entitled, "New Concepts in the Biology and Biochemistry of Ascorbic Acid" (published in the April 3, 1986 issue of the *New England Journal of Medicine*, 314:892-902), Mark Levine, M.D. discussed Vitamin C, including the history of its discovery, chemistry, biochemistry, physiologic properties, recommended dietary allowance and data derived from animal studies. *(continued on next page)*

Yet, controversy continued to exist in the nutritional field and a number of vocal "establishment" spokesmen (including Steven Barrett, M.D. of Allentown, Pennsylvania and Victor Herbert, M.D. of New York) say, in effect, "Taking big doses of vitamins, minerals and other nutritional supplements is 'quack medicine'."

Evidence of the continuing controversy about vitamins can be found in an article by Dan Sperling, published in *USA Today* on May 7, 1986: DOCTORS DEBATE USE OF VITAMINS.

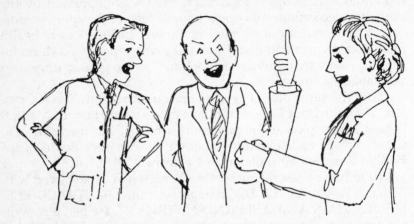

"For the 48 percent of us who take our daily vitamins, the growing controversy over their value and safety could be a bitter pill to swallow.

Dr. Levine also discussed the problem of the Recommended Daily Allowances (RDA) vs. the optimal amount of ascorbic acid and had this to say,

"The data in animals suggests even more strongly than the data in humans, that the RDA for the prevention of scurvy and the RDA for other measures of health are not similar . . . Studies in guinea pigs suggest that for growth and health, 10-16 mg/kg per day is necessary . . . For recovery from anesthesia, 50 mg/kg per day was optimal."

Based on Dr. Levine's observations, it seems to me that if a 130 lb. adult took a proportionate amount of Vitamin C, it would require 600 mg to 1000 mg per day for growth and health and 3 to 5 times that much during periods of stress. Here are other comments by Dr. Levine:

"Despite all the information available on ascorbic acid, we still do not know what the optimal dietary level is for human beings . . . I have come to explain my work today in order to change some of the preconceived notions many of us have about vitamins and cofactors. We don't really know how much of these entities the human body needs for optimal function."

I feel that Vitamin C, in doses larger than the RDA, helps many of my patients. Moreover, I feel it's a safe substance for people to take, yet, I realize it isn't a "cure all". Based on observations of Nobel prize winner Linus Pauling, Dr. Robert Cathcart and many others, I feel that Vitamin C helps people in ways we still don't understand. It seems to me that Dr. Levine's observations provide at least some support for things double Nobel prize winner Linus Pauling has been saying for many years.

That controversy took another turn this week when a panel of doctors asked colleagues to monitor patients' vitamin use.

The panel, sponsored by the American Dietetic Association, voiced concern over the rising use of vitamin and mineral supplements, citing possible toxic effects from "megadoses" taken by as many as 10 percent of us.

That concern isn't unanimous.

'There is no good scientific evidence that supplements taken at reasonable doses have caused a true toxin reaction,' says Jeffrey Bland, nutrition professor at the University of Puget Sound in Tacoma, Washington.

Except for such groups as pregnant and lactating women, some elderly and those on certain drugs, there's 'no justification for taking vitamins and minerals to cure or prevent disease,' says panel chairman Dr. David Heber, chief of nutrition at UCLA School of Medicine.

Not so, says Paul Lachance, nutrition professor at Rutgers University in New Brunswick, N.J. 'If a person isn't getting those nutrients in food, or if they're depleting them by such habits as smoking or drinking, then they probably should be using a supplement.'

Among the vitamins that may be toxic in high doses: vitamin A (liver damage); vitamin D (kidney damage); vitamin E (thyroid problems); and vitamin B6 (nerve damage)."[†]

Just before going to press, I received information about a new multilevel company, United Sciences of America, Inc. (USA), Dallas, Texas 75251. Since I use and prescribe nutritional supplements, I was pleased to see this material. Moreover, I was impressed by the Scientific Advisory Board listed in this company's literature. Included was the world-famous immunologist, Robert A. Good, M.D., Ph.D., Chairman of the Department of Pediatrics, University of South Florida, Tampa. In his position as Chairman of the Scientific Advisory Board of USA, Dr. Good commented:

"An explosion of new information shows that the proper combination of nutrients, combined with the reduction of caloric intake will help fortify the body's immune system and aid in fighting disease—I'm proud to be a member, and I've endorsed both our program and this entire organization."

Other members of the Scientific Advisory Board include Christiaan Barnard, M.D., Ph.D., Julius Axelrod, Ph.D., of the National Institute of Mental Health (a Nobel prize winner), Alexander Leaf, M.D., Chairman of the Department of Preventive Medicine, Harvard Medical School, Andrew V. Schally, Ph.D., (another Nobel

---

Prize winner in medicine and physiology-1977), and C. Norman Shealy, M.D., Ph.D., founding president of the American Holistic Medical Association plus a number of other scientists with impeccable credentials. *I was fascinated to see that the supplements promoted and marketed by this company, resembled those I had been recommending for my patients during the past several years.* Moreover, their Master Formula® is very similar to the Basic Preventive® multiple supplement first formulated by Dr. Elmer Cranton some 5 years earlier.

With the research data, support, and recommendations of scientists with such impeccable credentials, it seems to me that supplementing the diet with vitamins, minerals and essential fatty acids has now gained scientific credibility. Moreover, in our free enterprise society, I feel that many companies will be making such nutritional supplements available.

Here's a list of companies that I'm familiar with whose vitamin and mineral products are yeast-free and sugar-free:

Allergy Research Group
400 Preda Street
San Leandro, CA 94577
(800) 782-4274
(415) 639-4572

Amni—Advanced Medical Nutrition, Inc.
2247 National Avenue
Hayward, CA 94545
(800) 356-4791
(415) 783-6969

Bio-Tech Pharmical
P.O. Box 1991
Fayetteville, AR 72702
(800) 345-1199
(501) 443-9148 (ask for Dale Benedict)

Bronson Pharmaceuticals
4526 Rinetti Lane
La Canada, CA 91011-0628
(800) 521-3322 (outside California)
(818) 790-2646

Cardiovascular Research, Ltd.
1061-B Shary Circle
Concord, CA 94518
(800) 888-4585
(415) 827-2636

Freeda Pharmaceuticals
36 East 41st Street
New York, NY 10017
(800) 777-3737
(215) 662-3329

Klaire Laboratories, Inc.
Vital Life Company
1573 West Seminole Street
San Marcus, CA 92069
(800) 648-4755
(619) 744-9680

Vitaline Formulas
7222 Jefferson Avenue
Ashland, OR 97520
(800) 648-4755
(503) 482-9231

Willner Chemists
330 Lexington Avenue
New York, NY 10016
(212) 685-0441

Other reputable companies who manufacture and produce vita-min and mineral products that you may find at your health food store include: Alacer, American Health, J. R. Carlson, Makers of KAL, Naturally, Nature's Plus, Nu-Life, Nutritional Factors, Plus Products, Radiance, Randal Nutritional, Rich Life, Schiff, Solgar, W. T. Thompson Company, and Twin Lab.

44
Other Topics of Interest

More About Children

During the 1950s all of my patients were children. Then during the '60s and '70s (as my interest in allergies increased), I began to see more and more adult patients. And during the '80s, since learning about the role of *Candida albicans*, my practice has changed dramatically. Today, 9 out of 10 of the patients who come to me seeking help are adults.

Yet, my interest in children continues. Moreover, many people have urged me to talk more about candida-related health problems in children. For example, Ricky Weiss, of Minneapolis told me about a youngster, Darren, who although exceptionally bright, had been developmentally delayed, aggressive and unhappy.

In a recent report published in the 1985 Spring/Summer issue of PMS/CANDIDA AIM (Vol. 2, No. 4), entitled "Candida Therapy Gave My Son Another Chance", Margie Wold wrote:

"Our son, Darren, has been a 'handful' since he arrived from Bogota, Colombia at 11 weeks of age. At eighteen months, Darren began to have symptoms of severe hyperactivity. By the age of three, he had become so violent and aggressive, we sought help. He was seen by every specialist imaginable. Ritalin didn't help; neither did the Feingold diet. Finally, because we were desperate and didn't know what else to do, we made arrangements to put him in an institution.

"Then while waiting for a place, we found *The Yeast Connection*. As it turned out, Darren was a prime candidate. He had thrush as an infant and received many antibiotics for ear and throat infections.

"A few days after being put on the diet, Darren showed marked improvement. In less than one week his stuttering improved—he dressed himself and put away his toys. He seemed more reasonable and manageable. After a week on the diet, nystatin was added. Although he had ups and downs on nystatin, especially when the dose was increased, he improved significantly."

In a follow-up report published in the PMS/AIM newsletter[†], Darren's mother reported,

"Darren is usually cooperative in following his dietary program. He takes nystatin each day and, for a short period of time, he also took Nizoral®. He occasionally has a difficult day, but he has more good times than bad. He is still "behind" in his social relationships; however, children, who had previously refused to play with him, now accept him.

"Darren's academic progress has been 'fantastic'. He has been in a pre-kindergarten class for children with problems, but his teachers now recommend that he be mainstreamed into regular kindergarten next year with no special program. He is learning well, able to make mental connection, to follow directions and complete tasks. All of these were impossible for him a year ago.

"Now Darren responds normally to attention and affection. He likes to be cuddled and held, whereas previously, he rejected everyone. He isn't normal yet—it's an up and down kind of thing. But by comparison to a year ago, he is excellent."

Then at the San Francisco Conference on Human-Yeast Interaction in March 1985, I happened to have breakfast with Robert Payne, M.D. of Salt Lake City who told me a fascinating story about one of his patients who had responded to antifungal therapy. In May 1986 he sent me a full report on this patient. Here's a summary of her story:

"Susie (not her name) developed pneumonia at the age of 10 days. She received massive doses of antibiotics. Subsequently she developed severe asthma and the sleep apnea syndrome. She failed to thrive and weighed only about 15 pounds at the age of 1 year. Susie was unable to do anything. She was very unresponsive, sort of like a glob of clay. She didn't move around and wasn't interested in things. She also experienced continual respiratory infections and repeated asthma attacks.

"In evaluating Susie's problems, I sent blood specimens to immunopathologist, Edward Winger, M.D.[‡] She showed high levels of candida specific IgM and IgG antibodies. We put her on nystatin. Within a week, she showed a dramatic improvement and stopped having asthma attacks. She started to grow, thrive and become vigorous.

"Since antifungal treatment was started, Susie has had only one infection. We documented that with a strep culture. She's been happy, vigorous and her weight is normal. She's still taking nystatin. We tried to take her off of it after about a year . . . that was when she got her infection.

"Susie's mother noticed an observable change in her general physical vigor and her breathing rate. It was almost like she was going to become

†PMS/CANDIDA AIM, P.O. Box 6291, Minneapolis, MN 55406, (612) 724-4425. Director: Ricky Weiss.

‡Immunodiagnostic Lab, 400 29th Street, Oakland CA 94609.

asthmatic again. We counseled together and put her right back on the nystatin again. We've kept her on it now. She takes ⅛ teaspoon four times a day. Her health is excellent and her development is normal. She is active and into everything like any normal 3½ year-old child.

"Although I'm not claiming that a special diet and nystatin will cure every child with recurrent infections and failure to thrive and other difficult and frustrating problems, my experience with this patient has been an exciting one. Moreover, I've treated at least a dozen youngsters with a similar program who have shown good to excellent response."

Another favorable report came to me in a letter from a State Chairman of the American Academy of Pediatrics who recently wrote:

"I have a patient with autistic behavior which began after an extended course of antibiotics at age two. He is responding to high dosage nystatin therapy."

Then in May 1986, David Harbrecht, M.D., a Bountiful, Utah ear, nose and throat specialist, told me of his exciting experiences in treating several children with behavior and learning problems. Here's a summary of Dr. Harbrecht's comments:

"In recent months, I've seen three or four 6-8 year-old children with behavior and learning problems where I felt there was definitely a connection to candida. *Each child had received repeated courses of antibiotic drugs* during earlier childhood for respiratory infections.

"The nervous system symptoms in these children included *decreased attention span, behavior problems* at home and *disruptive conduct* at school. In addition, the parents all emphasized *irritability*.

"All four of these children were also bothered by *year-round nasal congestion and drainage*—and this was the main reason these children were brought to me. Food sensitivities occurred in these children, especially sensitivity to milk, wheat and corn. Sugar craving also was present in each youngster.

"In treating them, I changed the diets although getting the child to stick to the diet wasn't always easy. In addition, I've prescribed oral nystatin and all are showing significant improvement. My usual dose: ¼ teaspoon of the powder 4 times a day.

"One child has been on this program for four months and the response has been extremely gratifying. Moreover, if he misses even a single dose, his mother can tell the difference. For example, if he gets only three doses in a day, there will be a slight deterioration in his school work the following day. As long as he gets his medication, he does fine."

As I've already discussed, it seems to me that the youngsters who are at risk include especially: (1) Those who receive long-term antibiotic drugs for ear infections, sinus infections or bladder infections and (2) Teenagers who take long-term tetracycline for acne.

Clinical and research studies by Iwata, Truss, Witkin and hundreds of other physicians clearly show that: (1) Long-term antibiotic usage alters the bacterial flora of the gut; (2) When the bacterial flora of the gut is changed, *Candida albicans* tend to proliferate; (3) Under such circumstances, candida can and does put out toxins; (4) Such toxins affect many metabolic processes (Truss). They also affect the immune system (Iwata and Witkin).

Accordingly, if your child has received repeated courses of antibiotic drugs and . . .

1. continues to be bothered by infections
2. is irritable, hyperactive and hard to manage or depressed
3. experiences trouble in paying attention and learning and/or shows signs of developmental delay and/or regression
4. exhibits autistic behavior

. . . *I urge you to look for a possible "yeast connection"*.

Candida Affects Animals, Too

Although researchers often study animals to learn more about human disease, it hadn't occurred to me that candida could be causing significant problems in veterinary medicine.

Then at the 1985 San Francisco conference (see chapter 36), I met John Whittaker, D.V.M. of Springfield, Missouri and found that he had been interested in candidiasis for many years. In discussing candidiasis, Dr. Whittaker commented,

> "Candida has been recognized in the poultry industry for some time. Yet most people felt it was only an upper digestive tract invader and few recognized that it could wreck the immune system and serve as a 'door opener' for other diseases. For example, I see candida and gram positive bacterial infections go hand in hand.
>
> "I also feel that candida lowers resistance to protozoan diseases such as coccidiosis. It also makes animals more susceptible to internal parasites. It seems to me that improper use of antibiotics and sulfa drugs promotes the growth of candida in poultry and swine in the same way as they do in humans.
>
> "Frankly, candida is still a sort of 'ho-hum' disease agent in poultry and is totally overlooked in swine production. Moreover, most people in veterinary medicine ignore the role of candida in cats and other small

animals. Yet I feel they're often made ill by an insidious attack of candida. In addition, breeding problems in horses and other large animals often stem from candida infections of the uterus.

"Admittedly, much more research is needed in this field, but today . . . right now . . . sick patients, including both animals and humans, need relief administered by experienced doctors. And please remember, the physician, veterinary or medical, is *first* trained in the art of clinical medicine."

In April 1986, I had a visit with Dr. Whittaker and I asked him to tell me more about symptoms in remote organs of animals which he felt were candida related. Here are further comments:

"I've seen irritable . . . even "hysterical" . . . chickens with nervous system symptoms of all sorts. Some of these chickens would engage in feather picking and others would be unusually quiet as though depressed. And I've seen both conditions reversed with antifungal therapy.

"In addition, I've seen swine with candida-related skin and respiratory problems. Admittedly, these observations are empirical or 'anecdotal' and haven't been researched."

I also talked with John Thorman, a Canadian who works in the animal feed industry, who made the following comments:

"We began to notice some 3½ years ago that our pigs were not doing well and we identified candidiasis as a cause of these problems. The most common symptoms included behavioral symptoms. The pigs became excited and irritable. In addition, there was apparent suppression of the endocrine system so that labor did not come on after a normal time.

"We haven't seen impaired menstrual cycles in the sow but we've seen a lot of suppression of appetite and vaginal discharge. We've also seen pale color, skin problems and many secondary infections. We feel that candida suppresses the immune system in pigs, including certain white blood cells."

In an article in the January, 1986 *Hog Guide*, entitled, "Candidiasis: A Disputed Disease," reporter Marilyn Crabbe had this to say:

"Some claim this insidious yeast infection may be causing major losses in the hog industry. Others dismiss it, contending production losses, if any, are insignificant. . . .

"Veterinarian Carl Middlebrook doesn't need convincing. He's detected candidiasis-related problems in his large-animal practice in Monkton, Ont. 'It's a subtle sort of thing,' allows Middlebrook, who suspects some producers may unknowingly be feeding yeast problems to hogs in the form of spoiled grain.

"Once hogs are infected, he notes, the immune system breaks down, leaving the animal prone to an onslaught of other diseases. Consequently, the secondary diseases are recognized and treated, while the more subtle problem, candidiasis, is overlooked."

In treating animals with candidiasis, Whittaker and Middlebrook both emphasize the importance of building up the hemoglobin level and using supportive therapy to correct nutritional deficiencies. In the U.S. and certain foreign countries, Whittaker often includes lactobacillus products as supportive therapy, along with chelated or "complexed" minerals.

Human health effects of drugs in livestock and poultry feed were also discussed by Allen Magaziner, D.O. at the 19th Advanced Seminar of the American Academy of Environmental Medicine at Phoenix, Arizona in November 1985.

Dr. Magaziner talked about the antibiotics given to animals to promote weight gain and thus bring a higher price. Although he acknowledged that some animal diseases may be prevented, the wholesale use of antibiotics has produced antibiotic resistant bacteria. Moreover, he told of adverse effects in humans from antibiotics given to animals including effects on the endocrine system.

Since candida also affects the endocrine system, I felt that Dr. Magaziner's remarks on another group of drugs being given to animals would interest you. Among the things he talked about were premature sexual development in children noted by a Puerto Rican physician. Such side effects developed in children who had been eating meats containing hormones. When these children were put on a diet containing no meat, poultry or egg products, 58% of them improved.

In addition, he told of the work of another Puerto Rican physician who described a group of infants with enlarged breasts. When their diets were modified, and hormone-containing milk was avoided, 87% of the children improved.[†]

Here's still more: In a cover story article ("Animal Drugs") in the May 1986 issue of *Nutrition Action*, (published by the Center for Science in the Public Interest) Leslie Goodman-Malamuth commented:

"Back in 1949, a researcher working for the American Cyanamid

---

†Adapted from a report in the Winter 1985/1986 issue of *The Human Ecologist*, published by the Human Ecology Action League, Inc., 7330 N. Rogers Avenue, Chicago, IL 60626.

Corp. found that aureomycin helped baby chicks and piglets to gain weight rapidly. Since the early 1950s, farm animals in the United States have been dosed routinely with antibiotics. . . .

"Today, an estimated 50 percent of the antibiotics manufactured in the United States are fed to, injected to, or applied to livestock. And the manufacture of medicated feed additives is big business. The Animal Health Institute estimates that in 1984, American farm animals consumed $292.4 million worth of antibacterial additives . . .

"The medical use of antibiotics . . . promotes the spread of antibiotic-resistant bacteria."

The article also quoted Tufts University microbiologist Stuart Levy, M.D., who described his studies carried out on chickens which had been given tetracycline-supplemented food. *Within a few months, they found a dramatic increase in antibiotic-resistant bacteria in the intestines of the people caring for the chicks and their families!!*

They also noted "an alarming," rapidly rising resistance to six other antibiotics in three members of the farm family. Moreover, a number of reports have shown that outbreaks of antibiotic-resistant gastrointestinal infection develop in both animals and humans who have been treated with antibiotics.

This article makes no mention of candida-related health problems. Yet, it points out clearly the wide-spread use of antibiotics (and other drugs) in animals and describes some of the side effects which follow the use of these drugs. And they urge the FDA and other government agencies to devote more of their resources to dealing with animal/drug-related problems.†

The article concluded:

"How can you tell if the meat and milk your family consumes is tainted with drug residues? Regrettably, it's not possible.

"Until the FDA enforces the laws more rigorously, the consumer has three courses of action: to eat fewer animal products, to seek out meat, eggs and poultry grown without the use of drugs, or to eat the foods and just accept the slightly increased risk of illness from the drug residues."

"Alternative" or "Complementary" Diagnostic Tests and Therapies

Since the publication of the first and second editions of THE YEAST CONNECTION in 1983 and 1984, I've learned a lot I didn't know before. And I try to keep an open mind so I can keep on learning.

---

†Center for Science in the Public Interest has mounted a campaign aimed at cleaning up our food supply. For more information, write to Americans for Safe Food, CSPI, 1501 16th St., N.W., Washington, D.C. 20036.

Some of the new information I've received (such as Dr. Steven Witkin's immune system studies at Cornell University Medical School and Dr. Moses Adetumbi's studies on garlic at Loma Linda University) have been reported at scientific conferences and/or published in the scientific literature.

Other material I have acquired from various sources, including some which have been termed "alternative" or "complementary" medicine. (See also chapter 35) And most of this latter information hasn't been confirmed by scientific studies.

Nevertheless (to use a phrase I've used before), we live in a "future shock" world. Today, things all round us change more rapidly in a week than they changed in a year a few decades ago. Accordingly, I felt I should pass along to you information about candidiasis I've received from these "alternative sources" (even though some of the tests and therapies in this section may prove irrelevant or worthless). Yet, as pointed out by E. William Rosenberg, M.D., of the University of Tennessee, "It's very unscientific not to have an open mind." So here goes:

A controversial blood test for candidiasis: In the past two years, I've received a lot of information about a new and controversial test developed by Phillip Hoekstra, Ph.D. of Michigan and marketed by a California company. It's name: LIVCELL® Analysis. In a letter to me dated February 21, 1986, Bill Shaddle, General Manager of LIVCELL® Analysis had this to say,

> "Dr. Phillip Hoekstra has completed research which shows that *Candida albicans* in a cell wall deficient state can be detected in many patients. Obviously, if true, this would answer a great deal of questions in the medical field surrounding the . . . important work you've been involved in. Equally true, his work flies in the face of currently accepted medical science and has come under considerable interest and no little controversy."

Because I'd run into several health professionals who were using this LIVCELL® test including Walter Stoll, M.D. of Lexington, Kentucky, I called Dr. Stoll in May 1986, to learn more about this controversial test. Here's what Dr. Stoll had to say,

> "I've used the LIVCELL test on five hundred patients in the past six months and I've found it extremely helpful in helping me make a diagnosis of candidiasis. As you know, the technique requires the use of a special dark field microscope. Moreover, it's important for the technician to be trained to identify these candida organisms in the blood.
>
> "What we're seeing are cell wall deficient candida organisms in the blood of most of our candida patients. By contrast, we've run the same

study on a number of asymptomatic individuals and no more than 5% to 10% of them show candida in their blood smears.

"The test is simple to do and requires only a drop or two of blood. The drop is then put on a slide. A cover slide is applied and then an experienced technician examines the preparation under the dark field microscope.

"Of course to carry out the test, you first have to buy a dark field microscope which costs about $10,000, then you have to make sure your technician is properly trained."

In December 1985, I asked Jeffrey S. Bland, Ph.D. about the LIV-CELL® Test. This is what he had to say:

"This is a technique using dark field microscope to evaluate the presence of various unusual forms of candida within the blood. Dr. Phillip Hoekstra has been doing research on cell wall mutant forms of *Candida albicans* which he feels he has identified in the blood of the candida patients by fluorescence techniques. There seems to be quite a bit of literature on this topic, yet, the research is still in its infant state. I don't yet have an opinion one way or another on the technique, but I do have some interest in seeing if, in fact, it might have clinical utility. Like you, I'll continue to strive for more information.

Professionals who feel the LIVCELL® technique has *no value* include mycologist John Rippon, Ph.D. of the University of Chicago, Edward Winger, M.D., immunopathologist of the University of California (Berkeley), and mycologist Stanley Bauman, Ph.D., formerly of the University of Oklahoma.

Does the LIVCELL® analysis contribute to the diagnosis of candida? I don't know. Time will tell.

Another new test for candidiasis: In May, 1986, I received a letter along with information from Elias Ilyia, M.S., Ph.D., President of Diagnos-Techs®, Inc., 912 North First, P.O. Box 963, Renton, WA 98057, (206) 235-7335. Here are excerpts from Dr. Ilyia's letter:

"The growing awareness of yeast-related health problems further emphasizes the need for an accurate, affordable diagnostic test to confirm your clinical observations.

"Diagnos-Techs® is pleased to introduce Candascan®, an objective diagnostic service for yeast detection and quantification. Candascan® will allow you to tailor the dose and duration of the most effective antifungal agent and to evaluate/monitor the overall success of the therapeutic modalities employed.

"Candascan® also allows you to differentiate those patients with candidiasis from those with diseases exhibiting similar symptoms . . . The cost for a Candascan® test kit is only $17.50 which includes the collection and mailing kit, laboratory processing and reporting . . . This test provides you with important additional data not available through blood testing. Presently, Candascan® is available only in the state of Washington. However, it will soon be marketed nationwide."

Is this test worth doing? Does it help with the diagnosis? I don't know.

Homeopathic Extracts. During the past three years, I've received a number of letters and phone calls from people who tell me that homeopathic extracts helped them. Moreover, in the summer of 1985 I talked to several hundred women at the International Conference of the LaLeche League in Washington. During the question and answer session, a woman in the audience said,

> "I've been taking 500X homeopathic dilutions of sublingual candida extract and it helped me overcome my recurrent vaginitis."

Another woman in the audience gave me a similar report. A few weeks later, I received an unpublished report from Murray Susser, M.D. and associates entitled, "Preliminary Study on Homeopathic Candida Dilution Extract." In their report, they describe their results in treating patients with this extract. Here are excerpts from their report:

> "Dosage was based on clinical evaluation and the patient's history. Homeopathic candida dilutions of 6X strength were used for patients with intense symptoms arising from an acute exacerbation of their problems. 12X was administered to subacute cases; 30X was given to chronic patients. Standard doses were 5-10 drops three times a day . . . The best results were seen in patients with skin and vaginal complaints.
> "The homeopathic candida dilution offers a prompt, painless and relatively inexpensive alternative to nystatin and yeast restriction. In particularly severe cases, these therapies can be combined."

I don't understand homeopathic treatment, although it has been used (and continues to be used) by countless physicians and patients during the past 200 years. However, some of the dilutions are so weak that it's like putting a teaspoon of instant coffee in a swimming pool at one end and dipping out a cup at the other end and finding coffee molecules present. How could such therapy be effective? I simply do not know. Yet, it would seem to be safe. For more information write to Seroyal, 31648 Rancho Viejo Road, San Juan Capistrano, CA 92675.

Herbal remedies. During the past several years, I've received letters and phone calls from people who are drinking Pau d'Arco or taheebo tea, a material derived from the inner bark of two South American trees—the Lapacho Colorado and/or the Lapacho

Marado. These hardwood trees and their leaves are said to contain antifungal substances. Tea from these trees has apparently been used for centuries because of its supposedly curative powers.

Some of my patients have tried this tea and have reported favorable responses. However, since all of these patients were also using other methods of anticandida therapy, it has been impossible for me to evaluate the possible value of the tea. Moreover, Dr. C. Orian Truss presented studies at the Birmingham Conference showing candida colonies growing freely in culture media which contained the taheebo tea.

So if this tea helps—and many people feel that it does—it must help in ways that we do not yet understand. Does it possess value in helping patients with candida-related health disorders? Possibly yes. But I don't really know. Again, time will tell.

Another medicinal herb, "Feverfew", has been used since ancient times in self-treatment for migraine, arthritis and other complaints.

In a recent survey reported in the *British Medical Journal* (Vol. 291, August 31, 1985), it was noted that migraine victims who had eaten Feverfew leaves every day for prolonged periods claimed that the herb decreased the frequency of the attacks or caused them to be less painful, or both.

Moreover, another article in *Lancet* (Vol. 1, May 11, 1985) described the biological pathways which may explain the effectiveness of this herb. Apparently, it is both antispasmodic and anti-inflammatory and also acts as a mild sedative.

Like all treatments for migraine, Feverfew appears to work well for some and not at all for others. Moreover, although it brought relief to some 70% of 270 individuals with migraine who were studied at the University Hospital in Nottingham, England, side effects occurred occasionally.

Although I haven't used Feverfew in treating my patients, I found these reports fascinating. More information about this herb, including available preparations can be obtained from Cardiovascular Research, Ltd., 1061 Shary Circle, Concord, CA 94524, phones: (415) 827-2636 and (800) 351-9429.

Other candida remedies. In the past two or three years, many different preparations have come on the market which producers and marketers say help patients with candidiasis. Included is Cantrol® which according to the company producing the product (Nature's Way), has been designed to help you control *Candida albicans.* Three products are included in the Cantrol® pack as dietary supplements. The ingredients include Vitamin E, selenium, reduced glutathione, Vitamin C, beta-carotene, zinc, acidophilus, evening primrose oil, linseed oil and Pau d'Arco in capsules.

Another product, Candida-Cleanse®, manufactured by the Rainbow Light Nutritional Systems, provides tablets which contain a number of ingredients including Pau d'Arco powder, Pau d'Arco concentrate, acidophilus, biotin, and herbs of different types.

Still another product is Yeast Fighters® by Twinlab® contains *Lactobacillus acidophilus,* garlic extract, caprylic acid, biotin, and fiber in a "concentrated specially prepared herbal tea base".

Do these remedies help? Are they safe? Should I have mentioned them? Or should I have ignored them?

I deliberated over the answer to these questions for many weeks. And as you see, I decided to include them for these reasons:

1. I felt these remedies were safe.* Moreover, they're being advertised and distributed in compliance with current laws;

2. I recalled other remedies which had been "stumbled on" by ordinary folks or practicing physicians which worked and were used long before anyone knew why they worked. Examples include the successful use of foxglove tea (digitalis) for treating "dropsy" (heart failure) by "granny women" in England several hundred years ago. Moreover, this was a long time before physicians knew how and why this tea worked.

Another example: James Lind found that limes and other fresh fruits and vegetables prevented scurvy in English sailors 183 years before Nobel Prize winner Albert Szent-Györgi discovered vitamin C in 1929;

3. Countless people suffer from yeast-related health disorders who can't find a physician who will prescribe nystatin or Nizoral® and supervise their treatment program. And in such individuals, a trial of these "alternative" or "complementary" therapies would appear to be justifiable until they can find an interested, caring physician to help them (see also chapters 34 and 35).

---

*I've just come across a report describing severe adverse effects (pancreatitis) following the ingestion of 16 tablets of a homeopathic remedy (Kerr, H. D. and Yarborough, G. W., *New Eng. J. Med.,* 314: 1642-1643, June 19, 1986 (Correspondence). So any and every remedy, whether prescription or non-prescription, must be used with proper precautions.

I'm not saying that homeopathic remedies and the other tests and therapies listed are effective. And as pointed out by the British physician John Lister (chapter 35), it is important for the person with "vague symptoms" to make sure he or she isn't suffering from treatable organic disease (see also Chapter 38). And if such disease is ruled out, he or she may then use whatever methods are available and appropriate. Moreover, such methods should be considered as *complementary* rather than *alternative* to orthodox methods.

Could Your Dental Fillings Be Hazardous To Your Health?

Many of my teeth have been filled. Some with gold; some with porcelain or acrylic; some with mercury-containing silver/amalgam fillings. Some of these fillings have been in my mouth for years and so far as I know they haven't harmed me. Moreover, several of my good friends in the dental profession have commented,

> "All of this talk about the danger of amalgam fillings is exaggerated and overblown. The American Dental Society says they're safe."

Nevertheless, if I need fillings in my teeth, I'll tell my dentist to use something besides amalgam. I give my patients (especially those with yeast-related health disorders) the same advice. Here's why: *I'm worried about the possible toxic effects of silver/mercury (amalgam) fillings.* I've become more concerned because of additional information I have received on this subject from Michael F. Ziff, D.D.S.† and other dentists during the last several years.

In the fall of 1984 one of my candida patients (I'll call her Ella) (who had been improving on nystatin and a special diet for 6 months) experienced a major setback immediately after silver/mercury fillings were put in her mouth. A short time later another patient who had been improving on anticandida therapy experienced an even greater relapse when such fillings were put in her teeth.

Did these fillings play a part in causing a relapse? I don't know.

---

†Ziff, S. "Silver Dental Fillings, The Toxic Time Bomb". Aurora Press, New York, 1984. Price: $8.95 plus $1.00 postage and handling.
Ziff, S., Ziff, M. "The Hazards of Silver/Mercury Dental Fillings." Published by Bio-Probe, 4401 Real Ct., Orlando, FL 32808. Price: $2.50 including postage and handling.

Moreover, even though Ella had her fillings removed, she continued to experience problems so I was uncertain of the silver/mercury-illness relationship.

Then in April 1986 Alfred V. Zamm, M.D., a specialist in allergy, environmental medicine and candida-related health problems of Kingston, New York who has long been interested in environmental illness and anticandida therapy, called me. He also sent me folders he had prepared for his own patients entitled, "Mercury and Dentistry" along with a 16-page carefully referenced monograph entitled, "Anticandida Albicans Therapy: Is There Ever An End To It? Dental Mercury Removal: An Effective Adjunct." In addition he sent me a copy of a new book by Guy Fasciana, D.D.S. entitled, *Are Your Dental Fillings Hurting You? The Hazards of Having Mercury in Your Mouth*. (Keats Publishing Company, 27 Pine St., P.O. Box 876, New Canaan, CT 06840 (203) 966-8721. Price: $12.95 plus $2.00 postage and handling)

In the material he sent me and in phone conversations Dr. Zamm said, in effect,

> "Candida plays an important part in making people sick. But candida isn't the whole story. The problem with these patients is immunological dysfunction. While nystatin and a special diet helps them, many patients have to stay on the suppressive medicine indefinitely unless attention is paid to other things that could be weakening their immune system.
>
> "I have found two relatively new modalities to be helpful in treating my patients with immunological dysfunction: the use of supplemental selenium which enhances a person's ability to withstand petrochemical onslaught as pointed out by a number of observers including Stephen Levine, Ph.D. Then the second thing I do is to selectively have some of my patients remove their silver/mercury dental fillings.
>
> "Moreover, *I have found that, in many severely ill, sensitive patients (including those with candidiasis) who exhibit allergic and other manifestations, removal of silver/mercury dental fillings is a most important and effective way of improving their health."*

Here are excerpts from the 8-page folder, "Mercury and Dentistry"[†] which Dr. Zamm prepared for his own patients.

[†]Zamm, A. V. *Mercury and Dentistry. A brief overview of the mercury issue.* A patient instructional pamphlet designed to answer many questions that have been posed by patients, dentists, and other physicians. It covers how to make an educated guess as to whether removal of mercury fillings will have an overt benefit as well as the preparations the patient and dentist should make for a successful mercury removal. Price: $2.00. Send check made out to Alfred V. Zamm, M.D., together with a *self-addressed stamped* business sized envelope to: Staff, Alfred V. Zamm, M.D., 111 Maiden Lane, Kingston, NY 12401.

Question: How can I know in advance whether removal of my mercury fillings will help me?

Answer: You can't. There is no way to predict because:

1. Allergy to mercury is not the problem in question; hence, doing skin tests to prove someone is not allergic to mercury is irrelevant. . .

2. The patients most likely to obtain benefit are those who are most sensitive. Any lessening of any sort of metabolic load, however small, may be significant to these ultrasensitive patients.

Question: What has been the experience of other patients who have removed their mercury fillings?

Answer: The national data on this is limited. It is being collected via a variety of studies in the hope of determining whether a pattern exists.

In his continuing discussion Dr. Zamm described experiences with some of his patients. He also told of conversations with Theron Randolph, M.D. who reported that 20 of his patients had mercury fillings removed from their teeth and the results were mixed, i.e. there was benefit in many patients, but not in every one. Zamm pointed out that the removal of mercury fillings is *not* a "cure-all"; he also cited the example of one of his patients who is a universal reactor with severe sensitivity to many chemicals in his environment who has no teeth. (He wears full dentures, no fillings!)

Immune system change in people with amalgam fillings: In a May 1984 report (pages 617-619) in *The Journal of Prosthetic Dentistry,* entitled, "Effect of Dental Amalgam and Nickel Alloys on T-lymphocytes: Preliminary Report," David W. Eggleston, D.D.S.[†], told of changes in T-lymphocyte percentages before and after the insertion and removal of dental amalgam and nickel based alloys. He described tests which were carried out on three different patients.

In summarizing his findings, Dr. Eggleston made the following comments:

> "Both dental amalgam and nickel alloys have been considered relatively safe based on research and clinical observation over many years. Nevertheless, any chemical or dental material used for people must be subjected to new immunologic procedures as they become available.
>
> *"Preliminary data suggests that dental amalgam and dental nickel alloys can adversely affect the quantity of T-lymphocytes*—Further research may determine the frequency and magnitude of T-lymphocyte reduction and alterations by dental materials."

Should you have your dental fillings removed? I don't know. Yet, if

†Clinical Associate Professor, Department of Restorative Dentistry, University of Southern California, School of Dentistry, Los Angeles, California.

you suffer from chronic health disorders which haven't improved in spite of all of your efforts and those of your physicians, I feel a silver/mercury-illness relationship should be considered.

Colon Cleansing

I grew up in the pre-antibiotic days. Fortunately, I was a healthy youngster. I rarely missed school. Yet, from time to time, I can remember my father checking me and my siblings for some minor complaint. A part of the examination I remember most clearly had to do with my tongue. My father would say, "Son, stick out your tongue."

I would obey. Then after a moment's inspection, he'd be apt to say, "Just as I thought, you're bilious." I didn't know what bilious meant but the treatment for this condition included broth soup, clear juices and a dose of castor oil (ugh!). I loathed it. Yet, when I complained my father would say, "Son, that will clean the toxins out of your body."

I graduated from medical school in the '40s and I looked back on my father's early therapies with a benign smile. And I said to myself, "Doctors in those days felt they had to do something and (since they had few other medications that worked) they'd usually give laxatives." Yet, I knew of no scientific reason why laxatives would help anybody.

Through my many years of practice, I'd usually tell parents, "Forget about your child's bowel movements. Unless he suffers from hemorrhoids, it makes no difference whether he has a bowel movement twice a day or once a week. So-called toxins from the colon are a myth."

But gradually, in the last decade, I've become more interested in bowel movements and their possible relationship to overall health. My interest was especially piqued by a lecture Dr. Denis Burkitt (a famous English physician) gave to our local medical society in 1980. Dr. Burkitt spent 25 years studying health problems of Africans. Moreover, he found that Africans who ate their native diets with lots of vegetables, fruits and whole grains had two to four bowel movements a day. And those Africans were a lot healthier than their contemporaries who ate western diets. . . . loaded with fat, sugar and meat.

The unhealthy Africans tended to be constipated and to show what Dr. Burkitt called a prolonged "transit time" in getting rid of waste material in the intestinal tract.

In the last four or five years, I've read a number of reports in medical journals which have confirmed the Burkitt observations. Moreover, it seems that "toxins" of various sorts are absorbed from the intestinal tract of people who eat too much protein and fat, and too few fiber-containing foods.

Moreover, in the last three or four years, I've seen and heard reports from the American Cancer Society recommending broccoli, brussel sprouts, cauliflower, cabbage and other foods to help prevent cancer.

Here's more: Through "networking" with friends in the health food industry, I've received information about the importance of what is called "colon cleansing." And a letter I received from a California friend in June, 1986 said in effect,

> "Many symptoms of so-called candida infestation are caused by colon dysfunction as the primary culprit and secondarily by candida. When a person's colon is loaded with impacted fecal material, candida thrives. So any treatment which ignores the colon is going to be incomplete and often ineffective.
>
> "Overcoming the problem isn't too difficult, if a person consumes a high fiber, low animal fat diet. An excessively high level of proteins also can be harmful, especially if continued over a long period of time. And if dietary measures don't rid the colon of accumulated wastes, regular enemas and colonic irrigations may be essential."

I don't really know whether you need enemas or colonic irrigations. Yet, there's growing scientific evidence from many sources that my father and grandfather may have known something in the '20s that I didn't know until recently.

More on Sugar Substitutes

According to a report in the December 1985 *Pediatric News*, ". . . the sugar substitutes, saccharin and aspartame (a compound of phenylalanine, aspartic acid and methanol), appear safe at the concentrations that are normally consumed."

In a report presented to a conference on diet, nutrition, and cancer sponsored by the American Cancer Society, Paul M. Newberne, Ph.D., Professor of Pathology at Boston University School of Medicine, reviewed the various substances which are used to sweeten food. Three sweeteners, sucrose, corn syrup and dextrose account for 85% by weight of all substances that are intentionally used to sweeten foods. And if all of these sugary substances used in the typical American diet were replaced with aspartame, an individual's daily consumption would still be well below the apparently safe level of consumption.

Dr. Newberne concluded that there was no evidence of adverse effects among any individuals consuming such levels of aspartame, except those with defective phenylalanine metabolism.

About saccharin: According to the *Pediatric News* report, "Saccharin . . . has shown no evidence of carcinogenic potential in 20 human studies and 14 single-generation animal studies. Saccharin has been associated with the development of bladder cancer in rats after exposure at high levels in utero and throughout life, but the manner in which this occurs is not known."

To get other opinions on the artificial sweeteners, I consulted a number of my colleagues who gave me varying points of view. Here's a consensus of their thoughts and feelings, along with my own:

Most individuals with candida-related disorders have impaired immune systems. And they're more apt to react to environmental chemicals of any type, including those they touch, breathe, eat or drink. Accordingly, the person with a candida-related health disorder may experience adverse reactions to the artificial sweeteners.

Yet, candida patients . . . like most folks . . . like and even crave sweet foods. So they're caught in a trap, since sugar, corn syrup, maple syrup and honey all encourage yeast growth. What then is the answer? Here are suggestions:

1. Use whole complex carbohydrates (fruits) to sweeten foods after the first three weeks of your diet.

2. Use an artificial sweetener but don't go overboard. Use it in moderation and avoid packets of powder which contain sugar and corn sugar.

3. Rotate both your fruits and any artificial sweeteners you use. By so doing, you accomplish two things: First, by rotating, you lessen the amount of the particular substance (food or sweetener) that you consume. Then by rotating, you can more easily detect possible adverse reactions to the dietary ingredients you're consuming.

4. Make an effort to eat and enjoy foods that aren't sweet. I know that isn't easy. Yet, lots of people do it successfully (like those who take their coffee or tea "black" rather than loading it with sugar and corn syrup containing "whitener."

5. Do the best you can and as the weeks and months go by and as your immune system and your health improve, you can experiment. And perhaps you can relax a bit and follow a less rigid diet program.

Yeast Connected Weight Problems and Insomnia

Millions of Americans are plagued by weight problems. And I don't claim to be able to help all of them. Yet, many of my overweight patients have found that a comprehensive anticandida treatment program has enabled them to lose weight and keep it off.

For example, Ellen, a 38-year-old real estate agent commented:

> "My weight had fluctuated between 200 and 250 for years. I tried diets of many types. Although I'd lose weight for a month or two, it would always come back. I also suffered from headaches, hives, recurrent vaginal yeast infection and PMS. Since taking nystatin, following the anticandida diet and taking nutritional supplements, my life has been changed. I've lost 70 pounds; my sugar cravings have disappeared and I feel like a new person."

In June, 1986, I received a letter from Barbara Dewey of Michigan who commented,

> "*The Yeast Connection* saved my life. It helped me conquer many of my previously disabling symptoms. I'm now teaching diet workshop classes to help more people with candida-related problems. And I'm also lecturing to groups all over the state who want to learn more about the role of yeast in making people sick.
>
> "My major health problems included sugar cravings and overweight. I took diet pills on a doctor's prescription for 22 years, but obviously they didn't really help. Now, with nystatin and an anticandida diet, overweight no longer troubles me. Moreover, many people who attend my classes and who are on the anticandida treatment program report similar good results. So when you revise your book, please include overweight in your list of yeast-connected problems.
>
> "Here's another candida-related symptom: insomnia. For years, I'd wake up four or five times a night. Guess what? After taking nystatin for six weeks, my sleep problem has almost completely disappeared."

I was delighted to get this report from Barbara and I wasn't surprised to hear what she had to say.

Here's more: In their 1986 book, *Dr. Langer's Mega-Weight Loss Diet Revolution* (Thorson Publishers), Stephen E. Langer, M.D. and James F. Scheer describe a number of overweight patients who lost 25 or more pounds by following an anticandida treatment program. These authors also noted that various other ailments, some of which were subtle, contributed to weight problems in many people, including low thyroid function, low blood sugar, food allergies and a weakened immune system.

As pointed out by C. Orian Truss, M.D., individuals with candidiasis develop significant metabolic and biochemical abnormalities. Moreover, Truss and many other observers have noted that nervous system symptoms and hormone dysfunction occur commonly in individuals with candida-related disorders.

So it's easy to see how and why both weight problems and insomnia may be yeast connected.

Another Possible Cause of Chronic Illness—Limax Amoeba

In the last couple of years, I've received reports from a number of physicians who've become interested in chronic health problems including rheumatoid disease and a whole host of other symptoms which are said to be due to a tiny parasite, limax amoeba. Apparently the first observations of the relationship of this "little critter" to human disease were made by a British physician, Roger Wyburn-Mason.

A not-for-profit foundation, The Rheumatoid Disease Foundation, has now been established to carry on the work of Dr. Wyburn-Mason and to disseminate information about this new approach to human illness. Although I have no personal knowledge of this approach, a medical school professor I visited with recently said in effect,

> "Individuals with chronic illness which appear to be related to *Candida albicans* who aren't improving, should consider the possibility that this parasite is causing the problem."

For further information on the subject, write to The Rheumatoid Disease Foundation, Old Harding Road, Box 137, Franklin, TN 37064. Telephone: (615) 646-1030.

Are Toxic Chemicals Making You Sick?

Have you been exposed to odorous chemicals at work? Are insecticides sprayed inside of your home? Do you live or work in an improperly ventilated "tight building" which is loaded with paint, glue, formaldehyde and other chemical odors? Do you live near a heavily traveled road? Do you breathe in car exhaust and other chemical fumes while you're walking, jogging or riding your bicycle?

If you answered "yes" to any of these questions, you may have taken in toxic loads of all sorts of environmental chemicals.

How do you find out if you are a victim of such chemical poisoning? Until recently, doctors could only suspect it from your history. But now, John Laseter, Ph.D., formerly a professor at the University of New Orleans, has established a laboratory in Richardson, Texas where blood and fat tissue are examined for toxic levels of a number of different chemicals, including pesticides, herbicides, phenols, solvents, PCB's and heavy metals.

How do you get rid of these toxic chemicals? It isn't easy; however, several techniques and programs have been established to detoxify the individuals with these problems. One of these consists of nutritional supplements, vigorous exercise, sweating in a sauna bath and large doses of niacin. (These measures are designed to mobilize the poisons from your fatty tissues where they're stored and help you eliminate them from your body.)

Sulfite Sensitivity—Could It Be Related To Candida?

Many recent reports have appeared in both the medical and lay literature describing people with *"sulfite sensitivity"*. What is a *sulfite?* And where would a person run into this substance? According to a recent review article, (Simon, R. A. "Sulfite Sensitivity." *Annals of Allergy* 56:281-291) sulfites are widely used in the food and beverage industry. They're put in food containers to sterilize them.

They are also sprayed on foods including fruits, vegetables and other foods you'll find in grocery stores and salad bars to prevent foods from spoiling. The main way they're used seems to be to keep food looking crisp and fresh and to prevent it from turning brown.

Foods which are more apt to contain sulfite (in addition to those listed) include beer and wine, citrus drinks, shrimp and other seafoods, potatoes, avocados, fresh red meat and prepared vegetables in cellophane packages.

The first reports of sulfite sensitivity date back to 1973 and dozens of reports have appeared since that time. Symptoms in patients with sulfite sensitivity (or presumed sensitivity) include hives, asthma, swelling, dizziness, nausea, abdominal pain and even shock.

Could sulfite sensitivity be candida related? I don't know. However, in August, 1985, Constantine John Falliers, M.D., editor of the *Journal of Asthma* sent me the following report which appeared in the French medical literature (Drouet M. et al. *Allergie Immunol* 17:13, 1985):[†]

> "*Candida albicans* was isolated in numerous colonies from the saliva, feces, sputum, and urine of three asthmatic patients sensitive to meta-bisulfite oral challenges and is considered etiologically significant in that this and other molds can reduce *sulfates* to *sulfites*. Yeast infection may thus be associated with sulfite sensitivity in some cases."

More About Good Yeasts

In chapters 17 & 18, I pointed out that *not* all patients with candida-related health problems need to avoid the yeast-containing foods. To find out if you need to avoid these foods, follow a yeast-free diet for one week, then eat some yeast and see if it bothers you.

Here's more about the "good yeasts": In the July, 1986 issue of *Let's Live,* in an article entitled "Yeast: A Nutritional Good Guy," Frank Castellano commented,

> "We have perhaps besmirched the good name of a distant cousin (of candida) that can be very beneficial to our good health: nutritional yeast. . . . *All yeast is not the same. There are good guys and bad guys . . .*
>
> "Nutritional yeast is an excellent source of protein and amino acids and a superior source of natural B-complex vitamins, lacking only B-12 . . . Yeast contains many enzymes.
>
> "Sounds like something that you and I would like to have available to help us maintain optimum health . . . However, a controversy has grown within the natural food movement regarding yeast-related health problems. With all the attention focused on 'bad yeasts' such as *Candida albicans* . . . some people are throwing this nutritionally-rich baby out with the bath water by eliminating all yeast from their diets."

In his continuing discussion, the author quoted my good friend, John Rippon, Ph.D. of the University of Chicago, an authority on yeasts and molds, who said,

> "Not all yeasts contribute to yeast-related problems. *Candida albicans* . . . accounts for the vast variety of yeast-related health problems. On the other hand, *Candida utilis* yeast, the basic ingredient in the herbal yeast food supplement, Bio-Strath®, has been used beneficially for 35 years in over 35 countries. . . ."

[†]This brief report was also published in the *Journal of Asthma* (22 (5) 1985).

The International Health Foundation

During the past two years, I've received thousands of letters and phone calls from people seeking information and help. Here are excerpts from a typical letter:

> "I had suffered for years with fatigue, depression, headache and other symptoms affecting almost every part of my body. Six months ago, a friend gave me a copy of THE YEAST CONNECTION. Now, with the help and supervision of a knowledgeable, compassionate and interested physician, 90 percent of my symptoms have disappeared. I'm a happy, productive, healthy person. And through a candida support group, I'm working to help other people in my community."

But other letters come from people who've just learned about yeast-connected illness and who are desperately seeking a physician to help them. Although my staff and I have done our best to respond, our replies have often been delayed. Moreover, the yeast/human illness relationship hasn't been accepted by most American physicians. As a result, many people who feel they're troubled with such disorders experience difficulty in finding a physician who will listen empathetically to their pleas and help them.

To respond to this need the International Health Foundation was incorporated in the state of Tennessee in 1985. And in 1986 it was approved of by the Internal Revenue Service as a non-profit, tax exempt organization. During the past decade this foundation has received over 50,000 letters from people seeking information and help.

To respond, the foundation established an international roster of physicians who expressed an interest in yeast-related health disorders. In previous printings of *The Yeast Connection* appeared this statement:

> "If you'd like to receive a list of physicians in your area who are knowledgeable and interested in yeast-related health disorders, send $5 and a stamped, self-addressed envelope to Administrator, International Health Foundation, P. O. Box 3494, Jackson, TN 38303. However, the foundation cannot be certain that each physician listed will be able to help you."

Although many people who wrote to IHF were able to find physicians through our lists, we changed the program in the fall of 1993. Here's why: We had fewer than 1000 physicians in the United States on our referral roster. Although there were dozens of physicians in the more populous states, especially California, in many states there were only 3 to 5 physicians, and in 2 states there were none.

Moreover, many physicians on our list were so busy treating patients with candida-related health problems that the waiting period to obtain an appointment was six months or longer. Because of this situation we have developed a different approach which we feel will be more effective.

This approach features a 70-page packet which includes:

- A folder which briefly summarizes the candida/human interaction
- Information about the IRS-approved, nonprofit International Health Foundation.
- A candida questionnaire
- A potpourri of reprints, abstracts and comments which provide further information
- Comments of seven gynecologists and a dermatologist who found that anti-candida therapy and a sugar-free diet helped many of their patients with complex health problems
- New information about nonprescription antiyeast medications, including citrus seed extracts and mathake (a herbal tea), as well as notes on caprylic acid, *Lactobacillus* acidophilus, Bifidus (and other probiotics), garlic and aged garlic extract (Kyolic).
- Information about new prescription antiyeast medications Diflucan and Sporanox, as well as notes on nystatin and Nizoral.
- A 10-page treatment outline

This packet is available from the IHF, Box 3494, Jackson, TN 38303. A tax deductible donation of $20 (plus $2 postage) is requested to cover costs. If for any reason you aren't satisfied with the material in this packet, your donation will be refunded.

A letter which accompanies this packet says in effect, "If your physician is kind or caring (although skeptical of the yeast connection), show him/her all or part of the information in this packet."

Then you may wish to say to your physician, *Thank you for your interest and kindness, and for the help you have given me. Yet, I'm continuing to experience problems, and I feel that many of my symptoms may be yeast-related. Will you help me? If you would like further scientific support for the candida/human interaction, please write to IHF and they will be happy to send you additional information.*

45

Postscript

Can candida make people "sick all over"? Or is the candida-human illness relationship a "fad disease" which will soon be ignored by everyone including present day advocates and enthusiasts?

The answer to this question will depend on who you ask. Certainly I acknowledge that further scientific studies are needed. I also admit that candida isn't *"the"* cause—the only cause—of many of the chronic health disorders described in this book.

Yet, I know beyond any shadow of a doubt, based on my own experiences and the clinical and research studies of others including C. Orian Truss, M.D., Sidney M. Baker, M.D. (and others too numerous to mention), *that candida,* in ways that we still do not completely understand, *plays an important role in making many people sick.* I also know that when a comprehensive treatment program which includes antifungal therapy is pursued, countless chronically ill people regain their health.

I realize that the data presented in this book has been criticized as "anecdotal" and "unscientific" because much of it has been based on simple stories and reports from patients. Yet, in defending such an approach, I'd like to cite a recent editorial by Gene H. Stollerman, M.D., Professor of Medicine, Boston University School of Medicine entitled, "The Gold Standard"[†]. Here's a part of what Dr. Stollerman had to say:

> "As the insights of medical bioscience and technology increase our medical powers, I find renewed strength in my clinical skills. The medical history has become more focused and incisive as we learn better questions to ask . . . *Clinical experience is the gold standard on which patient care should be based.*"

[†]Stollerman, G. H., "The Gold Standard," *Hospital Practice*, Vol. 20, No. 1A. January 30, 1985, p. 9.

In making a diagnosis of many health disorders ranging from appendicitis, arthritis, or recurrent headaches, the medical history and the clinical experience and judgment of the physician examining the patient is more important than a barrel full of tests. And so it is with the health problems related to *Candida albicans* today . . . and perhaps even tomorrow.

Although new scientific studies may help confirm the role of candida in making people sick, we cannot and should not wait for such studies. Instead, we can learn "better questions to ask" our patients and continue to use our clinical experience and judgment in caring for them. In this way, we can help relieve the suffering of many sick people.

In caring for our patients, we must listen to them and learn from them. We also need to keep an open mind. In the words of Thomas Huxley, we should . . .

> "Sit down before fact as a little child, be prepared to give up every preconceived notion, follow humbly wherever and to whatever abyss nature leads, or you shall learn nothing".

46

References

1. Crook, W.G.: "The Coming Revolution in Medicine." Journal of the Tennessee Medical Association, 76:145-149, 1983.
2. Rippon J.W.: MEDICAL MYCOLOGY (2nd Edition). Philadelphia, W.B. Saunders, 1982.
3. Odds, F.C.: CANDIDA AND CANDIDOSIS. Baltimore, University Park Press, 1979.
4. Lucas, P.L., Macdonald, F., Peters, D.W. and Plumlee, L.A.: "Serological Identification of an Unrecognized Form of Candidosis with Acquired Immunodeficiency." (unpublished study).
5-a. Crook, W.G.: CAN YOUR CHILD READ? IS HE HYPERACTIVE? Jackson, Tennessee, Professional Books, 1977 (revised edition), pp. 150-155.
   b. Crook, W.G.: "Can What a Child Eats Make Him Dull, Stupid or Hyperactive?" Journal of Learning Disabilities, 13:53-58, 1980.
   c. Crook, W.G.: "Diet and Hyperactivity." Clinical Pediatrics (Letters), 68:300, 1981.
6. Cheraskin, E., Ringsdorf, W.M., Jr., Ramsay, R.R., Jr.: "Sucrose, Neutrophilic Phagocytosis and Resistance to Disease." Dental Survey, 52:46-48, 1976.
7. Prinz, R.J., Roberts, W.A., Hantman, E.: "Dietary Correlates of Hyperactive Behavior in Children." J. Consult. Clin. Psychol., 48:769, 1980.
8-a. Schoenthaler, S.: "The Effect of Sugar on the Treatment and Control of Anti-Social Behavior: A Double-Blind Study of an Incarcerated Juvenile Population." The International Journal for Biosocial Research, 3:1, 1982.
   b. Guenther, R.M.: "The Role of Nutritional Therapy in Alco-

holism Treatment." The International Journal for Biosocial Research, 4:5, 1983.

c. Warden, N., Duncan, M., Sommars, E.: "Nutritional Changes Heighten Children's Achievement: A 5-Year Study." The International Journal for Biosocial Research, 3:72, 1982.

9. PHYSICIANS DESK REFERENCE. Oradell, N.J., Medical Economics Co., 1983, p. 1942.

10. Mandell, M.: DR. MANDELL'S 5-DAY ALLERGY RELIEF SYSTEM. New York, Pocket Books, 1979.

11. Cheraskin, E., Ringsdorf, W.M., Jr.: "How Much Refined Carbohydrate Should We Eat?" Amer. Lab., 6:31-35, 1974.

12. Brody, J.: JANE BRODY'S NUTRITION BOOK. New York, W.W. Norton & Co., 1981.

13. Crook, W.G.: TRACKING DOWN HIDDEN FOOD ALLERGY. Jackson, Tennessee, Professional Books, 1980.

14. Sterrett, F.S.: "How Safe is Long Island Drinking Water?" Long Island Pediatrician, Summer 1982 (published by Nassau County Medical Center, 2201 Hempstead Turnpike, East Meadow, New York.)

15. Hippocrates. As quoted by Bell, I.R.: CLINICAL ECOLOGY. Bolinas, Calif., Common Knowledge Press, 1982, p.7.

16. Schroeder, H.: TRACE ELEMENTS AND MAN. Old Greenwich, Connecticut, Devon-Adair, 1973.

17. Higgs, J.M., Wells, R.S.: "Chronic Muco-Cutaneous Candidiasis: New Approaches to Treatment." British Journal of Dermatology, 89:179, 1973.

18-a. Whedon, G.D.: "Osteoporosis." (ed.) The New England Journal of Medicine, 305:397-399, 1981.

b. Spencer, H.: "Osteoporosis: Goals of Therapy." Hospital Practice, March, 1982, pp. 131-151.

c. Ulene, A.: "The Great Bone Robbery-Calcium: The Woman's Mineral." Family Circle, September, 1981, pp. 67-68, 120.

19. Cheraskin, E., Ringsdorf, W.M., Jr., Ramsay, R.R., Jr.: "Sucrose, Neutrophilic Phagocytosis and Resistance to Disease." Dental Survey, 52:46-48, 1976.

20-a. Horrobin, D.F.: "Alcohol—Blessing and Curse of Mankind!" Executive Health, Vol. XVII, #9, June, 1981.

b. Horrobin, D.F.: PROSTAGLANDINS: PHYSIOLOGY,

PHARMACOLOGY AND CLINICAL SIGNIFICANCE. Montreal, Eden Press, 1978.

c. Rudin, D.O.: "The Dominant Diseases of Modernized Societies as Omega-3 Essential Fatty Acid Deficiency Syndrome: Substrate Beriberi." MEDICAL HYPOTHESES, 8:241-242, 1982.

d. Rudin, D.O.: As quoted by Steven, L.J.: THE COMPLETE BOOK OF ALLERGY CONTROL. ("Looking at Your Essential Fatty Acids") New York, Macmillan, 1983.

21. Pauling, L.: "On Vitamin C and Infectious Diseases." Executive Health, Vol. 19, #4, 1983.

22. Cheraskin, E.: "The Name of the Game is the Name." In Williams, R.J. and Kalita, B.K.: A PHYSICIANS HANDBOOK ON ORTHOMOLECULAR MEDICINE, New York, Pergamon Press, 1977, pp. 40-44.

23. Cheraskin, E. and Ringsdorf, W.M., Jr.: PREDICTIVE MEDICINE. New Canaan, Connecticut, Keats Publishing, Inc., 1973.

24. Rea, W.: "Cardiovascular Disease Triggered by Foods and Chemicals." In Gerrard, J.W. (ed.): FOOD ALLERGY: NEW PERSPECTIVES. Springfield, Illinois, Charles C. Thomas, 1980, pp. 99-143.

25-a. Levin, A.S., McGovern, J.J., LeCam, L.L., et al.: "Immune Complex Mediated Vascular Inflammation in Patients With Food and Chemical Allergies." Annals of Allergy, 47:138, 1981.

b. McGovern, J.J., Lazaroni, J.A., Hicks, M.F., et al.: "Food and Chemical Sensitivity. Clinical and Immunological Correlates." Arch. Otolaryngology (in press).

26. Williams, R.: PHYSICIANS HANDBOOK OF NUTRITIONAL SCIENCE. Springfield, Illinois, Charles C. Thomas, 1975, Chapter 9.

27-a. Baker, S.M.: UPDATE, Vol. 1, #1, July, 1980. (A quarterly Digest of Information and Ideas on the Psychological and Biological Basis of Human Behavior and Development, published by The Gesell Institute of Human Development, 310 Prospect St., New Haven, Connecticut 06511.)

b. Baker, S.M.: UPDATE, Vol. 2, #5, December, 1982.

28. Schroeder, H.: "Pure Food is Poor Food." Prevention, July, 1975, pps. 124-136.

29. Cameron, E., Pauling, L.: CANCER AND VITAMIN C.

New York, New York, W.W. Norton and Co., 1979, pp. 108-111.

30. Anah, C., Jarike, L., Baig, H.: "High Dose Ascorbic Acid in Nigerian Asthmatics." Journal of Allergy and Clinical Immunology (Allergy Abstract Section), 62:5, 1981.

31. Cousins, N.: ANATOMY OF AN ILLNESS. New York, New York, W.W. Norton and Co., 1979.

32. Randolph, T.G., Moss, R.W.: AN ALTERNATIVE APPROACH TO ALLERGIES. New York, Lippincott & Crowell, 1980, p. 185.

33. Worthen, D.B.: Personal communication, March 29, 1983. (Chief of Information Services, Norwich Eaton Pharmaceuticals, Inc., Norwich, New York.)

34-a. Rowe, A.H., Sr.: "Allergic Toxemia and Migraine Due to Food Allergy." California West. Med., 33, 785, 1930.

   b. Randolph, T.G.: "Allergy as a Causative Factor of Fatigue, Irritability and Behavior Problems in Children." J. of Pediatrics, 31:560, 1947.

   c. Crook, W.G., Harrison, W.W., Crawford, S.E., Emerson, B.S.: "Systemic Manifestations Due to Allergy. Report of Fifty Patients and a Review of the Literature on the Subject (Allergic Toxemia and the Allergic Tension-Fatigue Syndrome)." Pediatrics. 27:790, 1961.

   d. Gerrard, J.W., Heiner, D.C., Ives, E.J., Hardy, L.W.: "Milk Allergy: Recognition, Natural History, and Management." Clinical Pediatrics, 2:634, 1963.

   e. Deamer, W.C.: "Pediatric Allergy: Some Impressions Gained Over a 37-year Period." Pediatrics, 48:930, 1971.

   f. Crook, W.G.: "Food Allergy . . . The Great Masquerader." Pediatric Clinics of North America, 22:227-238, 1975.

   g. Rapp, D.J., Fahey, D.J.: "Allergy and Chronic Secretory Otitis Media." Pediatric Clinics of North America, 22:259-264, 1975.

   h. McGovern, J.P., Haywood, T.J., Fernandez, A.A.: "Allergy and Serous Otitis Media." Journal of American Medical Association, 200:124, 1967.

   i. Deamer, W.C., Gerrard, J.W., Speer, F.: "Cow's Milk Allergy: A Critical Review." The Journal of Family Practice, 9:223-232, 1979.

35. Ogle, K., Bullock, J.D.: "Children with Allergic Rhinitis and/or Bronchial Asthma Treated with Elimination Diet: A

Five-Year Follow-up." Annals of Allergy, 44:273, 1980.

36. Speer, F.: ALLERGY OF THE NERVOUS SYSTEM. Springfield, Illinois, Charles C. Thomas, 1970.

37-a. Clein, N.W.: "Cow's Milk Allergy in Infants." Pediatric Clinics of North America, 1:949, 1954.

  b. Matsumura, T., et al.: "Significance of Food Allergy in the Etiology of Orthostatic Albuminuria." Journal of Asthma Research, 3:325, 1966.

38. McGee, C.T.: "How to Survive Modern Technology." Alamo, California, Ecology Press, 1979, p.11.

39. Crook, W.G.: "Adolescent Behavior." Clinical Pediatrics (Letters), 21:501, 1982.

40. Landers, A.: "Parents Should Give Help and Advice About Sex." Memphis Commercial Appeal, Section B, page 10, September 28, 1981.

41. Rosenberg, E.W., Belew, P.W., Skinner, R.B., Jr., Crutcher, N.: (Letters) The New England Journal of Medicine, 308:101, 1983.

42. Miller, J.B.: "Relief of Premenstrual Symptoms, Dysmenorrhea, and Contraceptive Tablet Intolerance." The Journal of the Medical Association of the State of Alabama, 44:1-4, 1974.

43. Mabray, C.R., Burditt, M.L., Martin, T.C., Jaynes, C.R., Hayes, J.R.: "Treatment of Common Gynecologic Endocrinologic Symptoms by Allergy Management Procedures." Obstetrics & Gynecology, Vol. 59, No. 5, 1982.

44. Kirkpatrick, C.H., Sohnle, P.G.: "Chronic Mucocutaneous Candidiasis." From IMMUNODERMATOLOGY, edited by Bigan Safai and Robert A. Good. Plenum Publishing Corporation, 1981, p. 495.

45. Hofstra, W., de Vries-Hospers, H.G., van der Waaij, D.: "Concentrations of Nystatin in Faeces after Oral Administration of Various Doses of Nystatin." Infection, 7:166-169, 179.

46-a. Miller, J.B.: "The Management of Food Allergy." In Gerrard, J.W. (ed.): FOOD ALLERGY: NEW PERSPECTIVES. Springfield, Ill., Charles C. Thomas, 1980, pp. 274-282.

  b. Sandberg, D.H.: "Renal Disease Related to Hypersensitivity to Foods." In Gerrard, J.W. (ed.): FOOD ALLERGY: NEW PERSPECTIVES, pp. 157-164.

  c. Rapp, D.J.: "Hyperactivity and the Tension-Fatigue Syndrome." In Gerrard, J.W. (ed.): FOOD ALLERGY: NEW PERSPECTIVES, pp. 201-204.

d. Hilsen, J.M.: "Dietary Control of the Hyperactive Child." The Long Island Pediatrician, Summer, 1982, pp. 25-32.

e. O'Shea, J., Porter, S.F.: "Double-Blind Study of Children with Hyperkinetic Syndrome", J. of Learn. Disabil., Vol. 14, #4, April, 1981.

47. Rinkel, H.J., et al.: "The Diagnosis of Food Allergy." Arch. of Otolaryngology, 79:71, 1964.

48-a. Krueger, A.P.: "Air Ions as Biological Agents" (Part I) Immunology & Allergy Practice, 4:129-140, 1982.

b. Krueger, A.P.: "Air Ions as Biological Agents" (Part II) Immunology & Allergy Practice, 4:173-183, 1982.

49. Soyka, F.: THE ION EFFECT. New York, E.P. Dutton, 1977.

50. Davis, D.R.: "Using Vitamin A Safely." Osteopathic Medicine, 3:31-43, 1978.

51-a. Truss, C.O.: "Tissue Injury Induced by C. Albicans: Mental and Neurologic Manifestations." J. of Ortho. Psych., 7:17-37, 1978.

b. Truss, C.O.: "Restoration of Immunologic Competence to C. Albicans." J. of Ortho. Psych., 9:287-301, 1980.

c. Truss, C.O.: "The Role of Candida Albicans in Human Illness." J. of Ortho. Psych., 10:228-238, 1981.

d. Truss, C.O.: "Metabolic Abnormalities in Patients with Chronic Candidiasis". J. of Ortho. Psych., 13:66-93, 1984.

52. Truss, C.O.: THE MISSING DIAGNOSIS. P.O. Box 26508, Birmingham, Ala. 35226, 1983.

53-a. Crook, W.G.: (Letters) J. of Ortho. Psych.,. 12:34-36, 1983.

b. Crook, W.G.: "PMS and Yeasts: An Etiologic Connection?" Hospital Practice (Letters), 18:21, 1983.

c. Crook, W.G.: "Plight of Imprisoned Youth". The Pharos (Letters), 46:39, 1983.

d. Crook, W.G.: "Depression Associated With Candida Albicans Infections". J. of Am. Med. Assn. (Letters), 251:2928, 1984.

54. Cathcart, R.F., III: "Vitamin C Function in AIDS". Medical Tribune, July 13, 1983.

55. Kirkpatrick, C.H., Alling, D.W.: "Treatment of Chronic Oral Candidiasis with Clotrimazole Troches." The New England Journal of Medicine, 299:1201-1203, 1978.

47

Reading List

(*Denotes books of special interest to Physicians)

Allergy, Immunology, Clinical Ecology and Environmental Medicine

*Bell, I.R.: CLINICAL ECOLOGY (A New Medical Approach to Environmental Illness). Bolinas, California, Common Knowledge Press, 1982.

Brostoff, J. and Shallacombe, (eds.), FOOD ALLERGY AND INTOLERANCE. W. B. Saunders, to be published late 1986.

*Dickey, L.: CLINICAL ECOLOGY. Springfield, Illinois, Charles C. Thomas, 1975.

Faelten, S. and Editors of *Prevention* Magazine: ALLERGY SELF-HELP BOOK. Emmaus, Pennsylvania, Rodale Press.

Forman, R.: HOW TO CONTROL YOUR ALLERGIES. New York, Larchmont Books, 1979.

Frazier, C.A.: COPING WITH FOOD ALLERGY. New York, The New York Times Book Co., 1974.

*Gerrard, J.W. (Ed): FOOD ALLERGY: NEW PERSPECTIVES. Springfield, Illinois, Charles C. Thomas, 1980.

Glasser, R.T.: THE BODY IS THE HERO. New York, Random House, 1976.

Golos, N., Golbitz, F.: COPING WITH YOUR ALLERGIES (Revised paperback edition). New York, Simon and Schuster, 1985.

Golos, N., Golbitz, F.: IF THIS IS TUESDAY IT MUST BE CHICKEN, 1981. Available from: Human Ecology Research Foundation of the Southwest, 12110 Webbs Chapel Road, Suite 305 E., Dallas, Texas 75234.

*Hare, F.: THE FOOD FACTOR IN DISEASE. London, Longmans, Green and Co., Vols. 1 & 2, 1905.

Ilg, F.L., Ames, L.B., Baker, S.M.: CHILD BEHAVIOR. New York, Harper & Row, 1981.

Jones, M.: THE ALLERGY COOKBOOK, Emmaus, Pennsylvania, Rodale Press, 1984.

Levin, A., Dadd, D.L.: CONSUMER GUIDE FOR THE CHEMICALLY SENSITIVE. 1982. (Available from: Alan S. Levin, 450 Sutter, Suite 1138, San Francisco, CA 84105).

Levin, A.S. and Zellerbach, M.: TYPE 1/TYPE 2 ALLERGY RELEASE PROGRAM. Jeremy D. Tarcher, Inc., Los Angeles. Distributed by Houghton Mifflin Company, Boston, Massachusetts, 1983.

Mackarness, R.: EATING DANGEROUSLY. New York, Harcourt Brace & Jovanovich, 1976.

Mackarness, R.: CHEMICAL VICTIMS. London, Pan Books, 1980.

Mackarness, R.: LIVING SAFELY IN A POLLUTED WORLD. New York, Stein & Day, 1981.

Mandell, M., Scanlon L.: DR. MANDELL'S 5-DAY ALLERGY RELIEF SYSTEM. New York, Pocket Books, 1979.

Mandell, M.: DR. MANDELL'S LIFETIME ARTHRITIS RELIEF SYSTEM. New York, Coward-McCann, 1983.

*Miller, J.: FOOD ALLERGY (Provocative Testing and Injection Therapy). Springfield, Illinois, Charles C. Thomas, 1972.

Nichols, V.: COOKBOOK AND EATING GUIDE. Xenia, Ohio 45385, 3350 Fair Oaks Drive.

*Philpott, W.H. and Kalita, B.K.: BRAIN ALLERGIES. New Canaan, Connecticut, Keats Publishing, Inc., 1980.

Randolph. T.G.: HUMAN ECOLOGY AND SUSCEPTIBILITY TO THE CHEMICAL ENVIRONMENT. Springfield, Ill., Charles C. Thomas, 1962.

Rapp, D.J.: ALLERGIES AND THE HYPERACTIVE CHILD. New York, Cornerstone, 1980.

Rapp, D.J.: ALLERGIES AND YOUR FAMILY. New York, Sterling, 1981.

Rippere, V.: THE ALLERGY PROBLEM: Why People Suffer and What Should Be Done. Thorson Publishers, Ltd., Wellingborough, Northamptonshire, England, 1983.

Rockwell, S.: COPING WITH CANDIDA (A handbook of recipes). P.O. Box 15181, Seattle, Washington.

Small, B.: THE SUSCEPTIBILITY REPORT. Deco-Plans, Inc. P.O.

Box 870, Plattsburgh, New York, 12901 (in Canada, P.O. Box 3000, Cornwall, Ontario K6H 5R8).

Small, B&B.: SUNNYHILL. Goodwood, Ontario, Canada, Small & Associates, 1980.

Smith, L.H.: IMPROVING YOUR CHILD'S BEHAVIOR CHEMISTRY. Englewood Cliffs, New Jersey, Prentice-Hall, 1976.

*Speer, F.: ALLERGY OF THE NERVOUS SYSTEM. Springfield, Ill., Charles C. Thomas, 1970.

*Speer, F.: FOOD ALLERGY. Littleton, Mass., PSG Publishing Co., Inc. 1983 (2nd edition).

Soyka, F., with Edmonds, A.: THE ION EFFECT. New York, Bantam Books, 1980.

Stevens, L.J. and G.E., Stoner, R.B.: HOW TO FEED YOUR HYPERACTIVE CHILD. New York, Doubleday, 1977.

Stevens, L.J., Stoner, R.B.: HOW TO IMPROVE YOUR CHILD'S BEHAVIOR THROUGH DIET. New York, Doubleday, 1979.

Stevens, L.J.: THE COMPLETE BOOK OF ALLERGY CONTROL. New York, MacMillan Publishing Co., 1983.

Truss, C.O.: THE MISSING DIAGNOSIS. 1983. (Available from P.O. Box 26508, Birmingham, AL 35226.)

Yoder, E.R.: A GUIDE FOR AN ALLERGEN-FREE ELIMINATION DIET, 1982. (Available from: Healthful Living Publishers, P.O. Box 563, Goshen, IN, 44526.)

Wunderlich, R. and Kalita, D.: CANDIDA ALBICANS AND THE HUMAN CONDITION. New Canaan, Connecticut, Keats Publishing, Inc., 1984.

Wunderlich, R. and Kalita, D.: NOURISHING YOUR CHILD. New Canaan, Connecticut, Keats Publishing, Inc. 1984.

Zamm, A.V. with Gannon, R.: WHY YOUR HOUSE MAY ENDANGER YOUR HEALTH. New York, Simon and Schuster, 1980.

Nutrition and Preventive Medicine

Abrahamson, E.M., Pezet, A.W.: BODY, MIND, AND SUGAR. New York, Avon, 1951.

Banick, A.E. (with Carlson Wade): YOUR WATER AND YOUR HEALTH. New Canaan, Connecticut, Keats Publishing, Inc. 1981.

Bland, J.: NUTRAEROBICS: The Complete Individualized Nutrition and Fitness Program for Life After Thirty. San Francisco. Harper & Row, 1983.

Bland, J.: YOUR HEALTH UNDER SIEGE: Using Nutrition to Fight Back. Brattleboro, Vermont, Stephen Green, 1981.

Brewster L., Jacobson, M.F.: THE CHANGING AMERICAN DIET, 1978. Available from CSPI Publications, 1755 S Street, N.W., Washington, D.C. 20009.

Brody, J.: JANE BRODY'S NUTRITION BOOK. New York, W.W. Norton and Co., 1981.

Brody, J.: THE NEW YORK TIMES GUIDE TO PERSONAL HEALTH. New York, Harper & Row, 1982.

Burros, M.F.: KEEP IT SIMPLE: 30-MINUTE MEALS FROM SCRATCH. New York, William Morrow & Co., Inc., 1981.

Cameron, E., Pauling, L: CANCER AND VITAMIN C. New York, W.W. Norton & Co., 1979.

Cheraskin, E., Ringsdorf, W.M., Jr. and Brecher, A.: PSYCHO-DIETETICS. New York, Bantam Books, 1974.

Cheraskin, E., Ringsdorf, W.M., Jr., Sisley, E.L.: THE VITAMIN C CONNECTION. New York, Harper & Row, 1983.

Cleave, T.L.: THE SACCHARINE DISEASE. New Canaan, Connecticut, Keats Publishing, Inc., 1975.

Cousins, N.: ANATOMY OF AN ILLNESS. New York, Bantam Books, 1981.

Dufty, W.: SUGAR BLUES. Nutri-Books Corp., P.O. Box 358, Denver, CO 80217.

Durk, P., Shaw, S.: LIFE EXTENSION. New York, Warner Books, 1982.

EXECUTIVE HEALTH (a monthly newsletter). 9605 Scranton Road, Suite 710, San Diego, CA 92121.

Fredericks, C.: PROGRAM FOR LIVING LONGER. New York, Simon & Schuster, 1983.

Fredericks, C.: PSYCHO-NUTRITION. New York, Grosset & Dunlap, 1976.

Goldbeck, N. and D.: THE SUPERMARKET HANDBOOK: ACCESS TO WHOLE FOODS. New York, Harper & Row, 1973.

Goodwin, M., Pollen, G.: CREATIVE FOOD EXPERIENCES FOR CHILDREN, 1980. CSPI Publications, 1501 16th St., N.W., Washington, D.C. 20036.

Guenther, R.: A NUTRITIONAL GUIDE TO THE PROBLEM DRINKER. New Canaan, Connecticut, Keats Publishing, Inc.

Hall, R.H.: FOOD FOR NOUGHT. New York, Harper & Row, 1977.

Hausman, P.: JACK SPRAT'S LEGACY: THE SCIENCE AND POLITICS OF FAT AND CHOLESTEROL. (Richard Marek, 1981). Available from CSPI Publications, 1501 16th St., N.W., Washington, D.C. 20036.

Hoffer, A., Walker, M.: ORTHOMOLECULAR NUTRITION. New Canaan, CT, Keats Publishing Co., 1978.

Hunter, B.T.: FACT/BOOK ON FOOD ADDITIVES AND YOUR HEALTH. New Canaan, CT, Keats Publishing, Inc., 1972.

Hunter, B.T.: THE GREAT NUTRITION ROBBERY. New York, Charles Scribner's Sons, 1978.

Hunter, B.T.: THE SUGAR TRAP & HOW TO AVOID IT. Boston, Houghton Mifflin Co., 1982.

Jacobson, M.F.: THE COMPLETE EATER'S DIGEST AND NU-TRITION SCOREBOARD. (New York, Doubleday Anchor Books, 1985). Available from CSPI Publications, 1501 16th St., N.W., Washington, D.C. 20036.

Jones, S.: CRYING BABY, SLEEPLESS NIGHTS. New York, Warner Books, 1983.

Katz, D., Goodwin, M.: FOOD: WHERE NUTRITION, POLITICS AND CULTURES MEET, 1976. CSPI Publications, 1501 16th St., N.W., Washington, D.C. 20036. (Out of Print)

Keough, C.: WATER FIT TO DRINK. Emmaus, Pa., Rodale Press, 1980.

Kinsella, S.: FOOD ON CAMPUS, A RECIPE FOR ACTION (Emmaus, Pa., Rodale Press, 1978). Available from CSPI Publications, 1501 16th St., N.W., Washington, D.C. 20036.

Lansky, V.: THE TAMING OF THE C.A.N.D.Y. MONSTER. Wayzata, MN, Meadowbrook Press, 1978.

Lesser, M.: NUTRITION AND VITAMIN THERAPY. New York, Grove Press, 1980.

Mindell, E.: VITAMIN BIBLE. New York, Warner Books, 1979.

Montagu, A.: TOUCHING: THE HUMAN SIGNIFICANCE OF THE SKIN. New York, Harper & Row, 1972.

Newbold, H.L.: MEGA-NUTRIENTS FOR YOUR NERVES. New York, Wyden Books, 1978.

OUR BODIES, OURSELVES. The Boston Women's Health Book Collective, 465 Mount Auburn Street, Watertown, Maine 02172.

Ott, J.N.: HEALTH AND LIGHT. New York, Pocket Books, 1976.

Passwater, R.A.: EVENING PRIMROSE OIL. New Canaan, CT, Keats Publishing, Inc., 1981.

Pfeiffer, C.C.: MENTAL AND ELEMENTAL NUTRIENTS. New Canaan, CT, Keats Publishing, Inc., 1975.

Pfeiffer, C.C.: ZINC AND OTHER MICRO NUTRIENTS. New Canaan, CT, Keats Publishing, Inc., 1978.

Price, W.A.: NUTRITION AND PHYSICAL DEGENERATION. Price-Pottenger Foundation, P.O. Box 2614, La Mesa, CA 92014, 1983 (latest edition).

Schauss, A.: DIET, CRIME AND DELINQUENCY. Berkeley, CA, Parker House, 1981.

Schroeder, H.A.: THE POISONS AROUND US (Toxic Metals in Food, Air and Water). Bloomington, IN, University Press, 1974.

Schroeder, H.A.: TRACE ELEMENTS AND MAN, Old Greenwich, CT, Devon-Adair.

Sheinkin, D., Schacter, M. and Hutton, R.: FOOD, MIND & MOOD. New York, Warner Books, 1980.

Sloan, S.: NUTRITIONAL PARENTING. New Canaan, Connecticut, Keats Publishing, Inc., 1982.

Smith, L.H.: FEED YOUR KIDS RIGHT. New York, McGraw-Hill, 1979.

Smith, L.H.: FOODS FOR HEALTHY KIDS. New York, McGraw-Hill, 1981.

Stevens, L.J.: THE NEW WAY TO SUGAR FREE COOKING. New York, Doubleday, 1984.

THE WOMANLY ART OF BREAST FEEDING. Franklin Park, IL, La Leche League, International, 1981.

Williams, R.J.: NUTRITION AGAINST DISEASE. New York, Bantam Books, 1973.

Williams, R.J.: PHYSICIAN'S HANDBOOK OF NUTRITIONAL SCIENCE. Springfield, Illinois, Charles C. Thomas, 1975.

Williams, R.J.: A PHYSICIAN'S HANDBOOK ON ORTHO-MOLECULAR MEDICINE. Elmsford, New York, Pergamon Press, 1977.

Wolf, R. (ed.): EATING BETTER FOR LESS: A GUIDE TO MANAGING YOUR PERSONAL FOOD SUPPLY. Emmaus, PA, Rodale Press, 1978.

Wright, J.V.: DR. WRIGHT'S BOOK OF NUTRITIONAL THERAPY. Emmaus, PA, Rodale Press, 1979.

Wunderlich, R.C., Jr.: SUGAR AND YOUR HEALTH. St. Petersburg, FL, Good Health Publications, Johnny Reads, Inc., 1982.

INDEX

candida conferences and, 272, 276
on fatty acids, 360–61, 369
Baker's yeast, 75
Baldwin, Richard S., 349
Banana-Oat Cake (recipe), 112
Bananas, 79, 106, 296
Barkie, Karen E., 106, 118, 296
Barley, 287, 293
Barley or Rice Soup (recipe), 110
Barlow's syndrome (MVP), 346
Barnard, Christiaan, 371
Barnes, Broda, 244
Barrett, Steven, 370
Basements, as mold source, 58
Basic Preventive®, 372
Bathrooms:
  cleaners, 203
  as mold source, 58
Bauman, David S., 276, 288
Bauman, Stanley, 383
B-cells, 137, 158
Beans, 72, 366
Bedding, as mold source, 58
Bedroom, chemical containments in, 148
Beef, 216, 230. See also Meat
Beers, 103, 209, 395
  consumption of, 188
  yeasts in, 75
Beet sugar, 193
Belching, 314. See also Intestinal gas
Best Barley Soup (recipe), 111
Bestways (magazine), 298, 368
Beta carotene, 287, 367, 386
Better Butter (recipe), 113
Billings, F. Tremaine ("Josh"), 252
Bio-Strath®, 396
Biotin, 367, 386
Birmingham candida conference (1983),
  285, 288, 314, 360, 385
Birth control pills, 14, 19, 58, 136, 153,
  154–55, 174, 177, 178, 182, 184, 215,
  228, 292, 322, 328, 339
  avoidance of, 62–63, 260
  and difficult cases, 225
  teenagers and, 208–9
Bladder problems, 228, 339, 342, 343, 378
  and PMS, 335
  See also Urinary tract problems
Bland, Jeffrey, 256, 322, 371, 383
Blastopore, 320–21
Blender Mayonnaise (recipe), 112
Bloating, 24, 188, 225, 242n., 291, 314, 338,
  354
  and PMS, 334–35
  See also Swelling

Blood:
  antibody studies, 317
  sugar, low, 394
  tests, to determine vitamin levels, 367.
    See also LIVCELL® Analysis
Bluestone, Charles D., 197
Bodey, Gerald P., 321
Body is the Hero, The (Glasser), 158
Bolton, Sanford, 355–56
Bone meal supplements, 367
Bones, thinning of. See Osteoporosis
Boric acid, in douches, 322
Borrel, George, 355
Bowels:
  disease of, 218–19, 310
  disturbances, in children, 192
  symptoms in, 241
  "tolerance" test, 236, 280
  See also Colon; Constipation
Bradley, Cecil A., 191n.
Brain, connection with other body
  systems, 168
Brain/Mind Bulletin (newsletter), 256
Braun, Bob, 269n.
Brazil nuts, 287
Breads (yeast), 75, 106, 286
  consumption of, 188
Breakfast, ideas for, 115–16
Breast milk, 196, 202, 357. See also Milk
Breasts:
  enlarged, in infants, 380
  tenderness of, 291, 292, 335, 338
  underdeveloped, 173, 183
Brewer, Tom, 298
Brewer's yeast, 75
Bridges, Turner, 68–69
British Holistic Medicine Association, 264
British Journal of Dermatology, 290
British Medical Journal, 385
British National Health Service, 264
Broad-spectrum antibiotics. See Antibiotics,
  broad-spectrum
Broccoli, 391
Brodsky, James, 174, 279n.
Brody, Jane, 69
Bronchitis, 177, 182, 224, 283
  antibiotics for, 18
Bronchodilators, 237
Brown, Margot, 266–67
Brown, Rachel, 349–50
Brown-bagging, 107
Browne, M. B., 319
Brussel sprouts, 391
Burkitt, Denis, 242n., 390–91
Bursitis, 182

Buscher, Dave, 354
Butter, 287

—C—

Cabbage, 391
Cadmium, 133, 304
Caffeine, 335
  PMS and, 291
  soft drinks and, 366
Cakes, 209
Calcium, 132–33, 159, 216, 261, 292, 298,
    365–67, 369
  acetate, 367
  ascorbate, 236, 237
  carbonate, 367
  deficiencies, 238, 366–67, 369
  gluconate, 367
Campbell, Don G., 221, 291
Campbell, Dory, 191n.
Cancer, 13, 326
  foods to help prevent, 391
  saccharin and, 118
Candascan®, 383–84
Candida albicans, 2, 3–4, 75
  conferences on, 269–77
  content analysis of, 320–21
  role in causing illness, 17–26
Candida Albicans Yeast-Free Cookbook, 254
Candida and Candiosis (Odds), 4, 239, 249
Candida-Cleanse®, 386
Candida Control Diet, 71, 101–8
  food sources, 100
  foods you can eat cautiously, 82
  foods you can eat freely, 81–82
  foods you must avoid, 83–84
  meal suggestions, 85–98
  shopping tips, 99
Candida cystitis, 4. See also Cystitis
Candida Enzyme Immunoassay (CEIA)®,
    276
Candida extracts, 174, 248–49, 270n., 271,
    280, 290, 318–19, 323, 384. See also
    Immunotherapy
Candida Foundation, 262
Candida Group Therapy, 263
Candida Information Group, 263, 264
Candida krusei, 285
Candida Questionnaire, 29–33, 165
Candida Research and Information
    Foundation (Canada), 263
Candida Support Group of Bethesda, 263
Candida tropicalis, 285
Candida utilis, 75, 396

Candidiasis, defined, 239n. See also Vaginal
    yeast infections
Candidiasis (Bodey and Fainstein), 321
Candidiasis Connection, 263
Candies, 106, 209, 224. See also Sugar;
    Sweets
Candistat-300®, 353, 355
Canditoxin (CT), 273–74
Cane sugar, 193. See also Sugar
Canker sores, 215
Cantrol®, 385–86
Capricin®, 353, 354, 355
  side effects from, 354
Caprylic acid, 53, 261, 321, 352–55, 386
  preparations, 251, 284
Caprystatin®, 53, 353, 354
Carbohydrates, 131
  complex, 68, 131, 159, 270, 279. See also
    Fruits; Vegetables; Whole grains
  and diet recommendations, 67, 68, 70,
    71, 76–77. See also Low-carbohydrate
    diet
  "good," 299–300
  in infants' diets, 202–3
  refined, 67, 70, 131, 136, 194, 202, 270,
    299, 335. See also Sugar
Cardiograms, 229
Car exhaust, 394–95
Carlson, Eunice, 273, 276, 322
Carpets, as mold source, 58
Carrots, 59
Carter, James P., 358
Castellano, Frank, 396
Cathcart, Robert F., 236, 370
Cats, 378–79. See also Animals
Catsup, 286
Cauliflower, 391
"Cave man diet," 123, 190, 235, 279
CEBV virus. See Epstein-Barr virus (CEBV)
Ceclor®, 61, 178, 194, 198, 347
Celiac disease, 107–8, 293
  sprue (CS), 294
Center for Human Nutrition, 69
Center for Science in the Public Interest
    (CSPI), 255, 297–98
Centers for Disease Control, 328
Cereals, 105–6. See also Grains; Whole
    grains
CHEER (newsletter), 254
Cheeses, 286, 366
  aged, 58
  fatty, 364
Chemicals, 20, 133–34, 243, 249, 251, 327,
    344, 394–95

418

Electromyogram, 366
Electroshock therapy, 216
Elimination diet, 123, 190, 201, 251, 286,
      311, 337
Elman, Suzi, 269*n.*
Emotional factors, 12, 67, 261
   love and affection, 137.
   See also Psychological factors
Encephalitis, 186
Endocarditis, bacterial, 347
Endocrine system, 271, 277, 316
   animals and, 380
   connection with other body systems, 168
   glands, 208, 362
   problems, 244, 354, 359
   viral disorders, 330
   See also Hormones
Endocrinopathies, 276, 315
Endogenous Alcohol Syndrome (Swaart), 291
Endometriosis, 174
Endorphins, 253
Enemas, 227, 300, 391, 396
   nystatin in, 241–42
   Entamoeba histolytica (parasite), 304
Environment:
   chemicals in, 12, 304, 316. *See also*
      Chemicals
   control measures, 203, 223, 224, 231
   favorable, 136–38
   molds in, 270. *See also* Molds
Environmental Health Associations, 254,
      263, 330
Enzymes, 396
   digestive, 250, 293
Epidermophyton (mold), 270*n.*, 280
Epstein-Barr Virus (CEBV), 262, 304, 326,
      329–31, 332
Equal®, 117, 118, 296. *See also* Aspartame
Erythema, 219
Erythromycin®, 59, 61, 178, 200
Essential fatty acids (EFA's). *See* Fatty acids,
      essential (EFA's)
Estrogen, 62, 245
   pills, 60
   See also Birth control pills
Evening primrose oil (EPO). *See* Primrose
      oil, evening
"Evening Primrose Oil" (pamphlet), 239
Executive Health (magazine), 239, 256, 297,
      360, 368
Exercise, 137, 165, 249, 260, 294–95, 297,
      323
   poor tolerance for, 346
   and toxic chemicals, 395
Eye problems, 25, 225, 226, 249, 283, 344

—F—

Fabric shop odors, 230, 344
Fainstein, Victor, 321
Fainting, 292
Falliers, Constantine John, 396
Family Circle (magazine), 298
Fasciana, Guy, 388
Fasweet®, 296
Fatigue, 13, 57–58, 63, 182, 185, 188, 215,
      240, 242, 244, 246, 249, 282, 283,
      292, 293, 303, 309, 311, 328, 329,
      343, 397
   in children, 196
   difficult cases and, 224, 225, 227, 228,
      229, 230
   MVP and, 346
   nystatin for, 270
   PMS and, 334
   sexual dysfunction and, 339, 340, 341
   in teenagers, 208
   in women, 173
Fats:
   avoidance of, 363–64
   "bad," 132
   "good," 131–32
   hardened, 159
   low-fat diet, 391
   saturated, 366
Fatty acids, essential (EFA's), 105, 132, 135,
      144, 159, 212–14, 226, 238–39, 261,
      275, 288, 292, 299, 346, 360–64, 369
   deficiencies, 367
   food sources, 366
   Omega 3, 335, 362–63, 367
   Omega 6, 360, 362–63, 364, 369
   studies of, 290, 304, 314
   See also Caprylic acid; Linseed oil;
      Primrose oil, evening
Feingold diet, 375
Feldene®, 216
Feldman, David, 301
Ferguson, Marilyn, 256, 265
Fermented beverages, 58. *See also* Alcohol;
      Beers; Wine
Ferment-free diet, 286
Fever, prolonged, 329
Feverfew (medicinal herb), 385
Fillings (dental), 304, 387–91
Fish, 201, 364. *See also* Seafood
Fish Cakes (recipe), 109
Fish oils, 369
Flatus, 314, 320. *See also* Intestinal gas
Floor waxes, 203
"Floppy valve" (MVP), 346

sexual dysfunction and, 339, 340, 341
teenagers and, 206, 208
See also Migraine headaches
Healing Heart, The (Cousins), 251, 253, 265
Health Consciousness (magazine), 257
Health food magazines, 298
Heart:
  failure, 386
  "murmurs" (MVP), 345–47
  palpitations, 226
  pounding, 292
  transplants, 326
Heartburn, 24, 354
Heber, David, 371
Hedges, Harold, 122, 123, 245, 279n., 295
Hemophilia, and AIDS, 326, 327
Henderson, John A., 71
Hepatitis, 326–27
  B virus, 331
Herbal remedies, 384–87, 396. *See also*
  Taheebo tea
Herbert, Victor, 370
Herbicides, 395
Herpes viruses, 329, 330. *See also*
  Epstein-Barr virus (CEBV)
Herring, 364
High blood pressure, 67, 68
High fiber diet, 391
High protein diet, 221, 226
Hippocrates, 3, 121, 123, 355
Hives (*urticaria*), 186, 290, 393, 396
Hoekstra, Phillip, 382, 383
Hoffman-LaRoche (Switzerland), 222
Hog Guide, 379–80
Holistic medicine, 264–67, 369
Holti, G., 290
Homeopathic extracts, 384, 387
Homeopathic medicine, 271
Homes, source of mold in, 58–59. *See also*
  Environment
Homosexuality, 335, 341
  and AIDS, 326, 327
Honey, 77, 119, 193, 299, 300
Hormodendrum (mold), 227
Hormones, 292
  changes in, 183–84, 292, 333, 341
  depression and, 341–42
  dysfunction of, 174, 276, 341, 359, 394
  fatty acids and, 361–62
  imbalance in, 244, 271, 316, 337–38
  pills, 62. *See also* Birth control pills
  produced by yeasts, 301
  in teenagers, 206, 208–9
  See also Endocrine system; Premenstrual
    Syndrome (PMS)

Horrobin, David F., 239, 290, 292, 360, 369
Hosen, H., 318
Hospital Practice (Journal), 180, 260, 345
Household cleaners, 316
HTLV III virus, 327
Human Ecology Active League (HEAL), 262, 264
Human Ecology Foundation of Canada, 257
Humanistic Health Committee, 265–66
Humidifiers, as mold source, 59
Hunter, Beatrice Trum, 69
Hurley, R., 285, 290
Huxley Institute Symposium (1981), 191
Hyperactive Children's Support Group, 258
Hyperactive Help, 258
Hyperactivity, 189, 190–95, 198–200, 375, 378
  sugar and, 193–94, 195, 296
  support groups, 258
Hyperalimentation, 272
Hyperventilation, 346
Hypha, 320–21, 322
Hypoglycemia, 102, 176, 211, 229
Hypothyroidism, 244
Hysterectomy, 226

—I—

Ilyia, Elias, 383–84
Immune complexes, 9
Immune system, 9–15, 137
  antibodies and, 378
  candida conferences and, 271, 272
  connections with other body systems, 168
  dental fillings and, 389–90
  factors which weaken, 12–13, 231, 394
  hormone problems and, 338
  how it protects, 157–60
  problems in, 359
  studies of, 288–89, 315–17, 382
  viral disorders and, 330
  See also AIDS
Immunoglobins, 9, 137
  E (IgE), 246–47
  tests for, 303
Immunosuppression, 315
Immunotherapy, 224, 230, 237, 246–48, 270n., 280, 284, 286, 318–20, 323
  "build-up" method of, 271
  candida conferences and, 271
  with yeast and mold extracts, 165. *See
    also* Candida extracts

423

Nystatin (*continued*)
Nizoral® and, 351, 352
nose drops, 241
physicians and, 279, 280, 281
PMS and, 334–35, 336, 337
powder, 300, 350–51
reactions to, 283–84, 285*n.*
resistance to, 322, 323, 328–29
sexual dysfunction and, 339
sniffing or inhaling of, 240–41
for teenagers, 206
vaginal, 290
See also Mycostatin

—O—

Oat Griddle Cakes (recipe), 113
Oats, 287, 293
Oberg, Gary, 195*n.*, 279*n.*, 354
Ocean Mist Nasal Spray®, 240
Ochsner, Alton, 368
Clinic (New Orleans), 68
Odds, Frank C., 47, 72, 239, 249, 269
Ohishi, Kozo, 221–22
Oldstone, Michael, 330
OME (Otitis media with effusion), 197. *See also* Otitis
Omega Factor, The: Our Nutritional Missing Link (Rudin), 360
Omega 3 and Omega 6. *See* Fatty acids, essential (EFA's)
Once Daily (Mittleman), 257
Optic neuritis, 214
Optivite®, 335
Organ transplants, 272, 326
Orgasm, 339
Orr, A. Stephens, 181–82
Orthomolecular, defined, 296–97
O'Shea, James A., 250, 279*n.*
on caprylic acid, 353–54
Osler, William, 160
Osteoporosis, 133, 367, 369
Otitis, 177, 200, 202
media, 193, 197, 198, 199
Ott, John, 136
"Outgassing," 148
Ovaries, 208, 363
problems with, 276, 337

—P—

Packovich, M.J., 257
Painful intercourse, 174, 182, 292
Pain pills, 230
Paint, 394. *See also* Chemicals
Palacios, H.J., 319
Palpitations (heart), 346

Pancakes (recipe), 114
Pancreatin, 250
Pangborn, John, 293
Panmycin®, 207, 229
Pantothenic acid, 367
Paranoia, 334. *See also* Mental diseases
Parasites, 304
infections, 239*n.*
limax amoeba, 394
Parvovirus, 331
Passwater, Richard A., 239, 287, 368
Pau d'Arco, 384, 386
Pauling, Linus, 136, 159, 236, 296–97, 368, 370
Payne, Robert, 376
PCB's, 134, 395. *See also* Chemicals
Peabody, Francis, 252
Peanuts, 76
avoidance of, 106
Pediatric News (journal), 391, 392
Pediatrics (journal), 310
Pediazole®, 198
Pelvic pain, 174, 182. *See also* Abdominal pain
Penicillin, 59, 61
history of, 349
for respiratory infections, 194
V or G, 347
People's Doctor, The (newsletter), 257
People's Medical Society, 255
Perfumes, 20, 215, 224, 228, 243, 316
children and, 203
soaps, 187
Periactin®, 186
Pesticides, 395. *See also* Chemicals
Petrochemicals, 316. *See also* Chemicals
Phagocytes, 134, 137, 202, 315
Pharmacological Basis of Therapeutics (Goodman and Gilman), 283
Pharyngitis, exudative, 199
Phenobarbital, 153
Phenols, 395
Phenylalamine, 391, 392. *See also* Aspartame
Phil Donahue Show, 208
Phosphate-containing foods, 365
Phosphorus, 365
Physical diseases, 163–65
Physician's Desk Reference, 281, 285*n.*
Pilar, Saul, 322
Pistachio nuts, 76
Pistey, Warren R., 272, 285
Pituitary gland, 208, 362
Pizza, 61, 209
Plaquenil®, 216

Soy allergy, 202
Spaciness, 338
Specialization, medical, 127–28
Speck, Marvin L., 243n.
Speer, Frederic, 201
Sperling, Dan, 370–71
Spices and condiments, 105, 286
Sporanox, 53–54
Spores, 320
Sprouts, 75, 78
Sprue, 107–8, 293
Squibb, E R. & Sons, 350
Squibb Institute for Medical Research, 281, 285
"Staph" germs, 322
Staphyloccus aureus, 273, 355
Steroids, 225, 237, 272, 283, 301. *See also* Corticosteroids; Cortisone
Sterrett, Frances S., 104
Stevens, Laura Jane, 296
Stewed Okra (recipe), 111
Stiehm, E. Richard, 309–10
Stir Fried Vegetable Scramble (recipe), 112
Stoll, Walter, 382–83
Stollerman, Gene H., 399
Stomach pains, 294, 338. *See also* Abdominal pain
"Stone Age" Diet, 279
Straus, Stephen, 329, 332
Strep throat, 136
Streptoccus faecium (C68), 261, 358
Streptomycin, 349
Substance abuse, 206. *See also* Alcohol
Sucrose, 391
Sugar, 70, 176, 216, 299, 300, 327
   avoidance of, 77–78, 117, 134, 159, 235, 363
   as cause of hyperactivity, 193–94, 195, 296
   children and, 199
   craving for, 192, 292, 344, 377, 393
   metabolism of, 275, 301, 314
   problems caused by, 102
   refined, 291, 296
   substitutes, 391–93. *See also* Aspartame; Saccharin
   in twentieth-century diets, 14
   See also Candies; Carbohydrates, refined; Sweets
Sugar-Free, Yeast-Free Recipes, 109–14
Sugar-Free Diet, 187, 190, 199, 200, 201, 212, 214, 294
Suicide, 294
   teenagers and, 206, 343
   See also Depression, suicidal

Sulfa drugs, 214, 378
Sulfites, sensitivity to, 395–96
Sulfonamide, 60, 62, 315
Summertime Salad (recipe), 111
Sumycin®, 207
Sunflower Crackers (recipe), 113
Sunflower oil, 364
Sunlight, 136
Support groups, 253, 261, 262–64
Susphrine®, 186, 237
Susser, Murray, 384
Swaart, Charles M., 191n., 221–22, 285, 290–91
Sweeta®, 296
Sweet and Sugar Free (Barkie), 106, 118
Sweetened foods, 224. *See also* Sugar
Sweeteners, 117–19, 391–93. *See also* Aspartame; Saccharin
Sweet 'N Low®, 296
Sweets:
   consumption of, 188
   craving for, 225, 292, 294
   teenagers and, 206, 207
   See also Candies; Sugar
Swelling, 396
   of ankles, 292
   See also Bloating; Joints
Swiss Steak (recipe), 109
Symposium on Candida Infections (Winner and Hurley), 285, 290
Symposium on Preventive Medicine, 265–66
Systemic disease, 4
Szent-Gyorgi, Albert, 368, 386

—T—

Tachycardia, paroxysmal, 229
Tagamet®, 188
Taheebo tea, 103, 250, 251, 384–85
   caprylic acid and, 353
T-cells, 137, 158, 244, 288
Tea, 103
   foxglove (digitalis), 386
   See also Taheebo tea
Teenagers:
   depression in, 195, 205–6
   problems of, 205–10
   suicide among, 206, 343
   See also Acne
Teeth. *See* Dental work; Fillings
Teich, Morton, 76, 106, 192, 201, 279n.
   on caprylic acid, 354
Temper tantrums, 199
Tension, 291. *See also* Anxiety; Premenstrual Syndrome (PMS)

Tenosynovitis, 215
Terramycin®, 178, 229
Testicles, 208, 362
Tetanus, 246
Tetracycline, 175, 186, 194, 216, 315
  for acne, 60, 62, 184, 207–8, 378
  Amphotericin B and, 281, 282, 284
  for animals, 381
Texas Medicine (journal), 318
Thiamin, 367
Thorman, John, 379
Throat infections, 213, 375. *See also* Sore
  throat
Thrombocytopenic purpura, 217
Thrush, 3, 189, 192, 198, 246, 321, 375
Thyroid, 208, 230, 244, 362
  problems, 276, 303, 337–38, 371, 394
Thyroiditis, 244
Time (magazine), 221
Tingling, 22, 212, 213, 215, 217, 226. *See*
  also Numbness
T-lymphocytes, 272, 389
Tobacco smoke, 20, 149, 187, 188, 215, 231,
  243, 316
  children and, 203
  See also Smoking
Toffler, Alvin, 307
"Tomato Effect, The" (Goodwin and
  Goodwin), 312–13
Tonsils, removal of, 197, 229
Touch, 137. *See also* Emotional factors
Toxic Shock Syndrome, 273
Toxic substances, 11, 14, 133–34, 195. *See*
  also Chemicals
Toxins. *See* Toxic substances
Trace Elements, Hair Analysis and Nutrition
  (Cranton and Passwater), 287, 369
Trace minerals (elements), 76, 132, 159, 298
  in nuts, 106
Tracking Down Food Allergy (Crook), 122,
  123, 235–36
Traffic accidents, 206
Tranquilizers, 230
Trichomycin, 222
Trichophyton (mold), 270*n.*, 280
Trubo, Richard, 331
Truss, C. Orian, 4, 155, 161, 176, 201,
  216–17, 248, 253, 259, 260, 269, 288,
  290, 304, 310, 313, 327–28, 339, 397,
  399
  on antibiotics, 378
  at candida conferences, 275, 276, 325,
  360, 385
  on early adolescence, 192

  on fatty acids, 369
  metabolic studies of, 313–15, 394
  on MVP, 346
  on PMS, 181, 182
  "The Role of Candida Albicans in
    Human Illness," 191
  See also Missing Diagnosis, The (Truss)
Tuberculosis, 160
Tuna, 364
"Twentieth Century Living" (newsletter),
  254, 330
Twinlab®, 386

—U—

Ulene, Art, 105–6
Under-achievement in school, 206. *See also*
  Learning disabilities
United Sciences of America, Inc. (USA),
  371
Unreality, feelings of, 21
Unrefined carbohydrates, 67. *See also*
  Carbohydrates; Whole grains
Update (journal), 253–54, 360–61, 368
Urethritis, 62, 184
Urinary tract problems, 23, 184
  in children, 194
  infections, 18, 60, 62, 292
  frequent urination, 215
  See also Bladder problems
Urticaria. *See* Hives
USA Today (newspaper), 370–71
"Using Vitamin A Safely" (Davis), 249

—V—

Vaccines, 54, 246. *See also* Candida extracts;
  Immunotherapy
Vagina, pH of, 322
Vaginal yeast infections (Candidiasis), 3–4,
  13, 23, 175–76, 181, 215, 216, 250,
  393
  difficult cases and, 224, 225, 226–27, 229,
  230
  PMS and, 334, 337
Vaginitis, 63, 174, 177, 178, 179, 182, 240,
  277, 292, 294, 313, 321, 343, 346
  candida extract injections for, 318–20, 384
  douches for, 322, 357
  monilial, 319
  nystatin and, 350
  sexual dysfunction and, 340
  yogurt for, 243–44
  See also Vaginal yeast infections
Vaponefrin®, 238
Vaporizers, as mold source, 59

ABOUT THE AUTHOR

WILLIAM G. CROOK, M.D. received his medical education and training at the University of Virginia, the Pennsylvania Hospital, Vanderbilt and Johns Hopkins, and has been caring for patients since 1949. He currently specializes in allergy, environmental and preventive medicine.

He is a Fellow of the American Academy of Pediatrics, the American College of Allergy and Immunology, the American Academy of Environmental Medicine and a member of the American Academy of Allergy and Alpha Omega Alpha.

Dr. Crook is the author of numerous scientific articles and eleven other books. For 15 years he wrote a nationally syndicated newspaper column (General Features and Los Angeles Times Syndicate).

Dr. Crook has been a popular guest on local, regional and national television and radio programs. He has addressed professional and lay groups in 35 states, 5 Canadian provinces, Mexico, Venezuela, England, Australia and New Zealand and has served as a Visiting Professor at Ohio State University and the Universities of California (San Francisco) and Saskatchewan.

Dr. Crook has presented his observations to physicians at the following medical schools: Georgetown, Johns Hopkins, University of Texas at San Antonio, University of California at San Francisco, University of South Florida at Tampa, University of California at Torrance, Vanderbilt University, the University of Minnesota and Thomas Jefferson University in Philadelphia.

Doctor Crook has been referred to as a preventive medicine "crusader" who says, "The road to better health will not be found through more drugs, doctors and hospitals. Instead, it will be discovered through better nutrition and changes in lifestyles."

Dr. Crook lives in Jackson, Tennessee, with his wife, Betsy. They have three daughters and four grandchildren. His interests include golf, oil painting, and travel.